Bone Tumors

Jaime Paulos • Dominique G. Poitout

Editors

Bone Tumors

Diagnosis and Therapy Today

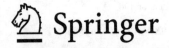 Springer

Editors
Jaime Paulos
Pontifical Catholic University of Chile
Santiago, Chile

Dominique G. Poitout
Unité d'Orthopédie
CHU de Marseille Hôpital Nord
Marseille, France

ISBN 978-1-4471-7499-8   ISBN 978-1-4471-7501-8   (eBook)
https://doi.org/10.1007/978-1-4471-7501-8

This Springer imprint is published by the registered company Springer-Verlag London Ltd.
part of Springer Nature.
The registered company address is: The Campus, 4 Crinan Street, London, N1 9XW, United Kingdom

Preface

The volume's two editors have dealt with patients with bone tumors for more than 40 years; Dominique G. Poitout in Marseille, France, and Jaime Paulos in Chile.

The aim of this book is to offer clinical and surgical knowledge from the simplest to the most advanced approach in bone tumors. It provides an actual knowledge for beginners in orthopedics to the most advanced surgical techniques of resection and reconstruction. To complete this aim, collaborators of great experience in bone tumors have contributed chapters in helping to reach our purpose.

We hope this book will assist orthopedic surgeons and residents for teaching and learning about bone tumors.

We must agree that the final decision in the diagnosis and treatment of a particular patient must come from the doctor him/herself or the team in charge of the patient.

Santiago, Chile   Jaime Paulos
Marseille, France   Dominique G. Poitout

Acknowledgements

We would like to thank all the people who made this book possible.

Our deepest appreciation goes to our patients, who while receiving all our support, effort, knowledge and dedication, relied on us and allowed us to carry out diagnosis and treatments of their bone tumor disease.

Our gratitude also goes to Oscar Contreras MD, Professor of Radiology at the Clinical Hospital of Universidad Católica, Chile, who facilitated a great number of images of cases submitted to surgery in the above mentioned institution.

A special word of thanks goes to Prof. Juan Fortune, who with his teachings initiated Prof. Jaime Paulos into the study of bone tumors from the very beginning of his residency.

Finally, we would especially like to thank each and every one of the authors of the chapters, who together with their experience and knowledge contributed to the edition of this book.

Prof. Jaime Paulos, M.D.
Prof. Dominique G. Poitout, M.D.

Contents

Part I Introduction

1 **Introduction** 3
Jaime Paulos

Part II Tumors Forming Bone Tissue

2 **Osteomas** 19
Dominique G. Poitout

3 **Osteoid Osteoma** 21
Dominique G. Poitout

4 **Osteoblastoma** 27
Eduardo N. Novais and Franklin H. Sim

5 **Osteosarcoma** 35
Dominique G. Poitout

Part III Lesions Forming Cartilage

6 **Osteochondroma and Hereditary Multiple Osteochondromas** 47
Franklin H. Sim

7 **Enchondroma** 57
Tomas Zamora

8 **Chondromyxoid Fibroma** 63
Dominique G. Poitout

9 **Chondroblastoma** 67
Franklin H. Sim

10 **Chondrosarcoma** 73
Jaime Paulos

Part IV Giant Cell Tumor

11 **Giant Cell Tumors** 87
Dominique G. Poitout

Part V Ewing's Sarcoma

12 **Ewing's Sarcoma** 97
Jean Camille Mattei and Dominique G. Poitout

Part VI   Vascular Bone Tumors

13   Hemangioma 115
Jaime Paulos

14   Hemangiosarcoma or Angiosarcoma 117
Eduardo Botello

15   Hemangiopericitoma 121
Jaime Paulos

Part VII   Bone Tumors of Conjunctive Tissue

16   Desmoid Fibroma 125
Antonieta Solar

17   Fibrosarcoma 127
Antonieta Solar

18   Lipoma 129
Antonieta Solar

19   Liposarcoma 131
Antonieta Solar

20   Fibrous Dysplasia 133
Jaime Paulos

21   Osteofibrous Dysplasia 137
Jaime Paulos

22   Non Ossifying Fibroma 139
Jaime Paulos

Part VIII   Pseudotumorals Lesions

23   Aneurysmal Bone Cyst 143
Pierre-Louis Docquier and Christian Delloye

24   Unicameral Bone Cyst 157
Dominique G. Poitout

25   Langerhans Cell Histiocytosis 163
Pedro Valdivia and Cristián Carrasco

26   Bone Hydatidosis 169
Jaime Paulos

27   Osteomyelitis 171
Jaime Paulos

28   Bone TBC 173
Jaime Paulos

29   Osteopoikilosis 175
Jaime Paulos

30   Paget's Disease of Bone 177
Jaime Paulos

31   Hyperparathyroidism 179
Jaime Paulos

Part IX   Other Tumors

32   Chordoma   183
Franklin H. Sim

33   Adamantinoma   189
Jaime Paulos

34   High Degree Undifferentiated Pleomorphic Sarcoma   193
Pedro Valdivia and Cristián Carrasco

35   Glomus Tumor   195
Sergio Morales

Part X   Bone Metastasis

36   Bone Metastasis   199
Jaime Paulos and Dominique G. Poitout

Part XI   Specific Surgeries for Bone Tumors

37   Application of Biomechanic Principles to Oncology   209
Dominique G. Poitout

38   Adjuvant Therapy in Bone Tumors   215
Jaime Paulos

39   Reconstruction with Bone Graft and Porous Titanium   217
Dominique G. Poitout

40   Sacral Surgery   229
Peter Rose

Index   237

Introduction

Jaime Paulos

Abstract

This chapter discusses the low frequency of bone tumors present in a general hospital, the importance of knowledge about them, their classification and methods of diagnosis, and the complementary study tests.

Keywords

Bone tumors · Orthopedic surgery

This book is focused on bone tumors. We will examine:

- the diagnosis
- the clinical and radiological aspects
- the therapy.

Sometimes it is very difficult to precisely diagnose a bone tumor, and so especially for children we have an obligation to always consider it and to give a diagnosis only when we are sure of it. Also the adapted treatment is given only if we are totally sure of our diagnosis. The diagnoses with their differences and numerous images have been included to explain them. We must have the results of the surgical biopsy.

The clinical study, the radiological exams, can only give an orientation but no more than that. Many different tumors have very similar aspects. We have insisted on their differences.

We have chosen the usual histological classification: the Jaffe and Lichtenstein classification, [1, 8] which is an histological one, but it could be more interesting to use a genomic classification, especially for certain types of tumors such as giant cell tumors or Ewing's sarcomas (World Health Organization Classification).

We have proposed different types of treatment following a perfect extracompartimental resection. Chemotherapy and/or radiotherapy can be used before the surgery and after

if it is necessary to destroy the tumoral cells which can be disseminated throughout the body.

Some years ago the only way to treat these malign tumors was by a major amputation; now, most of the time we can make, after a cancerological resection, a massive reconstruction with new techniques such as human cryopreserved bone stored in liquid nitrogen at $-196°$, or a massive metallic prosthesis made of titanium porometal directly cut in the operating room.

Bone tumors are a special chapter in orthopedics due to their high importance and low frequency of cases. Their high importance relates to the diagnosis of a bone tumor being always traumatizing for the patient. In a general hospital with orthopedic services no more than 3–5% of the orthopedic patients will be diagnosed with a bone tumor. Of course, centers dedicated to cancer and bone tumors concentrate this pathology and will develop the diagnoses, treatments and research on them.

Different levels of expertise about bone tumors in the physicians are necessary. General practitioners must know about the existence of the different types of bone tumors and it will often be the first physician to suspect a bone tumor in a patient and so, send the patient to an orthopedic surgeon. Orthopedic surgeons must know about the correct diagnosis and send this patient to a center or to a surgeon who treats bone tumors. And in addition to this, these centers must be carrying out research in this field.

In our personal experience, we see that very often the patient is not correctly oriented and is treated without a diagnosis and with unuseful treatments for his pathology, for example with anti-inflammatory drugs, physiotherapy, alternative therapies, etc.

Bone tumors have been studied at the Hospital of the Catholic University of Chile since 1962 with the formation of the National Register of Bone Tumors [4], where most of the bone tumors of the country were studied from the clinical, radiologic and anatomopathologic aspects, and providing guidelines for treatment when patients were not

J. Paulos (✉)
Pontificia Universidad Católica de Chile, Santiago, Chile
e-mail: paulos.jaime@gmail.com

© Springer-Verlag London Ltd., part of Springer Nature 2021
J. Paulos and D. G. Poitout (eds.), *Bone Tumors*,
https://doi.org/10.1007/978-1-4471-7501-8_1

treated in our own hospital. From this group of cases in the register, benign bone tumors made up 38% of cases, malignant bone tumors 20%, pseudotumoral lesions 35%, and metastasis 7% (the data exclude patients with known primary tumors). This data can give the reader an idea of the low frequency of bone tumors in a general hospital.

In our study approximately half of the total of primary bone tumors are malignant bone tumors and a third of the total are pseudotumoral lesions. In a study of 3345 bone tumors and tumor-like lesions, the distribution of them was the following:

Benign bone tumors

- Osteochondroma 544
- Chondroma 242
- Giant cell tumors 189
- Chondroblastoma 88
- Osteochondromatosis 50
- Hemangioma 49
- Chondromatosis 35
- Osteoma 34
- Fibroma 28

Malignant bone tumors

- Osteosarcoma 299
- Chondrosarcoma 130
- Ewing's Sarcoma 117
- Myeloma 107
- Malignant fibrous histyocitoma 37
- Limphoma primitive of bone 46
- Fibrosarcoma 23
- Parosteal osteosarcoma 19
- Adamamtinoma 11

Metastasis 269
Pseudotumoral lesions

- Unicameral cyst 303
- Osteomyelitis 300
- Metaphyseal fibrous defect 189
- Aneurysmal bone cyst 159
- Osteofibrous dysplasia 140
- Histiocytosis X 127
- Myositis ossificans 51

Others

- Osteopoiquilosis 2
- Hydatidosis osea 4
- Tumoral calcinosis 3
- Osteopetrosis 3

- Paget's disease 6
- Hyperparathyroidism 4
- Charcot arthropathy 2
- TBC (in bone) 4

Clinical Study of Bone Tumors

Bones can be affected with neoplastic lesions through three different mechanisms [1]:

1. Bone tumors which arise from cells or tissues of the bone considered like an organ. These are the primitive bone tumors.
2. Bone tumors coming from a non-osseous malignant tumor, called secondary bone tumors or metastasis.
3. Tumors that invade the bone like an extension of a malignant tumor around the bone.

Primitive Bone Tumors

The cells which form the different tissues of the bone like an organ have the capacity of forming a bone tumor as osteocytes, chondrocytes, fibroblastic cells, myeloreticular tissue, vascular tissue, fat cells, etc. These cells have the potential of forming bone tumors. On this basis Jaffe and Lichtenstein classified bone tumors according to a histogenetic classification. In that way bone tumors are classified like a series of osteogenetic, chondroblastic, fibroblastic, myeloreticular, fat, vascular, etc., bone tumors. However, there is not always only one type of cell present, and the histological diagnosis can become more complex.

Examples of this situation are the chondromyxoid fibromas, dedifferentiated osteogenic sarcomas, pleiomorfic sarcomas, etc. Sometimes the cells are so undifferentiated that the histologist cannot discover the origin of the tumor. Today, the best studies using histopathology, histochemistry techniques, and genetics studies can differentiate new lineages of bone tumors. Also sometimes the differentiation of a benign bone tumor and a malignant one is not easy, and the families of tumors whose origin are cartilage or fibrous cells or like the giant cell tumors are examples of this fact.

The basis of a final diagnosis depends on the conjunction of the clinical history of the patient, the imaging, and the histopathological study. It is necessary at this point to insist on this trio of methods for the diagnosis, and although sometimes one of them makes the final diagnosis the sum of these three elements are decisive for it. The clinical study depends on a good anamnesis and a physical examination and most of the time this tool provides a very good orientation to think in a bone tumor or not.

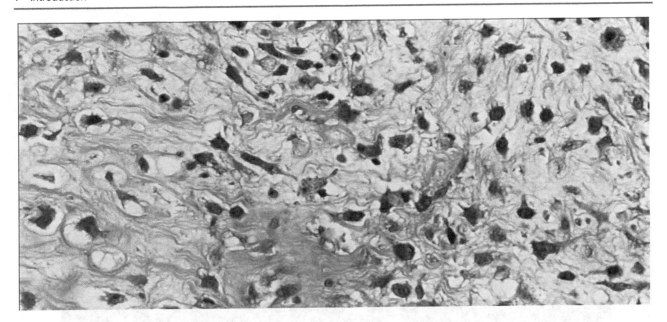

Fig. 1.1 Histology of a chondrosarcoma

Bone tumors in general are closely aligned to age. Specific bone tumors, most of them, appear between determined ages and only very occasional cases appear out of these age ranges. For example, a primitive osteosarcoma frequently appears in adolescents or young people and it is rarely seen over the fifth decade of life. When it appears in later life it is an osteosarcoma secondary to an irradiated bone, or Paget's disease, or varieties of it like parosteal osteosarcoma or a dedifferentiated sarcoma. Giant cell tumors are very rare before 15 years old, being more frequent between the third decade and fourth decade of life. Chondrosarcoma (Fig. 1.1) is more frequent between the fourth and fifth decade of life. Myeloma, like metastasis, is more frequent after the fifth decade. And so, each bone tumor is presented between determined ages and therefore is a great tool for the diagnosis.

A bone lesion of malignant aspect on a patient younger than 30 years is suspicious of a primitive bone tumor. On the other hand, in a patient older than 50 years the clinician must think of metastasis or myeloma (Fig. 1.2).

Symptoms and Signs of Bone Tumors

Symptoms that may be helpful for the diagnosis of a bone tumor are: (1) pain (2) swelling (3) functional disability (i.e., limping) (4) spontaneous fracture.

Although these signs are unspecific and can be found in many musculoskeletal diseases, clinical experience shows that patients with these findings appearing without a logical reason or a traumatic event may be affected by a bone tumor. In any of these cases the clinical physician must order an X-ray of the affected segment as the first laboratory examination.

Pain

Mostly the patient feels the pain on the site of the tumoral lesion. Sometimes the pain is related to a joint. In this case, it is representative of epiphysial bone tumors, for example giant cell tumors or juxtarticular bone tumors like osteosarcomas, typically located in the metaphysis of long bones. In the spine, metastasis, myeloma or hemangioma are most frequently presented with axial or radicular pain. Many times the pain is dull, not a heavy pain, and can be well tolerated by the patient for a long time. We very often see this kind of pain in benign tumors like osteochondromas (Fig. 1.1), enchondromas or also in the intraosseous growth of a malignant bone tumor. In those last cases, when the growth of the tumor reaches the periosteum, the pain becomes more intense and precise.

For this reason, bone tumors can be silent and ending in a late diagnosis.

Swelling

Benign bone tumors can grow slowly and without local signs. On the other hand, fast-developing tumors like

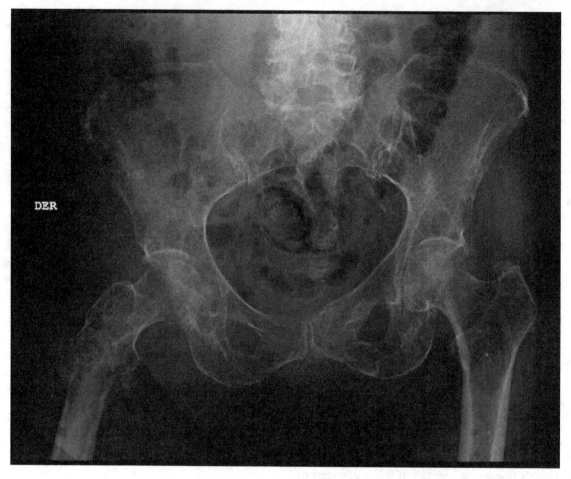

Fig. 1.2 Myeloma pelvis X-ray

Ewing's sarcoma or osteosarcoma quickly develop pain and swelling. This makes the patient seek clinical assistance sooner. In these cases the clinician must be aware of these signs as being suspicion of a tumor.

Disability

The disability produced by pain and sometimes by inflammatory signs can be clear signs of an aggressive bone tumor (i.e., bone tumor of giant cells or Ewing's sarcoma).

The diagnosis of bone tumors is frequently made late because these findings and symptoms may not be present, or only with a very low intensity. For these reasons the patient does not look for medical attention and on the other hand, the physician does not take in to consideration the signs and symptoms of the patient or doesn't think of a bone tumor as a differential diagnosis.

Sometimes bone tumors are found on an X-ray made for another reason (Fig. 1.3).

Spontaneous Fractures

These are produced by a weak structure of bone typically seen in osteoporotic fractures and bone tumors and pseudotumoral bone lesions (Fig. 1.4). There is no relationship between the energy involved and the resulting fracture. Usually the energy involved would be insufficient to achieve this fracture. An example of this is a patient that throws an object and suffers a humeral fracture or a patient that walking or by jogging suffers a lower extremity fracture. We can see this in children with bone cysts or osteolytic bone tumors in adults [7].

Diagnosis of Bone Tumors

The efficiency of the final diagnosis with only the clinical behavior of bone tumors in general is poor. However, the suspicion of the existence of a bone tumor should be very high.

Fig. 1.3 Asymptomatic
chondrosarcoma found after a hip
contusion **a** radiological aspect
b macroscopic aspect

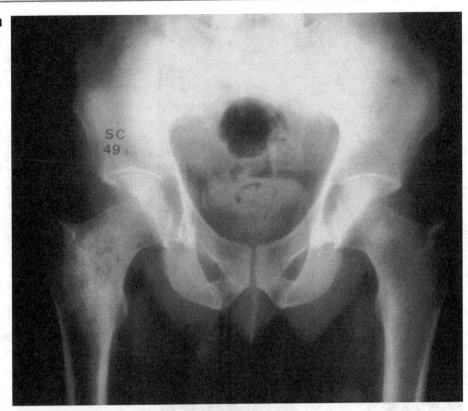

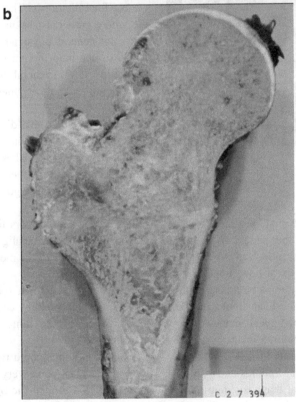

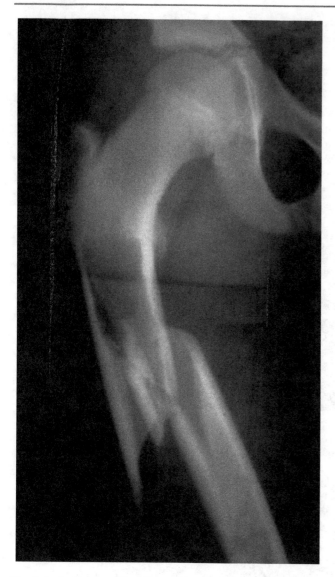

Fig. 1.4 A 12 year old patient with pathological fracture in an unicameral bone cyst

tomography), MRI which will give precise data about intraosseous extension and soft tissues around the tumor (Fig. 1.6). Scintigraphy (with Tc 99) or PET-CT (positron emission tomography) will be useful for the study of polyostotic lesions or the spreading of bone metastasis.

However, the histology studies must also be correlated with clinical and radiological findings.

A classic sample of this is the histopathological finding in myositis ossyficans (Fig. 1.7) and osteosarcoma. Both microscopic features can be very similar and for the final diagnosis of the patient's clinical history will be definitive for making the diagnosis. In brief, the final diagnosis must be made with the participation of the clinical orthopedic surgeon, the radiologist and the pathologist.

Brief of the Procedure of Diagnosis

The suspicion of the diagnosis of a bone tumor begins with the physician that has contact with the patient for the first time; then a radiological study must be done and finally the biopsy study by the pathologist. The physician, not the specialist, should be able to think of the diagnosis of a bone tumor and then send the patient to the correct place for the correct final diagnosis. The biopsy and the interpretation of the whole case must be in the hands of a specialist; however, the general physician must think in a tumoral bone lesion to continue the correct process. A lot of time could be wasted if the general physician would not consider a bone tumor and so the patient would not receive the correct diagnosis.

Then, the radiologist discovers the presence of a lesion and gives its description, proposes if it is a benign or malignant lesion and makes a diagnosis (Fig. 1.8).

A specialist surgeon dedicated to bone tumors must do a correct biopsy, taking a good piece of tissue to identify the tumor lesion.

Malignant bone tumors like Ewing's Sarcoma, osteosarcoma, fibrosarcoma, malignant fibrous histiocytoma and myeloma are some of the most malignant bone tumors of our body.

We cannot wait for a spontaneous change in the lesion since almost always they continue to grow, and perhaps the identification of the tumor does not reflect its potential growth rate (Fig. 1.9).

Some conditions could reflect a more severe bone tumor lesion. There are some very aggressive bone tumors which are a condition of their biological behavior, for example, the aggressiveness of giant cell bone tumors, although they are classified as benign bone tumors.

If the general physician is the first person to see the patient, he must correctly drive the patient to the final diagnosis.

The second step for the diagnosis of bone tumors is the imaging studies [9]. The first image must be a conventional X-ray of the segment where the physician thinks the bone tumor is located. There are a lot of typical images of bone tumors, but there are no pathognomonic images of a bone tumor. Also a false image can be found (Fig. 1.5).

With these two elements, clinical findings and X-rays, it is possible to achieve a hypothetical diagnosis, but the final diagnosis must be confirmed with a bone biopsy. Secondary studies must also be made such as scanner (CT, computed

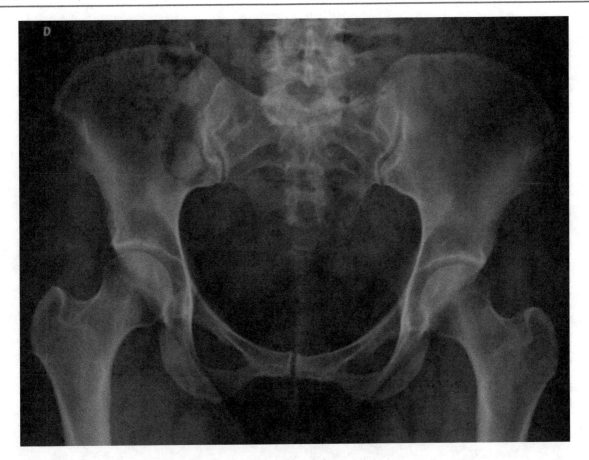

Fig. 1.5 False image of gas inside a bowel simulating an osteolytic bone lesion

The size of the bone tumor can also be a feature for prognosis condition. Big tumors are more difficult to remove.

The location of the tumor is also an important factor. A benign tumor in a critical place can be very dangerous for the patient. The invasion of the tumor is also a bad prognosis and making a resection very difficult or impractical.

Bone Biopsy

Two possible ways to make a bone biopsy are [5]:

(1) Open surgical biopsy
(2) A needle biopsy. The biopsy size must be the correct one for the histological interpretation (Fig. 1.10).

Inside a bone tumor it is possible to find different types of tumor tissues, for example, in a dedifferentiated sarcoma you can find tissues of a chondrosarcoma and also of an osteosarcoma. The incision of the biopsy must be made in such a way that it can be excised, when the definitive resection of the whole tumor is done.

The surgeon performing the biopsy must be familiar with incisions of limb salvage surgery.

Many surgeons prefer an open biopsy to be sure that they will take a good amount of tissue for the histological study. A biopsy can be done with a needle biopsy, but sometimes that can be insufficient. However, in experienced hands core biopsy can provide an accurate diagnosis in 90% of cases.

Classification of Bone Tumors

The World Health Organization (WHO) has made an effort to classify bone tumors. Nowadays, is the most useful classification as described below [6].

1. **Bone Tumors Forming Bone Tissue**
   – BENIGN Osteoma
     Osteoid osteoma
     Osteoblastoma

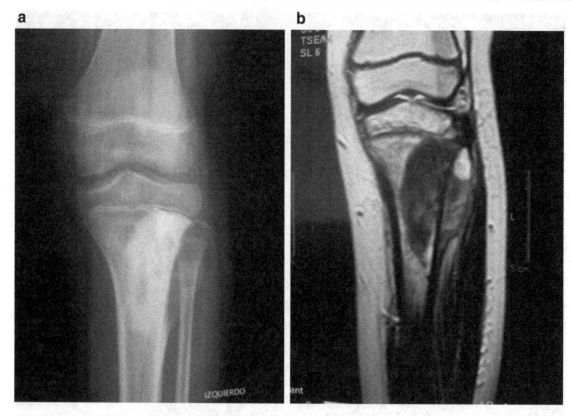

Fig. 1.6 Radiological aspect of an osteosarcoma **a** X-ray **b** MRI

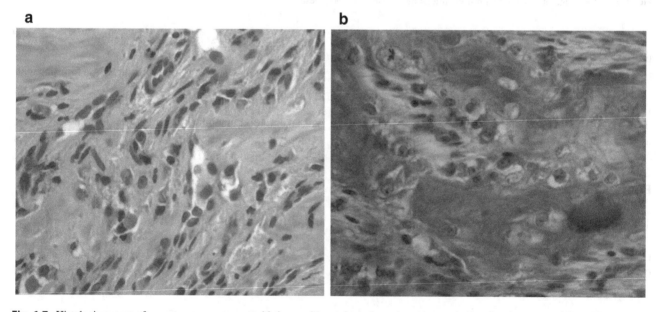

Fig. 1.7 Histologic aspect of an osteosarcoma: **a** osteoid tissue with cytological atypia without mitosis related to a myositis ossificans or an osteosarcoma **b** typical histopathology of an osteosarcoma with typical tumoral cells with mitosis

Fig. 1.8 Bone sarcoma showing periosteal reaction, radiated image and Codman's triangle, all signs of a malignant lesion

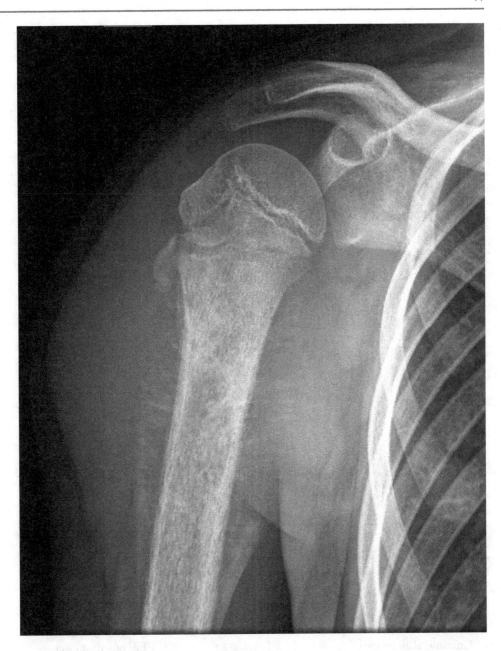

  – MALIGNANT
    Osteosarcoma
2. **Bone Tumors Forming Cartilagenous Tissue**
  – BENIGN
    Chondroma
    Osteochondroma
    Chondroblastoma
    Chondromyxoid fibroma
  – MALIGNANT
    Chondrosarcoma
3. **Giant Cell Tumors**
4. **Bone Marrow Tumors**
    Ewing's sarcoma and reticulosarcoma

    Lymphosarcoma
    Myeloma
5. **Vascular Tumors**
    Hemangioma
    Hemangiosarcoma
6. **Tumors of Connective Tissue**
    Desmoid fibroma
    Lipoma
    Fibrosarcoma
7. **Other Bone Tumors**
    Chordoma
    Adamantinoma
    Neurofibroma

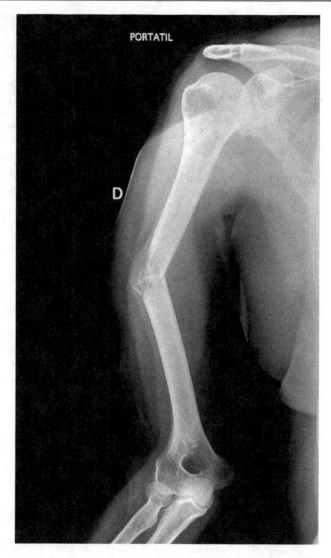

Fig. 1.9 Pathological humerus fracture on breast metastatic carcinoma

8. **Pseudo-Tumoral Lesions**
   Unicameral bone cyst
   Aneurysmal bone cyst
   Juxta-articular cyst
   Metaphyseal lagoons

   Eosinophylic granuloma
   Fibrous dysplasia
   Ossyficant myositis
9. **Secondary Cancer of Bone**
   Metastasis

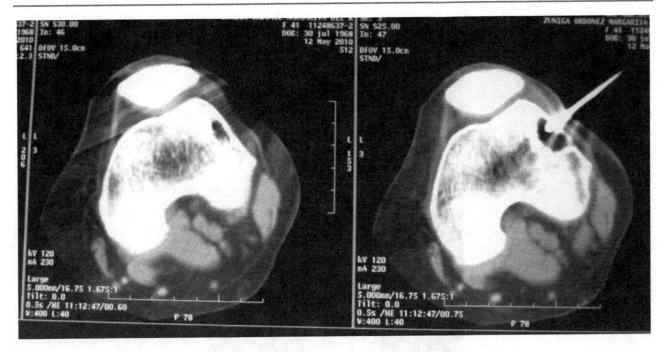

Fig. 1.10 TAC assisted biopsy

Staging

The most well-known staging of malignant bone tumors is the Enneking [2, 3] grading system, classifying it in three main stages:

Stage	Grade	Site	Metastasis
IA	low grade	intracompartment-T1	M0 (none)
IB	low grade	extracompartment-T2	M0
IIA	high grade	extracompartment-T2	M0
IIB	high grade	extracompartment-T2	M0
IIIA	Metastatic	intracompartment-T1	M1 (regional or distant)
IIIB	Metastatic	extracompartment-T2	M1 (regional or distant)

For example, Fig. 1.11 represents a humerus radiography, where a heterogeneous lesion that goes through the cortical bone can be seen; according to the Enneking classification it would be in stage IIB.

Another system for staging bone tumors is the AJCC (American Joint Committee on Cancer) or TNM System. This system is based on the origin and the tumor size, lymph node involvement and the presence or absence of metastasis as follows (Table 1.1):

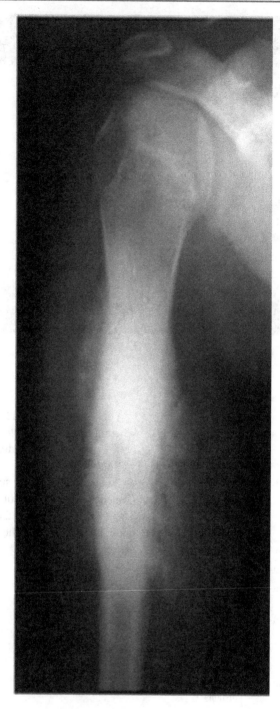

Fig. 1.11 Osteosarcoma stage IIB (high grade, extracompartment)

Table 1.1 Staging bone tumors (AJCC)

Stage	Grade	Size	Depth	Nodes	Metastasis	Survival 5 years
1A	low	<8 cm	any	none	none	98%
1B	low	>8 cm	any	none	none	
IIA	high	>8 cm	any	none	none	82%
IIB	high	>8 cm	superficial	none	none	82%
III	any		deep	none	none	52%
IVA	any	any			lung	
IVB	any	any		+	other than lung	30%

Note: Low grade tumors are grades G1 and G2
High grade tumors are grades G3 and G4
Size of tumors: T1 = < 8 cms, 2 = > 8 cms
Nodes: N0 = no regional nodes; N1 = with regional nodes
Metastasis = stage IV
The TNM stage system is better used in soft tissue tumors

References

1. Dahlin's Bone Tumors, 6th edn (August 2017), K. Krishnan Unni, Mayo Clinic, Lippincott Williams and Wilkins.
2. Enneking WF. A system of staging musculoskeletal neoplasms. Clin Orthop. 1986;204:9–24.
3. Enneking WF, Spanier SS, Goodman MA. A system for the surgical staging of musculoskeletal sarcomas. Clin Orthop. 1980;153:106–20.
4. Fortune J. Registro Nacional de Tumores Oseos (cl) Revista Chilena de Ortopedia y Traumatología. 1983: 24–1.
5. Mankin HJ, Mankin CJ, Simon HA. The hazards of the biopsy. J Bone Joint Surg Am. 1996;78:656–63.
6. OKU Director Lawrence R. Menendez. Tumores osteomusculares. American Academy of Orthopedic Surgeons-Musculoskeletal Tumor Society.
7. Paulos J. Fracturas en hueso patológico, estudio clínico radiológico e histopatología. Revista de la Sociedad chilena de Ortopedia y traumatología. 1976; XVII:28–36.
8. Schjowics F. Tumor and tumor-like lesions of bone, 2nd edn. Berlin; Heidelberg; 1994.
9. Özülker T. Atlas of PET-CT imaging in oncology: a case-based guide to image interpretation. Springer-Verlag; 2015.

Osteomas

Dominique G. Poitout

Abstract

Osteomas are rare tumors; most of them are found on the cranial bone of intramembranous ossification. The treatment is usually performed by neurosurgeons.

Keywords

Osteoma • Cranial bone tumor

These are the only lesions within a strictly bone-formation process, while in all other tumors or tumor-dystrophies, hyperplasia of bone tissue constitutes an epiphenomenon. Paradoxically, the true osteomas are among the rarest bone tumors. They are found mainly in the bones of the skull and face [1, 2] (Fig. 2.1).

In the limbs, primitive osteomas are extremely rare and should not be confused with chondromas or ossified osteochondromas.

Skull and Face Osteomas

These tumors are found on the frontal, temporal, occipital bone or maxilla. These are bones of intramembranous ossification and not cartilagineous. Orbital osteomas are the most frequent. It is very difficult to differentiate primitive from secondary osteomas related to the ossification of a chondroma, trauma or infection.

The clinical history (trauma, local infection) can help to distinguish between them. The effect of gender is not important. Lesions are observed in patients mainly between 20 and 30 years of age. From the pathological point of view, it is conventional to distinguish between the compact and spongy osteomas. Compact osteomas have a very similar structure than long bones cortex.

Histology: slats are arranged more or less regularly in the vicinity of Haversian canals and they are concentric in the ebony type.

The structure of spongy osteomas resembles the epiphyseal cancellous bone. The bays of uneven thickness are filled with a medullar tissue which may be fibrous, adipose or hemorrhagic. Symptoms of osteoma are generally discreet. Trauma or infections are often revealing elements.

Superficial osteomas are quickly recognized and as a hard tumors; they have a broad, irregular surface, usually painless and not adherent to the superficial plans.

The discovery of the profound osteomas can be made very late when they have attained significant dimensions (osteoma orbital) and are the cause of nerve compression or circulatory disorders [3].

On radiographs, the osteoma appears as a compact cancellous bone mass of variable dimensions with a wide base implantation. The therapy of skull osteomas belongs mainly to the field of neurosurgical disciplines.

D. G. Poitout (✉)
Aix Marseille University, Marseille, France
e-mail: Dominique.poitout@live.fr

© Springer-Verlag London Ltd., part of Springer Nature 2021
J. Paulos and D. G. Poitout (eds.), *Bone Tumors*,
https://doi.org/10.1007/978-1-4471-7501-8_2

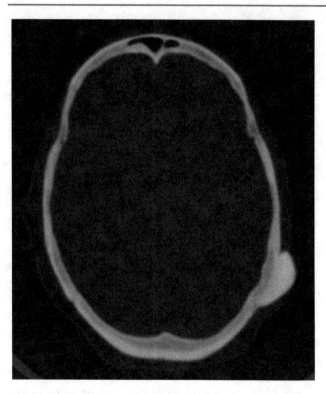

Fig. 2.1 Skull osteoma

References

1. Ishii T, Sakamoto Y, Miwa T, Yoshida K. A giant osteoma of the ethmoid sinus. J Craniofac Surg. 2018;29(3):661–2. https://doi.org/10.1097/SCS.0000000000004206.
2. Kakkar A, Nambirajan A, Suri V, Sarkar C, Kale SS, Singh M, et al. Primary bone tumors of the skull: spectrum of 125 cases, with review of literature. J Neurol Surg Part B Skull Base. 2016;77 (4):319–25.
3. Satyarthee GD, Suri A, Mahapatra AK. Giant spheno-ethmoidal osteoma in a 14-year boy presenting with visual impairment and facial deformity: Short review. J Pediatr Neurosci. 2015;10(1):48–50. https://doi.org/10.4103/1817-1745.154340.

Osteoid Osteoma

Dominique G. Poitout

Abstract

Osteoid osteoma is a benign bone tumor, painful and small sized, frequently found in the cortical of long bones, creating a typical nidus surrounded by compact bone. Surgery and radiofrequency are the most used methods of treatment.

Keywords

Osteoma osteoide • Nidus • Radiofrequency

Definition: This is a benign osteoblastic bone tumor composed of osteoid and atypical bone.

Etiology

The osteoid osteoma is a lesion of relatively high occurrence. Its growth is exceptional after 35 years of age. Half of all cases are found in the second decade of life. The influence of gender is significant; boys are affected twice as often as girls.

The lesion is mainly located at the long bones of the limbs, but also on the vertebrae (back arc), and the bones of the foot and hand. The femur and tibia are the main locations, which alone make up half of the cases. The lesions can occasionally be found in other locations [1–4].

On the long bones, the lesion may be located at the cortical diaphysis or at epiphyseal cancellous bone. The location is always unique.

Pathological Anatomy

The histology is essential to the diagnosis. The specific lesion, called a nidus, of any small volume, requires careful preoperative identification. It is surrounded, in a very large number of cases, with a perifocal condensation reaction with no specific character. The treatment consite in take the lesion as a whole, with its compact peripheral tissue, leaving the pathologist to discover the nidus himself, after cutting and decalcification (Figs. 3.1 and 3.2).

Macroscopic Anatomy

The lesion is extremely small, 2–3 mm to 1 cm, exceptionally higher. It forms the nidus, a small spherical or ovoid mass of reddish brown coloring of soft grainy appearance. This mass is surrounded by a thin layer of compact bone when the tumor is inside the spongy tissue. When the lesion is located in the cortex, the perifocal reactions are much more pronounced, bone hyper condensation sometimes extending to several centimeters of the nidus, reaching in some cases the entire diaphyseal circumference. When the nidus is superficial the cortical is thickened by periosteal bone apposition.

Microscopic Anatomy

The lesion consists essentially of osteoid tissue disposed in irregular tight spans, sometimes interlacing. Many cells occupy the spaces between the bays: osteoblasts, mesenchymal cells, spindle-shaped cells, probably representing transitional forms between fibroblasts and osteoblasts, osteoclasts, and finally, staying in contact with spans in the gaps.

The vascularization is rich. The histological appearance varies with the aging of the lesion due to the ossification center of the ring or osteoid tissue. The formed bone is an

D. G. Poitout (✉)
Aix Marseille University, Marseille, France
e-mail: Dominique.poitout@live.fr

© Springer-Verlag London Ltd., part of Springer Nature 2021
J. Paulos and D. G. Poitout (eds.), *Bone Tumors*,
https://doi.org/10.1007/978-1-4471-7501-8_3

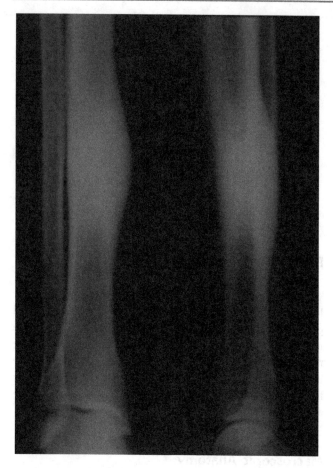

Fig. 3.1 Condensation cortical

atypical bone, non Haversian, consisting of dense and highly calcified spans.

These bays appear in purple on sections stained with hematoxylin-eosin, while the bays of osteoid tissue stain light pink (Fig. 3.3). This progressive ossification results in "a very dense osteosclerosis", made of lamellar bone closely applied to each other with a provision in mosaic, puzzle, or marquetry, reminiscent of pagetic layout and seems likely to be interpreted as a way of healing a lesion. It is noted that in contact with the nidus, densification of the bone may extend to more or less great distance. This condensation is due to the thickening of the spans between which the marrow is depleted and becomes fibrous. Beyond the normal cortical, it can be observe the display of concentric layers of newly formed bone, subperiosteal, increasing both the height and the circumference of the shaft.

Clinical Study

The pain is the essential clinical symptom. The pain is constant and often intense. At first, the pain is generally moderate and gradually, the pain intensity increases. This is

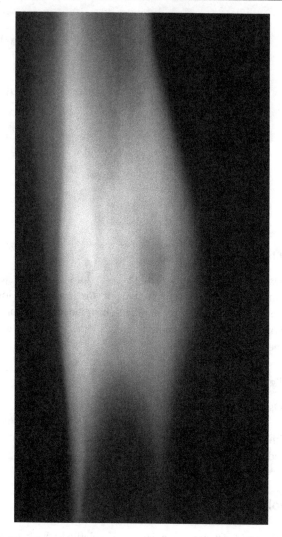

Fig. 3.2 Nidus intracortical (little lake)

when the patient comes to the doctor (two years on average after the first sign). The pain is sharp, and can in some cases take a lancinant character; nocturnal exacerbation is usual, waking the patient, urging him to stand up, to walk. The nocturnal pain is very characteristic. Classically it is said that the pain is ameilorated by the use of salicilates.

The physical exam reveals, in general, no change in appearance or temperature of the skin. Much more common is the recognition of a hypersensibility to pressure, to which constancy and topographic accuracy give a very evocative exquisite pain.

The general exam of the subject and the various biological investigations are negative. However, one can observe clinical forms that may by their atypical character mislead the diagnosis.

In the vicinity of a joint, the osteoid osteoma may manifest as pain on mobilization, limitation of movement or even a synovial effusion. Pain can sometimes sit away from the lesion, to the point that radiograph results may remain outside the affected area.

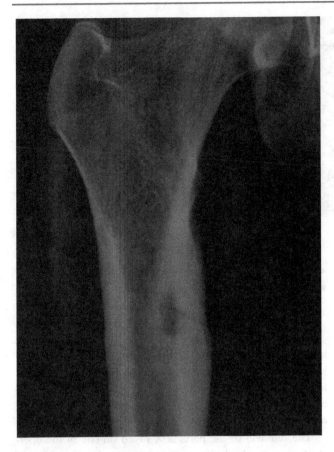

Fig. 3.3 Cortical osteoid osteoma

The topography of radicular pain may be also responsible for misdiagnosis [5].

In the lower limbs, one can observe a limp of order analgesic, sometimes caused by an elongation of the affected limb, as if the vicinity of the osteoid osteoma causes an excitation of the growth cartilage.

With the spine, osteoid osteoma can determine analgesic stiffness and simulate Pott's disease.

Radiology

Radiology, especially axial computer tomography, is used to specify the precise location of the tumor. With this knowledge the surgeon is guided to perform the correct excision of the lesion.

The study of the sequential shots must include study of the central lesion and perifocal reactions.

The nidus appears as a small bright spot, round or oval, a few millimeters in diameter, with a regular edge, sitting in a thickened cortical thickness or, conversely, in the epiphyseal spongy tissue. Its clarity is homogeneous in young forms.

In older lesions, they show granulation that consists of small intra-focal calcification, seedlings, or even a larger central opacity suggesting the existence of a small round receiver and performing a rounded image.

Sometimes calcification is annular, leaving a little clear central place, and realizes an aspect to target

The perifocal events are almost always significant, disproportionate to the smallness of the causal lesion. The hypercondensation outskirts of the nidus may be several centimeters, the transition to healthy bone taking place gradually. The periosteal hyperostosis manifests itself at first by a double outline periosteal that do not significantly alter bone morphology (Fig. 3.4).

Later, the osteoid osteoma causes a bone deformity of tumor aspect, spindle-shaped or oval. Sometimes the primitive cortical remains visible under successive periosteal apposition of bones, recognizable by their layered look.

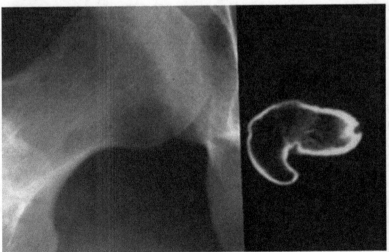
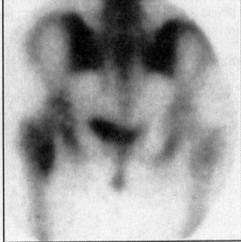

Fig. 3.4 RX, scan and scintigraphy of a femoral neck osteoid osteoma

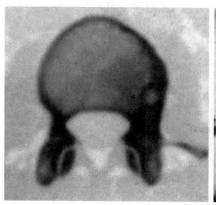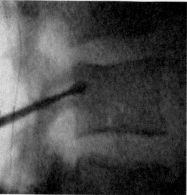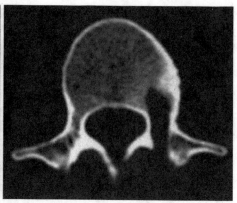

Fig. 3.5 Vertebral nidus; excision by transpedicular curettage

Thereafter, the sclerosis and the new bone formed and the opacity of the picture can no longer discern its structure.

Radiologically as pathologists, there is a striking difference between the osteoid osteoma developed in the thickness of cortical or within the epiphyseal spongy tissue.

For the latter, the perifocal reaction is generally moderate, marked only by a border of condensation. The nidus is often larger, up to 10–15 mm in diameter. The cortical osteoid osteoma, however, gives rise to an intense and extensive perifocal sclerosis.

The periosteal reaction is more important when the lesion is superficial, close to the periosteum. It is in these forms that the image of the nidus is particularly difficult to "extract" from a massive hypercondensation. This is the scanner that allow its discovery.

Bone scintigraphy gives a peak uptake located at the nidus which affirms its precise nature and topography. It is the capital exam with which to seek out this disease [6].

Because of the importance of its perifocal condensation, osteoid osteoma is more similar to an abscess than a tumor. It should be noted, moreover, that the lesion extension is linked to only the peripherical reactions, to the exclusion of any increase in the nidus itself, which is unusual in a tumor process.

Treatment

No malignancy was reported during the evolution of osteoid osteoma. Some cases of spontaneous cure are known.

The ossification of the nidus is a way of healing. Surgery is the best treatment. Its purpose is to remove the mass lesion: (Fig. 3.5)

- to permit histological identification;
- to avoid recurrences which can be responsible for some incomplete curettage.

The excision of the nidus imposes a meadow and precise intraoperative identification; in addition, resection of a small lesion must not cause damage functionally. It must be performed after identification, and involves complete removal of the tumor area and drilling with 3.2 drill bits at the periphery of the tumor which is then removed with a chisel.

The removal of the parts is X-rayed on-site in the operating room to check the reality of the complete excision of the tumor.

A reconstruction by autograft, armed or not by the osteosynthesis material may be necessary to prevent the occurrence of fracture.

Embolization of the tumor performed under a scanner has been proposed, but the result cannot be considered as reliable as surgery.

Treatment with radiofrequency: this is performed under CT guidance to produce a local zone of necrosis. It expects to achieve a success rate of 90% [7].

References

1. Abdelhafid D, Moncef E et al. L'Ostéome ostéoide de l' extremité inférieur du radius: á propos d'un cas,localisation rare et revue de la littérature. Pan Afr Med J. 2016; 24: 46.
2. Rosenthal DI, Hornicek FJ, Torriani M, Gebhardt MC, Mankin HJ. Osteoid Osteoma: percutaneous treatment with radiofrequency energy. Radiology. 2003;229(1):171–5.
3. De Filippo M. Radiofrequency ablation of osteoid osteoma. Acta Biomed. 2018: 19(89) (1–S): 175–185.

4. Raux S, Kohler R, Canterino I, Chotel F, Abelin-Genevois K. Ostéome ostéoïde de la fosse acétabulaire: À propos d'une série de cinq cas traités par résection percutanée. Revue de Chirurgie Orthopedique et Traumatologique. 2013;99(3):292–6. https://doi.org/10.1016/j.rcot.2013.02.002.

5. Sim FH, Dahlin DC, Stauffer RN, Laws Jr ER. Primary bone tumors simulating lumbar disc syndrome. Spine. 1977; 2:65–74.

6. Vigorita VJ, Ghelman B. Localization of osteoma osteoid: use of radionuclide scanning and autoimaging in identifying the nidus. Am J Clin Pathol. 1983; 79: 223–225.

7. Montañez-Heredia E, Serrano-Montilla J, Merino-Ruiz ML, Amores-Ramírez F, Villalobos M. Osteoid osteoma: CT-guided radiofrequency ablation. J Acta Orthop Belg. 2009; 75(1): 75–80.

Osteoblastoma

Eduardo N. Novais and Franklin H. Sim

Abstract

Osteoblastomas are benign bone tumors composed of well vascularized connective tissue stroma. This is a rare condition, affecting mostly younger patients. It may present in any bone but is most frequently found in the spine and may present with radicular compression symptoms. In the spine, CT scans are the imaging of choice. Differential diagnosis includes osteoid osteoma, aneurysmal bone cyst and giant cell tumor and osteosarcoma. Treatment alternatives include curettage or marginal to wide resection, depending on the location and stage of the tumor.

Keywords

Osteoblastoma • Spine tumor • Aggressive osteoblastoma

Definition

Benign osteoblastoma is a primary bone tumor composed of well-vascularized connective tissue stroma in which there is active production of osteoid and primitive woven bone. It was first delineated as a distinct entity by Jaffe and Mayer who in 1932 described an osteoblastic osteoid tissue-forming tumor. In 1954 it was designated as a "giant osteoid osteoma" by Dahlin and as an "osteogenic fibroma" by Golding. It was not until 1956 that osteoblastoma obtained its currently accepted name independently proposed by Lichtenstein and Jaffe.

E. N. Novais (✉) · F. H. Sim
Mayo Clinic, Rochester, MN 55905, USA
e-mail: eduardonilo@hotmail.com

F. H. Sim
e-mail: sim.franklin@mayo.edu

Epidemiology

Osteoblastoma is a rare tumor accounting for approximately only 1% of all bone tumors and for 3.5% of all benign tumors seen at the Mayo Clinic. Although the tumor has been reported in patients as young as 6 months and as old as 75 years the peak incidence is at around 20 years of age, and more than 70% of patients are younger than 30 years of age at time of diagnosis. Male patients are affected more commonly than female patients (male-to-female ratio is 2:1).

Locations

Osteoblastoma may affect virtually any bone, however it is most frequently observed in the vertebral column (Figs. 4.1 and 4.2) [1]. The spine and the sacrum were involved in 30% of cases and the long tubular bones were involved in 34% of patients, with the lower extremity being more commonly affected than the upper extremity. 15% of tumors occur in the skull, mandible or maxilla, and 5% involved the innominate bone. Osteoblastoma involved the small bones of the hands and feet in 10% of patients.

In the spine, the thoracic and lumbar vertebrae are the most common sites of involvement. The posterior elements, more typically the pedicle and the laminae are more commonly involved. 55% of the tumors are contained in the dorsal elements and 42% in both posterior elements and the vertebral body. Involvement of the vertebral body is unusual. When present in the appendicular skeleton, these lesions have a predilection for the diaphysis in 75% of cases with the reminder in the metaphyses. Epiphyseal location is extremely rare. The femur and the tibia are the long bones most typically affected by chondroblastoma. Multicentric osteoblastomas involving more than one bone are extremely rare but have been reported in the hand and leg.

© Springer-Verlag London Ltd., part of Springer Nature 2021
J. Paulos and D. G. Poitout (eds.), *Bone Tumors*,
https://doi.org/10.1007/978-1-4471-7501-8_4

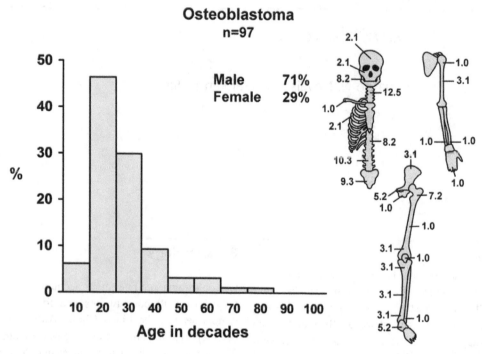

Fig. 4.1 Distribution of osteoblastoma

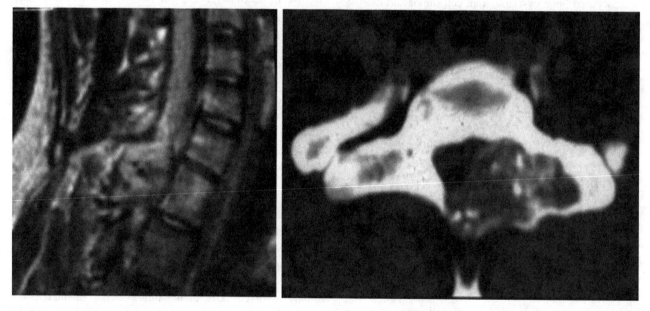

Fig. 4.2 Osteoblastoma: cervical spine C6

Genetics

Osteoblastomas have been associated with exhibited kary-otypic abnormalities, however no specific characteristic translocation has yet been identified. Chromosomal rear-rangements have been described with chromosome numbers ranging from hypodiploid to hyperdiploid. Involvement of chromosomes 1 and 14 appears to be recurrent in osteoblastoma.

Clinical Manifestation

Pain is the most common presenting symptom. Symptoms are typically present for a few months to two years. Pain is less localized, and accentuation at night and amelioration with salicylates are less constant when compared to the typical pain pattern of osteoid osteoma. Other prominent complaints are local swelling, tenderness, warmth and gait abnormalities. The clinical presentation of an osteoblastoma located in the spine may include neurologic deficit with muscle weakness or atrophy, hypoesthesia, and radicular nerve-root compression symptoms [2, 3]. Spinal deformity including progressive painful scoliosis and torticollis may develop. In rare occasions osteoblastoma may present with systemic symptoms such as weight loss, chronic fever, anemia and osteomalacia.

Imaging

Radiographic findings: the radiographic features of osteoblastoma are often nonspecific (Fig. 4.3). Based solely on radiographs, the indication of osteoblastoma was possible in 43% of cases in a review of 116 cases of appendicular osteoblastomas. In one-quarter of the cases the radiographic appearance was not considered specific for any particular diagnosis and in 17% of cases a diagnoses of osteoid osteoma was suggested. In the remaining cases many other diagnoses were suggested: chondroblastoma, osteosarcoma, aneurysmal bone cyst, fibrous dysplasia, chondrosarcoma, giant cell tumor and infection.

In the appendicular skeleton the lesion is often located within the cortex (65%) with a medullary location being less common (35%) (Fig. 4.4). The lesion is variable in size, ranging from 1 to 11 cm. The margins are most commonly well defined, however they can also be poorly defined or indefinite. In a study including 40 appendicular osteoblastomas, the lesion had a well-defined margin in only 33 cases and the remainer had an aggressive appearance. Osteolysis and osteosclerosis, alone or combined may be present. Cortical thinning, expansion of bone and a soft tissue mass are characteristics of an aggressive lesion that can be misinterpreted as evidence of a malignant tumor (Fig. 4.5). In the spine, a well-defined expansile osteolytic lesion, partially or extensively calcified, arising from the posterior elements suggest the diagnosis of osteoblastoma. Scoliosis has been reported in tumors of the ribs and the thoracic and lumbar vertebrae.

Other imaging techniques, such as bone scintigraphy, CT scanning and MRI may be useful tools to evaluate the local extension of the lesion and potential additional sites of involvement. Nevertheless these techniques cannot outline specific features that would allow the diagnosis. For the spine, a CT scan is the preferred imaging modality, since it can identify the lesion, degree of sclerosis, and extent of bony involvement. MRI may overestimate the extent of the lesion because of extensive reactive changes.

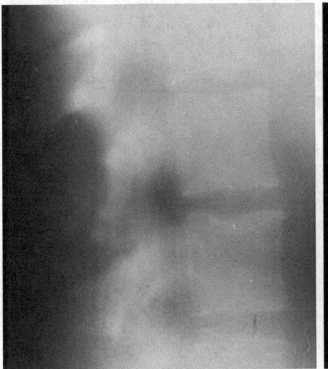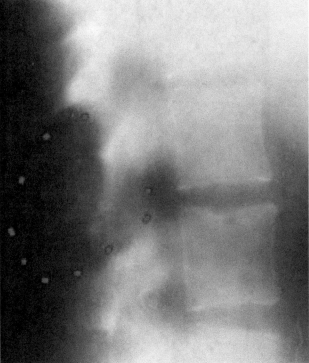

Fig. 4.3 Vertebral location is frequent (posterior arc)

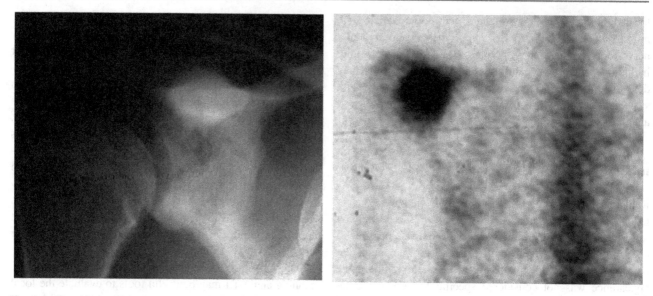

Fig. 4.4 Glenoid osteoblastoma

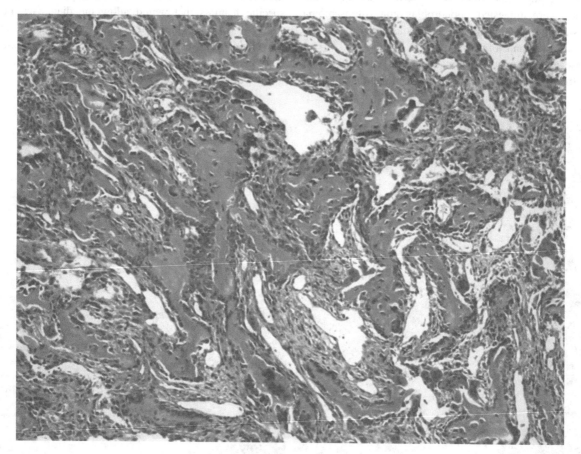

Fig. 4.5 Osteoblastoma is composed of numerous irregularly shaped bony trabeculae between which there is hypocellular fibrovascular connective tissue

Pathology

Macroscopical analysis of gross specimens obtained at surgical curettage reveals a red or red brown, hemorrhagic, granular, friable tissue with a sandpaper consistency due to the tumor bone. Analysis of resection specimens reveals a reasonably well-circumscribed lesion that frequently is intracortical with extensive surrounding sclerotic bone and a larger nidus than that of an osteoid osteoma. Spinal osteoblastomas often extend into paraspinal soft tissue; a feature that is less common in the appendicular osteoblastoma.

Microscopically, osteoblastoma is similar to osteoid osteoma, consisting of a well-vascularized connective tissue stroma in which there is active production of osteoid and primitive woven bone. The bony trabeculae are variably calcified and the osteoblasts may have small, inconspicuous nuclei with abundant cytoplasm or large vesicular nuclei with prominent nucleoli. The intertrabecular stroma is composed of capillary proliferation and loosely arranged spindle cells without atypia. Osteoblasts may show mitotic activity but they are not atypical. The vascularity is rich, often with extravasated red blood cells. Classic histologic features such as long interanastomizing trabeculae of osteoid or woven bone rimmed by a single row of osteoblasts within a loose fibrovascular stroma are not consistently present and osteoblastoma may show variations in its histologic features.

Classically the bone trabeculae are thick and well formed, however fine lacelike osteoid, a typical feature of osteosarcoma may be seen focally in up to 20% of cases. Cartilage is not considered a part of the histologic spectrum of osteoblastoma, however rare examples in which the tumor contained hyaline cartilage or chondroid matrix have been previously reported. Areas resembling secondary aneurysmal bone cyst may be seen in as many as 10% of cases. A multifocal pattern—the presence of more than one nidus within a single area of tumefaction may be identified.

Differential Diagnosis

Although a number of radiographic features may suggest a diagnosis, they usually do not allow for a correct diagnosis. In the spine, an expansile partially calcified lesion with osteolysis involving the posterior elements may be identified as osteoblastoma. Vertebral osteoblastoma should be differentiated from osteoid osteoma, aneurysmal bone cyst (ABC) and giant cell tumor (GCT). Unlike osteoblastoma and ABC, GCTs of the spine typically involve the vertebral body but may extend into the neural arch. Osteoid-osteoma of the spine is usually seen in patients between 10 and 20 years

old, while osteoblastoma tends to develop in patients who are slightly older. Histologically the lesions are similar; the primary difference between these lesions being the tendency of osteoblastoma to form a less sclerotic but more expansile mass. Osteoid osteomas are more sclerotic, are non-expansile, and become painful earlier in their development. McLeod et al. [4] arbitrarily defined lesions that were less than 1.5 cm in diameter as osteoid osteomas and lesions that were more than 1.5 cm in diameter as osteoblastomas. Aneurysmal bone cyst of the spine also usually arises in the posterior elements and can expand and extend into the pedicles, vertebral body, and spinal canal resulting in pathologic fracture and neurologic compromise. CT scanning may help in the differential diagnosis that must be confirmed by histological analysis of a biopsy prior to definitive treatment. In the appendicular skeleton the differential diagnosis should include osteoid osteoma, aneurysmal bone cyst, eosinophilic granuloma, enchondroma, fibrous dysplasia, chondromyxoid fibroma and solitary cyst. In rare instances an osteoblastoma may demonstrate radiographic features of local aggressiveness that are common to osteosarcoma such as destruction of the cortical bone, formation of Codman's triangle, and soft tissue extension. Histologic analysis may reveal a highly cellular tumor containing compact areas of osteoblasts that are larger and have more frequent mitoses than the osteoblasts in conventional osteoblastoma. There may be numerous multinucleated osteoclast type giant cells and abundant osteoid and trabeculae of woven bone, the so-called speculated tumor bone similar to that occurring in conventional osteosarcoma. Large sheets of osteoblasts approximately twice the size of conventional osteoblasts are evident and appear plump, with prominent nucleoli. These cells are termed epithelioid osteoblasts and are a hallmark of this more aggressive type of osteoblastoma. Lucas et al. however failed to identify a correlation between histopathologic features and clinical and radiographic aggressiveness of the tumor. According to the authors, aggressive behavior is within the spectrum of osteoblastoma. In their study 12% of the tumors had radiographic features that suggested malignancy and most of those were conventional osteoblastomas in histologic analysis (Fig. 4.6).

In the past the more aggressive pattern of osteoblastoma has been addressed under the terms "aggressive osteoblastoma" and "malignant osteoblastoma" however precise definition of these lesions are still not clearly established and the two have been regarded as either identical or different lesions. Bertoni et al. [1] and others have reported cases of osteosarcoma that on histologic analysis resembled osteoblastoma and recommended that these tumors were

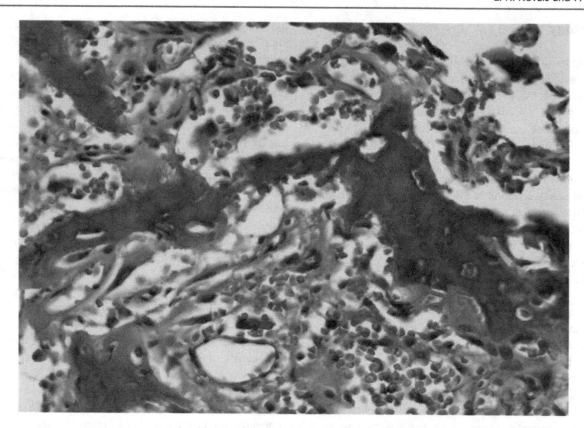

Fig. 4.6 Prominent osteoblastic rimming of the bony trabeculae are evident; vascular spaces are generally prominent

similar to the so-called malignant osteoblastoma. Whatever the term used, they postulated that it is important to recognize this small group of osteoblasts as rich lesions that resemble osteoblastomas but behave like osteosarcoma. Perhaps the most difficult and important task is to differentiate an aggressive osteoblastoma from a conventional osteosarcoma as it has major clinical implications. Histologically the most important criterion for differentiating osteoblastoma from osteosarcoma is permeation. Osteoblastoma are well-demarcated lesions with no tendency to permeate between pre-existing bony trabeculae.

Treatment

Treatment of osteoblastoma depends on the localization and stage of the tumor. In stage 1 (latent) or stage 2 (active) osteoblastoma, curettage (intralesional excision) and bone grafting is indicated. For stage 3 (aggressive) osteoblastoma the resection should be either marginal or wide. Independently of the method of treatment the goal should be complete excision of the tumor. Osteoblastoma of the spine may impose a more challenging problem than a tumor located in a long bone due to a more complex anatomy and the close proximity of neurovascular structures. In addition, tumor resection may jeopardize the structural stability of the vertebral column and may mandate spine instrumentation. Recurrence rates of spinal osteoblastoma are related to the type of surgical resection and stage. In aggressive osteoblastomas recurrence rates with incomplete resection are reported in up to 50% of cases, while for the less aggressive lesions the recurrence rate has been reported at between 10 and 15%. Accumulative review of the isolated aggressive spinal osteoblastomas showed recurrence rates of intralesional excision were 93%; marginal resection, 15%; and en bloc resection, 20% (1/5). In aggressive osteoblastoma of the spine (stage 3) characterized when a lesion breaks through the bone and has a soft tissue mass, en bloc resection is recommended when anatomically feasible, to minimize risk of local recurrence. Selective arterial embolization may be helpful immediately preceding surgery to reduce hemorrhage during the operation. The role of radiation therapy in recurrent lesions or in lesions that cannot be totally resected or due to anatomic constraints such as involvement of neurological structures is controversial, with the majority of reports demonstrating no advantage.

References

1. Bertoni F, Unni KK, Mcleod RA, Dahlin DC. Osteosarcoma resembling osteoblastoma. Cancer. 1985;55:416–26.
2. Wold M, Sim U. Atlas of orthopedic pathology. W.B. Saunders Company; 1990.
3. Nemoto O, Moser RP Jr, Van Dam BE, Aoki J, Gilkey FW (1990) Osteoblastoma of the spine: a review of 75 cases. Spine 1990; 15: 1272–1280.
4. McLeod RA, Dahlin DC, Beabout JW. The spectrum of osteoblastoma. Am J Roentgenol. 1976;126:321–35.

Osteosarcoma

5

Dominique G. Poitout

Abstract

Osteosarcoma, or osteogenic sarcoma, is a primary malignant bone tumor with a variety of histological subtypes grouped into three categories, each one with a different prognosis. As a malignant tumor, it has the capacity of making early metastasis, being the lung being the most frequent secondary location. The most common location is in either in the lower extremity around the knee or in the upper extremity in the proximal humerus. The diagnosis is made considering clinical aspects, radiology and histology. The therapy has evolved in the past decade and it includes a combination of radical surgery, chemotherapy and immunotherapy. The decision is made according to the histological subtype, size and the presence of metastasis. The main prognostic factors are location, histological type, size of the tumor and metastasis at the moment of diagnosis.

Keywords

Osteosarcoma • Osteogenic sarcoma • Bone tumor • Chemotherapy • Radical surgery

Osteogenic sarcoma or osteosarcoma: the definition is histological.

It is a malignant primitive bone tumor in wich the tumoral cells produce osteoid bone tissue [1].

The tumoral osteogenic cells are prevalent for the diagnosis, although it can be associated to any zone showing chondroblastic or fibroblastic tissue. It is necessary to identify these cells clearly within the group of osteosarcomas and this makes the difference between chondrosarcomas or fibrosarcomas.

D. G. Poitout (✉)
Aix Marseille University, Marseille, France
e-mail: dominique.poitout@live.fr

The histological, pathological, clinical and evolutive aspects are variable and must be considered both for the prognosis and the therapy. Because of the difficulties considering the study of series of similar ostesarcomas and their prognosis and as there are few number of cases using different therapeutic methods the comparison are not reliable.

The prognosis was considered very bad until not long time ago. Today, although it is still considered very severe thanks to the development of research in surgery and chemotherapy, the prognosis has improved a lot in the last years (Fig. 5.1).

Anato-Pathological Study

Anatomical aspects. Almost always when the diagnosis of osteogenic sarcoma is made with a biopsy, the X-ray study shows an extended bone sarcoma which has broken compromises not only the metaphysis but also partially the diaphysis. The slides, sometimes show invasion of the medular canal, this sometimes even without a radiological image.

There are multiple aspects of these sarcomas: osteogenics, others chondrogenics, others hypervascularized, others necrotics, some with few osteogenics, others hypercondensants. These different macroscopics or microscopics aspects, make the difference among the forms of osteosarcoma.

Histopathological aspects. There are multiple histological aspects of osteogenic sarcomas that can be helpful in their prognosis.

First Category (Type I) Prognosis Relatively Favorable

The well-differenciated osteoblastic sarcomas is sometimes mistaken with osteoblastomas. The healing in most cases obtained with a simple resection.

© Springer-Verlag London Ltd., part of Springer Nature 2021
J. Paulos and D. G. Poitout (eds.), *Bone Tumors*,
https://doi.org/10.1007/978-1-4471-7501-8_5

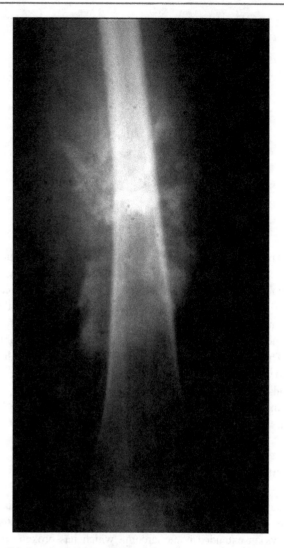

Fig. 5.1 Image of an osteogenic sarcoma

The juxtacortical sarcoma described by Geschickter and Copeland is localized in the external cortical which seems to be over it not invade the intramedular region.

The periosteal sarcoma is under the periosteo which separates it from the cortical.

These two tumors are of difficult histolological interpretation because the fusiform cells show very few mitosis and exceptionally monsters cells; the tumoral bone tissue looks of an organoid appearence with the risk of mistaking the real diagnosis.

We need to know that the osteoma, which is in the differential diagnosis has not atypical cells and sometimes between the trabeculaes, a little hematopoietic bone marrow can be found making it very different from finding fusiform cells of a juxtacortical sarcoma (Fig. 5.2).

Second Category (Type II)

These sarcomas are of bad prognosis. They represent in more or less 65–70% of cases of the common form of these sarcomas. The histology is very polyform and sometimes shows chondrogenesis or osteogenesis.

In young people, there is frequently a chondrogenic prevalence. In these sarcomas, three cytological types are distinguished: ostéoblastic, fibroblastic and chondroblastic.

The osteoblastic type is considered to be the most malignant form with the worst prognosis. This sarcoma represents the most frequent case of osteogenic sarcomas.

It is necessary to distinguish degrees of malignancy considering three elements:

- Frequency of mitosis
- The existence of anaplastics areas
- The existence of vascular embolism.

The anaplastic zones and the existence of many vascular embolisms are major pejorative factors. The number of mitosis is more artificial because of the poliformism of these tumors; the presence of poor zones of mitosis can exist with osteogenic zones and anaplastic zones sometimes without formation of osteoid or chondroid tissue.

Third Category (Type III)

They are sarcomas of a very bad prognosis.

The telangiectasic sarcomas frequently affect the metaphysis and the diaphysis. It is somewhat difficult to make differential diagnosis between an aneurismatic cyst and an angiosarcoma (Fig. 5.3).

The anaplastic sarcomas have many variable polymorfic cells in size and form due to chondrogenic or osteogenic production.

The anaplastic sarcomas of round cells set the differential diagnosis with an Ewing's sarcoma. A network of reticulina and the P.A.S. reaction show intracytoplasmic granulations, the nucleoli are more irregular, the chromatin is less fine. Frequently, there is a big nucleus, differentiating it from an Ewing sarcoma in which they are of little dimensions.

The anaplastic sarcomas have cells of irregular form. In some 30 year old patients, the invasion of the diaphysis has been found. This states the differential diagnosis with the metastasis of a Parker sarcoma. In this case, the osteogenesis is represented with some very fine spans forming an irregular maze.

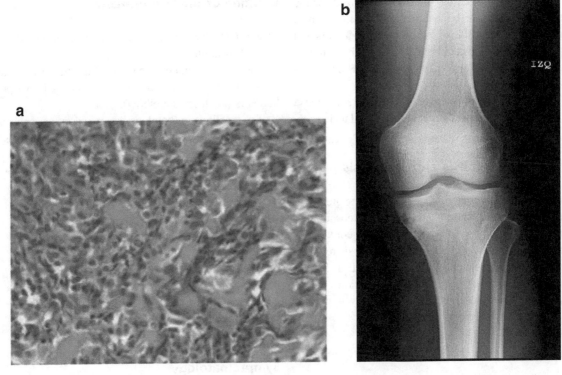

Fig. 5.2 Osteosarcoma **a** histological aspect, and **b** radiological aspect of osteosarcoma on proximal metaphyseal bone of tibia

Fig. 5.3 X-ray and MRI of a
telangectasic osteosarcoma

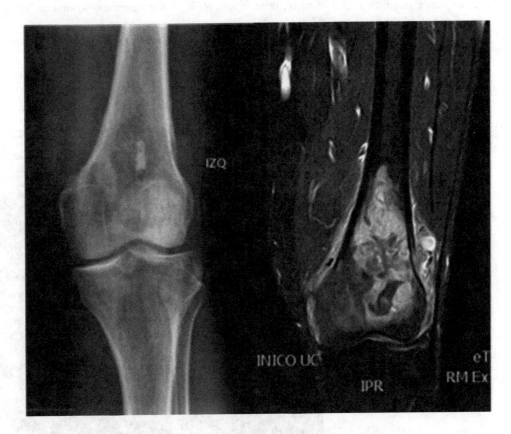

The sclerosant osteosarcomatosis is characterized for the existence of quite a lot of bone formation developed in a short time. The radiological image shows opaque tumors and the histology shows an osteoblastic tumor with abundant osteogenesis. This last form has a very bad prognosis (Fig. 5.4).

It is true that it is necessary to differentiate all these multiple forms. This requires a perfect histological technique.

Clinical Study, Diagnosis and Prognosis

The clinical aspects differ but most of the time there are some characters that would allow to suspect of an osteosarcoma. However, it is necessary to insist that the most convincing suspicion is not a certainty. Therefore, the diagnosis requires an histological confirmation. This means that a biopsy is mandatory before taking any therapeutic decision.

In opposition, the clinical aspects can be very important because they can have a prognostic value [2].

Sex

The frequency is a little higher in men (more or less 60%); more than half of the cases appear between 15 to 25 year old patients. The prognosis is especially severe in young children.

Location of the Osteosarcoma

It is a metaphyseal tumor and can also be found in a diaphyseal location.

The most frequent location is in the lower extremity around the knee and in the upper extremity in the proximal humerus (far from the elbow).

The locations in the plane bones and in the rachis are less frequent but they have a worse prognosis, sometimes with a difficult access to radical surgery.

The femoral location seems to be twice more severe than the tibial or the fibular one [3].

Development of the Tumor

The invasion of the soft tissue is constant.

The size of the tumor gives a prognostic value, being 40% of survival for tumors of less than 5cms, and only 4% for the ones over 10 cms.

Symptomatology

Two alarming symptoms are the pain and the existence of tumefaction.

The pain can be violent and at night but most of the time it is very slow delaying consulting the physician.

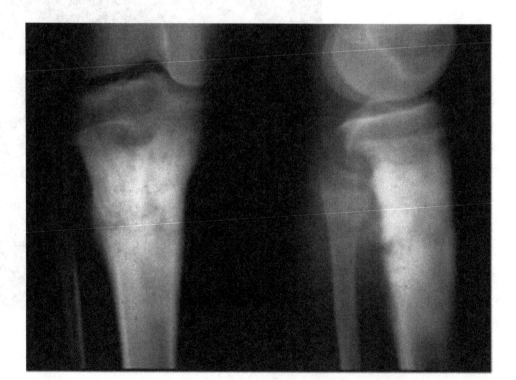

Fig. 5.4 Osteosarcoma, osteoblastic image on X-ray

The tumefaction is only detectable in some locations and in the developed cases. These signs need a radiological exam.

Radiological Aspects (TAC, MRI, Arteriography, Scintigraphy)

The radiological study is essencial for the diagnosis, preceding the biopsy.

In the developed forms, the malignancy signs are characteristics:

diffuse bone remodeling without precise limits, a zone of osteolysis or condensation, cortical breakage, periosteal reaction, invasion of the soft tissue and images of anarchic osteogenesis in blaze form. It is necessary to pay special attention to the less evident images (Fig. 5.5).

The scanner (TAC) will better show the calcified zones and can precise the intra and extra osteolytic bone extension.

The MRI will practically give an anatomical study about the intra and extra extension of the tumor and the soft tissue around the bone. It will be able to show the vascular and nerve compromise and overall the existence of "skip" metastasis. This means intramedullary locations far from the primitive tumor in the same bone.

A scintigraphy can show in evidence a debutant lesion or a discrete osteolytic central zone (hyperfixant) or with a little cortical erosion.

The arteriography will be requested systematically to determine in preop the aspect of the vessels around the tumor and considering intraop risks in the dissection of the tumor. This exam can also be asociated with the MRI which analyses the vascular walls and of the eventual invasion.

A biopsy must be requested in all the forms of presentation.

Biological Signs

Neither the VHS nor alkaline phosphatase has a diagnostic value.

Special Anatomoclinical Forms

The osteosarcoma in adult or old people can be less characteristic and can have a diaphyseal location.

It is necessary to know that radio-induced sarcomas that can appear many years after the irradiation of the bone. In same cases only a diligent bone biopsy can make the difference with a radio-necrosis.

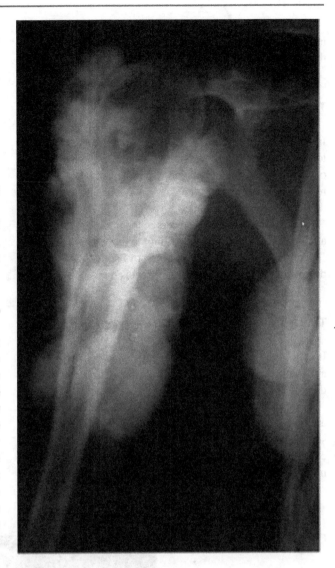

Fig. 5.5 Bone formation in osteosarcoma

The multicentrics osteosarcomas are less frequent in men but are often found in dogs. They are habitually present under condensant forms.

The osteosarcomas in a Paget or in a giant cell tumor with an osteolytic presentation has a very bad prognosis.

The Metastasis

From the prognostic point of view, it could be said that the osteosarcomas would have a lung presentation in whose records a bone lesion is found.

Death is the effect of a metastasic development even though the primitive bone sarcoma could have disapeared for example with a block resection.

Patients do not really die of a femur sarcoma but of a tumor in which the primitive bone location is secondary to the development of metastasis.

The Detectable Metastasis

In 98% of the cases metastasis are in the lungs. In other locations they are exceptional sometimes isolated but most of the time associated to lung metastasis. After the 20th month, a statistic survival curve without metastasis falls down very quickly to under 30%.

Most of the metastasis appears in the first two years giving afterwards a good chance of healing to the surviving patients.

The current therapy (chemotherapy) sometimes does not do much; it only slow down their eclosions.

The Non Perceptible Disease

It is necessary to distinguish the appearance of metastasis in an anatomical evolution so as to make a possible early diagnosis of its real existence.

The anatomical characteristics of the bone lesion, the arteriography findings and those of the electronic microscopy in the invasive process of early stages, the circulatory conditions facilitate embolic phenomenon setting the malignant cells into the circulatory blood.

The study of tumoral growing of lung metastasis established by the time of duplication, suggest that the metastasis can be seen under a subclinic stage in 60 or 80% of the patients when patients first examined. In fact the diagnosis is only made in 10% of these cases.

Earliness in the diagnosis of metastasis as an imperceptible sickness is utmost in programming todays current therapy.

Virologic and Immunologic Study

After the first sarcomatous virus was discovered by Rous in 1911, other sarcoma viruses have been isolated in the mouse, cat, and monkey, and there for special attention is given today to the research of viruses in human sarcomas.

Miriam Finkel in 1963 and Dmochowski's experience only found osteosarcoma viruses in rodents, but in men, not surely yet. The particles C representative of these viruses of type ARN have been exceptionally found in human cell cultures. They are characterized by the presence of a very special enzyme, the retrotranscriptase, that can copy the DNA, the viral RNA, stage necessary for its final integration in the genetic material of the infected cell. But the integration can only include a portion of the viral genome and it is necessary to detect the biochemical and immunological footprints of the viral components (Fig. 5.6).

Fig. 5.6 Lung metastasis

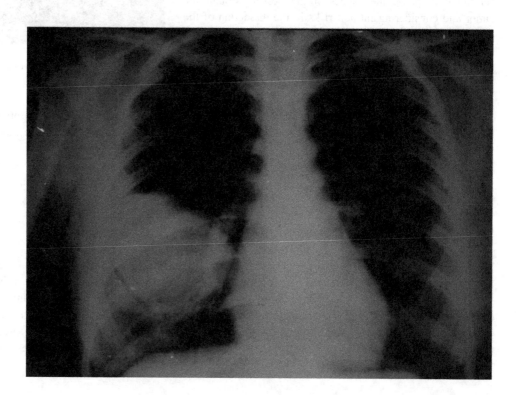

The existence of modified due to the activity of the retrotranscriptase of a viral RNA in the human sarcoma cells is not very convincing because its type of activity has been found in other human tissues and in embryonnary non-transformed cells cultures. In the absence of direct tests of the virus action, indirect tests have been tried:

- Find common antigens on the surface of tumoral cells and finding antibodies in the serum other human tissues and in embryonnary non transformed cells cultures.
- Find techniques of hybridation to detect and measure the sequence of genetic information in the core of nucleid acids of the cell, being wittness fraction of the existence of a viral genome. But these viral sequences cannot be bounded to the tumoral character.

So the viral hypothesis related with human sarcomas has not been proven till today. Although in the absence of a demonstration of an etiological viral agent, the antigenicity given by the tumoral cells could be used to stimulate the immunological defense of the organism against the tumor; the efficiency of vaccination using tumoral antibodies has not been demonstrated up to now.

Therapy

There are many therapeutical methods, but there is some facts to be considered: Exceeding the therapy of the local bone lesion, looking at the non-perceptible sickness and therefore the local therapy must be associated to the general sickness.

Direct Methods on the Bone: Radical Surgery

It is necessary to have a perfect knowledge of the tumoral limits and the zones in contact with the vessels and nerves. The MRI and the arteriography will give the best information for the tumoral resection, a near few centimeters away from the tumor. The tumoral resection has the same value as the amputation. If the vessels and nerves are invaded they must be resected. The surgical aproach for the biopsy must be imperatively resected with the tumor and together with it, to avoid a local recurrence.

The resection will be considered marginal when the tumor is not opened and is resected near its limits (less than 2 cms.) and considered intratumoral when the tumor is opened. Any doubt justifies an amputation considering the patients life risk.

The massive bone reconstruction with a massive bone graft or a prosthesis will not be possible after a complete carcinologic resection [4, 5].

Irradiation is not used today unless it allows a carcinologic resection [6].

Some Asian authors propose an irradiation in situ, intraop after the dissection. The series seem satisfactory from the carcinogenic point of view.

The Associated Methods to the Non Perceptible Sickness

The Chemotherapy. The discovery of effective products and the association of them allow to reach an important survival rate. The methotrexate used in increasing high doses with folic acid, adriamicine, cyclofosfamide, and cis-platinum have proved the demonstration of their effectiveness [7].

The combination of several chemotherapeutic agents has been very beneficial. The combination of methotrexate–folic acid and adriamicine, used for a long time has reached a survival near 60–75% without metatasis [8].

The protocol from Rosen (T10) with the combination of adriamicine, cyclophosphamide and methotrexate–folic acid has been a very interesting.

The promising results using the adjuvant chemotherapy must be aware of the complications of chemotherapy, sometimes deadful and even mortal. The therapy, the doses, the chronology and the overseeing must be very well checked [9].

Interferon

Discovered in 1957 by Isaacs and Lindenmann. The interferons are proteins with antiviral activity but are also anti-tumoral and immunomodulatory activity.

Immunotherapy

We can believe in it only if a sarcoma is produced due to a failure of the immunologic system and also thinking that if healing comes after an amputation it is due to the immunologic defense.

The results are uncertain and with only little series. No randomized essays have been published; the efforts are concentrated in comparing different chemotherapeutical protocols [10].

Therapy of Perceptible Metastasis

The irradiation of local metastasis is very disapointing; the reduction of the volume tumoral or its disappearence is very ephemeral [8].

In these cases, the chemotherapy has only a low answer and very rarely healing.

The least disapointing results can be obtained with the association of chemotherapeutic agents like adriamicine, methotrexate, folic acid, cyclophosphamide, mitomycine D, dacarbasine (DTIC) and cis-platinum.

Nevertheless it is necessary to know that considering the low efficacy and the morbidity of the chemotherapy, it is necessary to balance its benefit with the peacefullness of an expected death.

In opposition, the chemotherapy must be retaken when the lung metastasis are resecables. The prognosis is better when the metastasis appears later in the follow-up.

The systematic resection of lung metastasis is nowadays indicated and gives excellents results.

Schematic treatment of osteosarcoma:

- Diagnosis: clinic–image–histopathology
- Treatment:

  – Neoadjuvant chemotherapy [11]
  – Surgery
  – Adjuvant chemotherapy [12–14]
- Drugs most commonly used for osteosarcomas are:
  Doxorubicina (adriamycina), actinomicyna D, ifosfamida, ciclofosfamida, cisplatino, methotrexato HD; Protocols used in the Protocol T 10 from Rosen.
- Example of a protocol (must be managed by a chemotherapist):
  – neoadjuvant chemotherapy; 6 to 18 weeks:
  – adriamicina–cisplatino 4 weeks
  – 4–6 weeks; methotrexato HD + A.folico
  – adriamicyna–cisplatino 4 weeks
  – metotrexato HD 2 weeks
  – surgery:
    resection in block + reconstructive surgery; or amputation
  – study of tumoral necrosis of the tumor
  – chemotherapy adjuvant
    metotrexato HD + AF 1 week
    adriamicina-cisplatino 1 week
    repeat untill 28 weeks.

Fig. 5.7 Rx. juxtacortical osteosarcoma

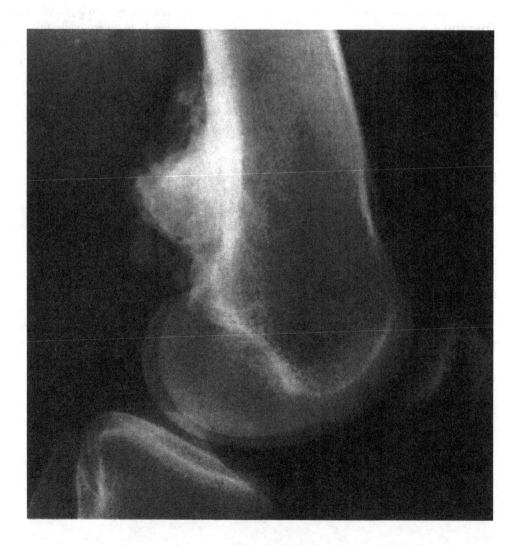

The Juxtacortical Osteosarcoma

This was described in 1951 by Geschikter and Copeland, its anatomo-clinical characteristics and overall having a more favorable prognosis requires to separate this tumor from other osteosarcomas (Fig. 5.7) [15, 16].

It is a well-differentiated histological type. Its topography is determined by a cortical implantation and an extraosseus development.

It is not very frequent with a low prevalence in women.

It appears later than the habitual osteosarcoma, mostly in the third or fourth decade of life.

The most frequent location is the posterior distal metaphysis of the femur.

Its painless presentation explain a late diagnosis which is only made when the tumoral volume appears.

The X-ray shows an extraosseus mass of regular limits without invasion of the soft tissues with an opacity similar to the cortex over which it is implanted and with a long implantation on it.

The scanner can give the exact zone of the implantation of the tumor in the cortical.

The MRI shows no invasion of the soft tissues.

The growing of the tumor is very slow and the metastasis appears very late.

The treatment is exclusively surgical. Irradiation and chemotherapy are not useful. The resection of the distal femur with reconstruction with a massive allograft, a masive endoprosthesis or allograft with endoprosthesis gives better functional results. The arthrodesis-reconstruction according to the Juvara technique improved upon by Merle D'Aubigné is sometimes proposed when there is no soft tissue to get a useful knee function. A complete resection of the tumor and the cortical must be made far from the implantation base.

If a recurrence occurs, an amputation is needed, because the risk of metastasis becomes possible.

The results, considering the slow evolution and the late recurrence and the late appearence of metastasis, must be judged with a long follow-up.

References

1. Misaghi A.Osteosarcoma: a comprehensive review. SICOT J 2018; 4:12. https://doi.org/10.1051/sicotj/2017028. Epub April 9, 2018.

2. Rosen G, Marcove RC, Caparros B, Nirenberg A, Kosloff C, Huvos AG. Primary osteogenic sarcoma: The rationale for preoperative chemotherapy and delayed surgery. Cancer. 1979;43(6): 2163–77.

3. Ozaki T, Flege S, Kevric M, et al. Osteosarcoma of the pelvis: experience of the cooperative osteosarcoma study group. J Clin Oncol. 2003;21(2):334–41.

4. Malek F, Somerson JS, Mitchel S, Williams RP. Does limb-salvage surgery offer patients better quality of life and functional capacity than amputation? Clin Orthop Relat Res. 2012;470(7):2000–6.

5. Nystrom LM, Morcuende JA. Expanding endoprosthesis for pediatric musculoskeletal malignancy: Current concepts and results. Iowa Orthop J. 2010; 30:141–149.

6. DeLaney TF, Park L, Goldberg SI, et al. Radiotherapy for local control of osteosarcoma. Int J Radiat Oncol Biol Phys. 2005;61(2): 492–8.

7. Brosjö O. Surgical procedure and local recurrence in 223 patients treated 1982–1997 according to two osteosarcoma chemotherapy protocols: The Scandinavian Sarcoma Group experience. Acta Orthop Scand Suppl. 1999;285:58–61.

8. Moore DD et al. Advances in targeted therapy for osteosarcoma. Zhou W. et al. Discov Med Cancer Treat Res. 2014;162: 65–92. https://doi.org/10.1007/978-3-319-07323 PMID: 25070231, https://doi.org/10.1007/978-3-319-07323-1_4.

9. Hawkins DS, Conrad EU III, Butrynski JE, Schuetze SM, Eary JF. [F-18]-fluorodeoxy-D-glucose-positron emission tomography response is associated with outcome for extremity osteosarcoma in children and young adults. Cancer. 2009;115(15):3519–25.

10. Wang D, Tang L, Wu H, Wang K, Gu D. MiR-127-3p inhibits cell growth and invasiveness by targeting ITGA6 in humanosteosarcoma. IUBMB Life. 2018; 70(5):411–419. https://doi.org/10.1002/iub.1710. Epub March 23, 2018, PMID: 2957311.

11. Bacci G, Bertoni F, Longhi A, et al. Neoadjuvant chemotherapy for high-grade central osteosarcoma of the extremity: Histologic response to preoperative chemotherapy correlates with histologic subtype of the tumor. Cancer. 2003;97(12):3068–75.

12. Picci P, Bacci G, Campanacci M, Gasparini M, Pilotti S, Cerasoli SF, Bertoni F, Guerra A, Capanna A, Albasinni U. Histologic evaluation of necrosis in osteosarcoma induced by chemotherapy. Cancer. 1985; 56: 1515–1521.

13. Harrison DJ, Schwartz, MD. Osteogenic sarcoma: systemic chemotherapy options for localized disease. Curr Treat Options Oncol. 2017;18:24.

14. Eilber FR, Rosen G. Adjuvant chemotherapy for osteosarcoma. Semin Oncol. 1989;16(4):312–22.

15. Unni KK, Dahlin DC, Beabout JW, Ivins JC. Paraosteal osteogenic sarcoma. Cancer. 1976;37:2466–75.

16. Claude L, Rousmans S, Bataillard A, Philip T. Fédération nationale des centres de lutte contre le cancer (FNCLCC); Fédération hospitalière de France (FHF); Fédération nationale de cancérologie des CHRU (FNCCHRU); Fédération française de cancérologie des CHG (FFCCHG); centres régionaux de lutte contre le cancer (CRLCC); Société française de lutte contre les cancers de l'enfant et de l'adolescent (SFCE). Standards and Options for the use of radiation therapy in the management of patients with osteosarcoma: Update 2004. Cancer Radiother. 2005; 9(2): 104–121. Review. French. PMID:1588088.

Part III
Lesions Forming Cartilage

Osteochondroma and Hereditary Multiple Osteochondromas

6

Franklin H. Sim

Abstract

Osteochondroma is the most common bone tumor, mainly affecting patients under 20 years of age. It presents in 90% of the cases as a solitary lesion. The remaining cases are part of the multiple hereditary osteochondromas syndrome. The pathogenesis is not entirely clear. Osteochondromas usually develop at the metaphysis of long bones. Malignant transformation is rare in solitary lesions, but more common in hereditary syndromes. Solitary osteochondromas are asymptomatic and may be diagnosed incidentally through X-rays. Differential diagnosis includes benign and malignant lesions.

Keywords

Osteochondroma • Cartilage • Exostoses • Bone tumor • Benign bone lesion

Definition

The World Health Organization defines osteochondroma as "a cartilage capped bony projection arising on the external surface of bone containing a marrow cavity that is continuous with that of the underlying bone." The generic term exostosis indicates any outgrowth of bone and should not be mistakenly used as a synonym of osteochondroma. Solitary osteochondroma occur as non-familial, sporadic lesions. The terms hereditary multiple osteochondromas (HMO), hereditary multiple exostosis (HME), diaphyseal aclasis, multiple cartilaginous exostosis and hereditary multiple exostosis have all been used to characterize growth of multiple osteochondromas.

F. H. Sim (✉)
Mayo Clinic, Rochester, MN 55905, USA
e-mail: sim.franklin@mayo.edu

Epidemiology

Osteochondroma is the most common neoplasm affecting bone, however its true prevalence is difficult to define as many patients are asymptomatic and the tumor is never identified. Nevertheless it is estimated that osteochondromas comprise around 35% of all primary benign bone tumors and 10% of all tumors. In the pediatric population the occurrence of 35.2 per million inhabitants per year has been reported.

Approximately 90% of all osteochondromas present as solitary lesions. The remaining cases are part of the multiple hereditary osteochondromas syndrome.

The majority of osteochondromas affect children and adolescents, with approximately 80% of lesions occurring in the first two decades of life. Around 60% of the patients are male.

Locations

Osteochondromas usually develop in bones that are formed through the process of enchondral ossification. Most often the metaphysis of a long tubular bone is affected, rarely the diaphysis. The most commonly involved sites, in descending order, are the distal femur, proximal humerus, and proximal tibia (Fig. 6.1).

The pelvis is involved in approximately 5% of cases [1] while the involvement of the spine is around 3% [2]. The posterior elements of the lumbar and cervical spine are most often affected. Involvement of the spine has been reported to be associated with development of spinal cord compression and subsequent neurologic deficit [3–8]. The small bones of the hand and feet may be involved in the context of multiple osteochondromas [9–12]. Osteochondroma may involve the scapula in up to 5% cases and it can lead to snapping syndrome and pseudowinging of the scapula [13,14]. Rarely a lesion may involve the ribs or the sternum (Figs. 6.2 and 6.3) [15]

© Springer-Verlag London Ltd., part of Springer Nature 2021
J. Paulos and D. G. Poitout (eds.), *Bone Tumors*,
https://doi.org/10.1007/978-1-4471-7501-8_6

Fig. 6.1 Epimediology and location on skeleton osteochondroma

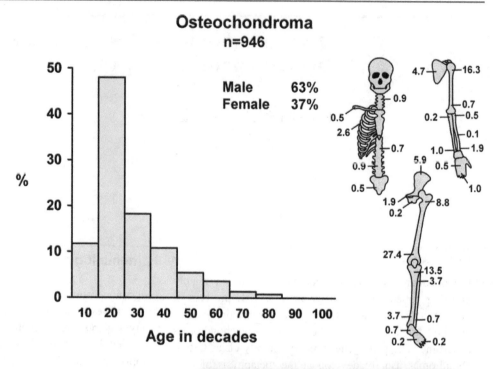

Osteochondroma
n=946

Male   63%
Female   37%

%

Age in decades

Etiology and Pathogenesis

There has been an increasing debate about the true nature of osteochondromas. Some authors consider osteochondromas a growth disturbance) [16] (developmental aberration hypothesis) while others defend it is a true benign neoplasm. In the past, the typical justaphyseal location has led to the hypothesis that osteochondromas arises from a portion of the physeal cartilage and its growth [17]. Cartilage metaplasia, defective bone remodeling [18], dysfunction of the periosteum [19] have all been suggested to play a role in the pathogenesis of osteochondromas. The alteration in the direction of normal bone growth resulting from aberrant epiphyseal development has been suggested as the main cause of osteochondromas [16, 20]. Secondary osteochondromas have been reported after radiation therapy [21, 22] and after fractures involving the growth plate [23]. However, cytogenetic studies have identified two loci and subsequent mutation in genes suggested that loss or mutation of EXT1 and EXT2 genes are important in the pathogenesis of both solitary and multiple osteochondromas, therefore compelling evidence of the neoplastic origin of these lesions [24–26].

Hereditary multiple osteochondromas is the most common genetic skeletal dysplasia, with an estimated prevalence of 1/50 000 and is inherited as an autosomal dominant disorder with full penetrance [27] (Fig. 6.4).

HMO has been associated with mutations in the EXT1 gene on chromosome 8q24.11–q24.13) and in the EXT2 gene on chromosome 11p12-p11. To date, there have been

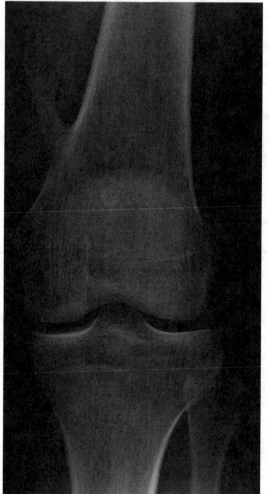

Fig. 6.2 Pediculated osteochondroma: typical aspect on X-ray

Fig. 6.3 CT showing osteochondroma of the sternum

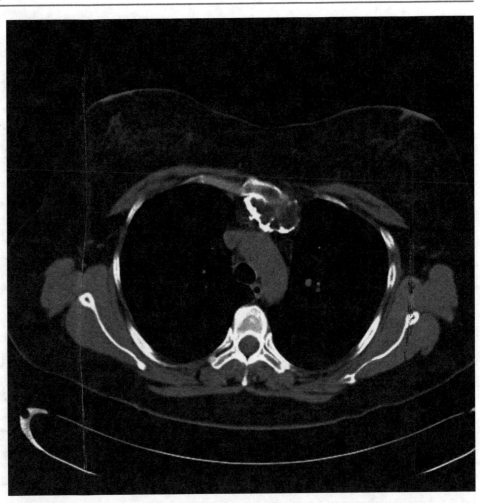

close to one hundred different EXT1 and fifty different EXT2 mutations reported [26, 28, 29]. Inactivating mutations (frame shift, nonsense and splice-site) represent approximately 80% of the causing mutations of HMO [26]. Missense mutations are less common [30]. In solitary osteochondromas mutation on these genes are reported mainly in the cells from the lesion itself [31].

Pathology

The macroscopic features of an osteochondroma depend whether the lesion is pedunculated or sessile (Fig. 6.5). Sessile osteochondromas are usually round with a thin cartilage cap while pedunculated lesions resemble a mushroom with a bony stalk and a cartilage cap. The cap has a smooth surface and usually ossifies in the skeletal maturity when it should measure no more than a few millimeters. Overlying the cap often a bursa is found.

Microscopically a thin periosteal layer covers the cartilaginous cap. The thin cartilaginous cap is composed of chondrocytes in lacunae arranged in clusters with abundant chondroid matrix. The base of the cartilaginous cap resembles the appearance of the physeal growth plate with maturation via endochondral ossification to regular bone trabeculae. The intertrabecular space is usually filled with fatty or hematopoietic marrow.

Natural History

Osteochondroma usually grow and ossify during skeletal development (Fig. 6.6). Although rare, spontaneous regression of a solitary osteochondroma has been reported.

The lesions should stop growing with skeletal maturity. Lesions that continue to grow after skeletal maturity must be carefully evaluated for the possibility of malignant transformation. Malignant transformation is extremely rare in solitary osteochondromas (less than 1%).

In hereditary multiple osteochondromas malignant transformation is more frequent. Clinically based studies report rates ranging from 0 to 5%.

The most common tumor associated with osteochondromas and HMO is peripheral chondrosarcomas, however

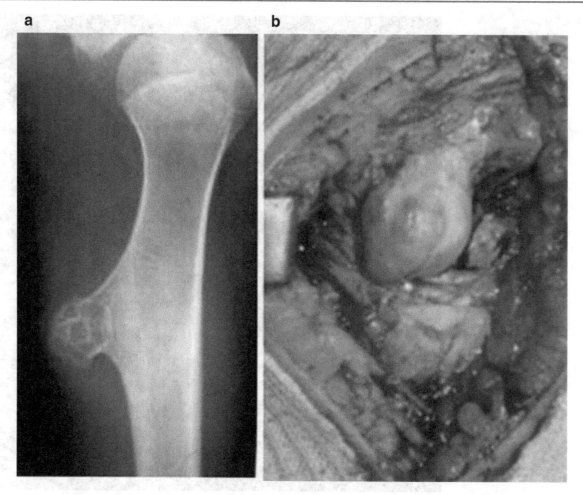

Fig. 6.4 Femur osteochondroma: **a** radiological aspect **b** intraoperative aspect

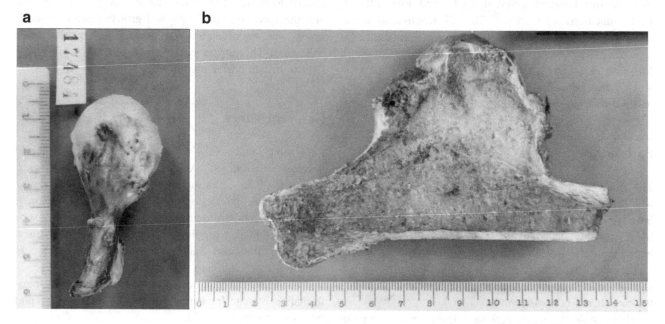

Fig. 6.5 Macroscopic aspect of osteochondroma **a** pediculated osteochondroma **b** sesile osteochondroma

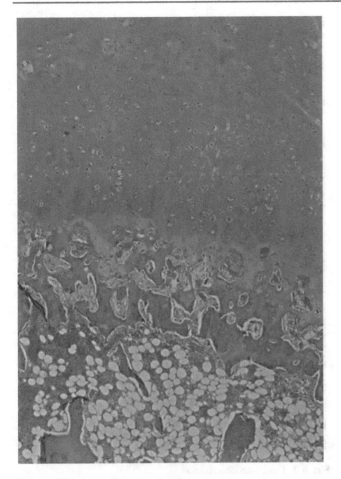

Fig. 6.6 Histology of an osteochondroma

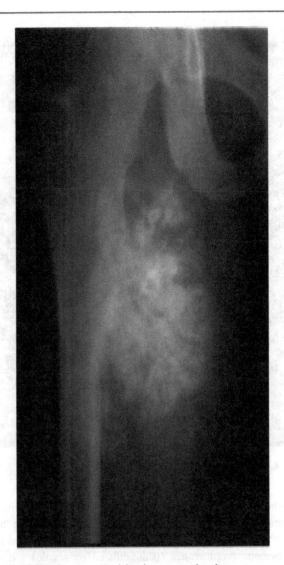

Fig. 6.7 Chondrosarcoma arising in an osteochondroma

osteosarcoma has also been reported. Chondrosarcoma arising in an osteochondroma is typically a low-grade neoplasm (Fig. 6.7).

The diagnosis of malignant transformation is challenging and requires clinical, imaging and histologic information. Growth beyond skeletal maturity and radiographic and advanced imaging evidence of an enlarged cartilaginous cap (greater than 2 cm) are features associated with malignant transformation. Histologically the columnar pattern of the chondrocytes is lost. There is permeation of the bone and nodules of cartilage extending into soft tissues with mitotic activity, atypia and necrosis.

Clinical Manifestation

A large number of solitary osteochondromas are asymptomatic and may be diagnosed incidentally. Initial presentation may be related to a painless palpable mass. Mechanical irritation of the surrounding tissues may result in the development of a bursa around the cartilaginous cap. Overlying tendons and muscles can also be irritated, resulting in pain and reduced range of motion. Occasionally

an osteochondroma can produce symptoms due to pressure on nearby nerves. This is specially true for osteochondromas arising in the proximal fibula. Rarely venous thrombosis and pseudoaneurysms of arteries may result from direct pressure from a osteochondroma.

A fracture of the osteochondroma stalk may produce acute pain. Osteochondroma of the spine may cause spinal cord or nerve root compression and patients may present with neurologic deficit.

In hereditary multiple osteochondromas there is a wide clinical variation on the number of lesions. Multiple deformities of both upper and lower extremities have been reported in association with HMO. These include ankle valgum, genu valgum and ulnar deviation of the wrist with relative shortening of the ulna. Most often there is bilateral symmetric involvement of the extremities. Unusual sites for solitary osteochondromas (Fig. 6.8), such the pelvis are more commonly affected in HMO.

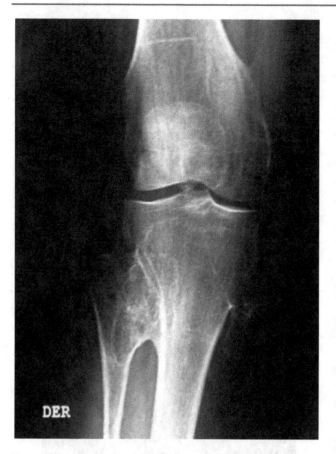

Fig. 6.8 Osteochodromatosis

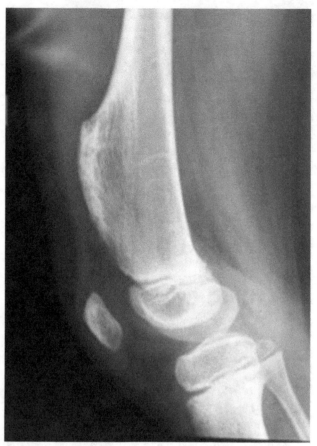

Fig. 6.9 Cesil osteochondroma

The radiographic appearance of a solitary osteochondroma is highly suggestive and usually sufficient for the correct diagnosis (Fig. 6.9). Typically it is characterized by an osseous protuberance (pedunculated or sessile) arising from the external surface of a metaphysis of a long tubular bone. The medullary cavity of the lesion should be continuous with the medulla of the affected bone. These slow-growing lesions will classically point away from the nearest joint and towards the diaphysis. In HMO the metaphysis of the tubular bone is usually widened due to failure of normal tubulation. The surface of an osteochondroma expands in a mushroom shape to form the cartilage cap. The tip of the osteochondroma may not be visible on plain radiographs. A large and poorly defined cartilaginous cap that contains irregular calcification is worrisome for malignant transformation.

Other Imaging Techniques

Although radiographs may be enough for the diagnosis of an osteochondroma of the extremities both CT scans and MR imaging have an important role in the evaluation of a lesion in areas where the anatomy is more complex (i.e., the pelvis

and spine). In addition, a CT scan is helpful to examine the medullary continuity between the lesion and the host bone. This feature is important in order to differentiate a benign osteochondroma from juxtacortical lesions like peripheral chondrosarcoma and periosteal chondromas.

MR imaging has a definitive role in evaluating the cartilaginous cap of an osteochondroma. The high signal intensity on T2 weighted images allows measurements of the cartilaginous cap of an osteochondroma supplying additional information about the likelihood of sarcoma transformation.

Differential Diagnosis

Benign lesions:

– Subungueal exostosis: Usually found on the distal phalanx of the great toe (Fig. 6.10).
– Bizarre parosteal osteochondromatous proliferation (Nora's lesion).

The medullary portion of the exostosis is not directly in continuity with the medulla of the host bone. Usually involve small bones of the hands and feet.

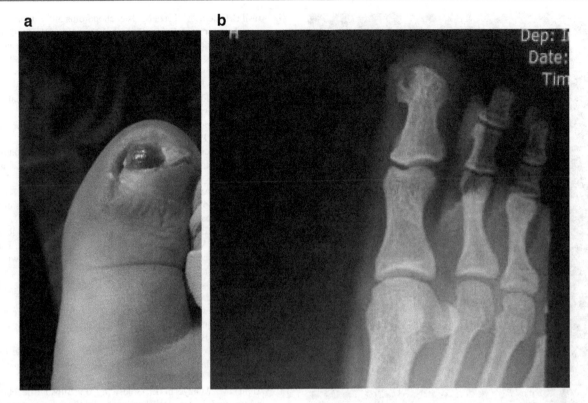

Fig. 6.10 Subungual exostosis: **a** clinical aspect **b** radiological aspect

– Metachondromatosis:

Autosomal dominant disorder characterized by multiple osteochondromas and intraosseous enchondromas mainly involving the digits. Unlike HMO rarely the multiple lesions cause lower limb deformities.

– Langer–Giedion syndrome – trichorhinophalangeal syndrome, type 2

Combined features of multiple exostoses with those of trichorhinophalangeal syndrome. Patients have a wide spectrum of mental retardation and deformities of the craniofacial bones and digits.

– Potcki–Shaffer syndrome

Patients present multiple exostosis, enlarged parietal foramina, craniofacial abnormalities and congenital deformities of the hand. Mental retardation may be present.

Malignant lesions:

– Parosteal osteosarcoma (Fig. 6.11)

Osteosarcoma of the surface of bone that radiographically has the appearance of a heavily mineralized mass. Most

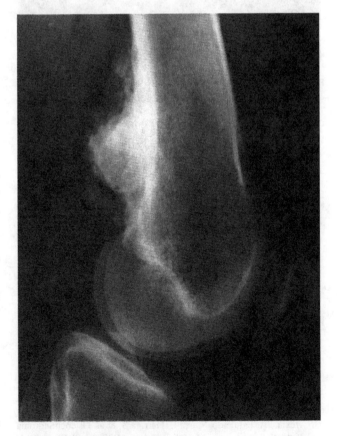

Fig. 6.11 Parosteal osteosarcoma

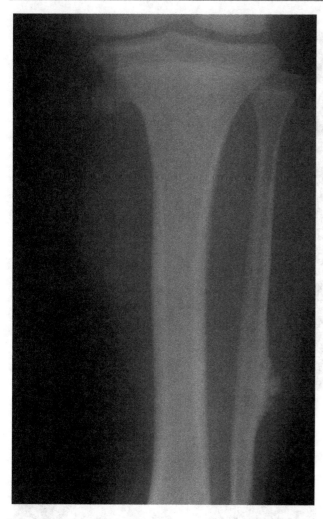

Fig. 6.12 Periosteal chondrosarcoma

commonly involves the posterior cortex of the metaphysis of the distal femur.

– Periosteal chondrosarcoma (Fig. 6.12)

Predominantly chondroblastic located on the surface of bone soft tissue invasion and without medullary involvement.

– Chondrosarcoma arising in an osteochondroma.

References

1. Unni KK, Inwards C, Bridge J, Wold LE, Kindblom L-G. Tumors of the bones and joints. AFIP Atlas of tumor pathology series IV. 1st ed. 2005. p. 37–59.
2. Albrecht S, Crutchfield JS, SeGall GK. On spinal osteochondromas. J Neurosurg. 1992;77:247–252.
3. Mexia, JA, Izquierdo Nunez E, Garriga S, et al. Osteochondroma of the thoracic spine and scoliosis. Spine. 2001;26(9):1082–1085.
4. Arasil E, Erdem A, Yüceer N. Osteochondroma of the upper cervical spine. A case report. Spine (Phila Pa 1976). 1996;21:516–518.
5. Morikawa M, Numaguchi Y, Soliman JA. Osteochondroma of the cervical spine: MR findings. Clin Imaging. 1995;19:275-278.
6. van der Sluis R, Gurr K, Joseph, MG. Osteochondroma of the lumbar spine. Spine. 1992;17(12);1519–1521.
7. Cohn R, Fielding JW. Osteochondroma of the cervical spine. J Pediatric Surg. 1986;21(11):997–999.
8. Malat J, Virapongse C, Levin A. Solitary Osteochondroma of the spine. Spine (Phila Pa 1976). 1986;11(6):625–628.
9. Karr M, Aulicino P, DuPuy T, Gwanthmey F. Osteochondromas of the hand in hereditary multiple exostosis: Report of a case presenting as a blocked proximal interphalangeal joint. J Hand Surg. 1984;9A:264–268.
10. Wood VE, Molitor C, Mudge MK. Hand involvement in multiple hereditary exostosis. Hand Clinics. 1990;6(4):685–692.
11. Fuselier CO, Binning T, Kushner D, Kirchwehm WW, Rice JR, Hetherington V, Kahl RL, Hanley DC, West A, Gray J, et al. Solitary osteochondroma of the foot: an in-depth study with case reports. J Foot Surg. 1984;23(1):3–24.
12. Smithuis A. Osteochondroma of the foot. Report of a case. J Bone Joint Surg Br. 1965;47(4):748.
13. Fageir M, Edwards M, Addison A. The surgical management of osteochondroma on the ventral surface of the scapula. J. Pediatr. Orthop., Part B. 2009;18(6):304–307.
14. Cooley LH, Torg JS. "Pseudowinging" of the Scapula Secondary to Subscapular Osteochondroma. Clin Orthop. Relat Res. 1982;162:119–124.
15. Wright JM, Matayoshi E, Goldstein AP. Bursal osteochondromatosis overlying an osteochondroma of a rib. A case report. JBJS, 79(7):1085–1088.
16. D'Ambrosia R, Ferguson AB, Jr. The formation of osteochondroma by epiphyseal cartilage transplantation. Clin Orthop. 1968;61: 103–115.
17. Milgram JW. The origins of osteochondromas and enchondromas. A histopathologic study. Clin Orthop Relat Res. 1983;(174): 264–284.
18. Keith A. Studies on the anatomical changes which accompany certain growth-disorders of the human body: I. The nature of the structural alterations in the disorder known as multiple exostoses. J Anat. (1920); 54(Pt 2–3):101–115.
19. Jaffe HL. Hereditary multiple exostosis. Arch Pathol. (1943);36: 335–357.
20. Huvos AG: Chondrosarcoma including spindle-cell (dedifferentiated) and myxoid chondrosarcoma; mesenchymal chondrosarcoma. In: Huvos AG (ed). Bone tumors: diagnosis, treatment, and prognosis. 2 ed. Philadelphia: WB Saunders Company; 1991. p. 343–393.
21. Milde T, Alamo, L, Stadelmann, C, Schweigerer, L, Witt, O. Multifocal osteochondroma after repeated irradiation in a boy with Hodgkin disease. J Pediat Hematol/Oncol. 2005;27(6):344–345.
22. Jaffe N, Ried HL, Cohen M, McNeese MD, Sullivan MP. Radiation induced osteochondroma in long-term survivors of childhood cancer. Int J Radiat Oncol Biol Phys. 1983;9:665–670.
23. Mintzer CM, Klein JD, Kasser JR. Osteochondroma formation after a Salter II fracture. J Orthop Trauma 1994;8:437–439.
24. Cook A, Raskind W, Blanton SH, Pauli RM, Gregg RG, Francomano CA, Puffenberger E, Conrad EU, Schmale G, Schellenberg G, Wijsman E, Hecht JT, Wells D, Wagner MJ. Genetic heterogeneity in families with hereditary multiple exostoses. Am J Hum Genet. 1993;53:71–79.
25. Mertens F, Rydholm A, Kreicbergs A, Willen H, Jonsson K, Heim S, Mitelman F, Mandahl N: Loss of chromosome band 8q24 in sporadic osteocartilaginous exostoses. Genes Chromosom Cancer 1994;9:8–12.

26. Wuyts W, Van Hul W: Molecular basis of multiple exostoses: mutations in the EXT1 and EXT2 genes. Hum Mutat. 2000;15:220–227.

27. Pierz KA, Stieber JR, Kusumi K, Dormans, JP. Hereditary multiple exostoses: One center's experience and review of etiology. Clin Orthop Relat Res. 2002;(401), 49–59.

28. Dobson-Stone C, Cox RD, Lonie L, Southam L, Fraser M, Wise C Bernier F, Hodgson S, Porter DE, Simpson AH, Monaco A. Comparison of fluorescent single-strand conformation polymorphism analysis and denaturing high-performance liquid chomatograph for detection of EXT1 and EXT2 mutations in hereditary multiple exostoses. Eur J Hum Genet. 2000;8:24–32.

29. Bernard MA, Hall CE, hogue DA, Cole WG, Scott A, Snuggs MB, Clines GA, Ludecke HJ, Lovett M, Van Winkle WB, Hecht JT. Diminished levels of the putative tumor suppressor proteins EXT1 and EXT2 in exostosis chondrocytes. Cell Motil Cytoskeleton. 2001;48:149–162.

30. Cheung PK, McCormick C, Crawford BE, Esko JD, Tufaro F, Duncan G. Etiological point mutations in the hereditary multiple exostoses gene EXT1: a functional analysis of heparan sulfate polymerase activity. Am J Hum Genet. 2001;69:55–66.

31. Alman, BA. Multiple hereditary exostosis and hedgehog signaling: implications for novel therapies. J Bone Joint Surg. 2009;91 (Supplement 4):63–67.

Enchondroma

7

Tomas Zamora

Abstract

Benign cartilaginous neoplasms are among the most common bone lesions. Enchondromas are the classical presentation of them and are usually found incidentally. Their clinical presentation can range from an asymptomatic lesion in an adult to multiple lesions as part of a syndrome in a younger patient. If the clinical and radiological presentation is characteristic, enchondromas can be treated non-operatively with observation alone. However, in certain circumstances, the differential diagnosis among a benign enchondroma or an atypical cartilaginous neoplasm/low-grade chondrosarcoma can be difficult and might need further investigations and a multidisciplinary approach. In cases of symptomatic lesions, diagnostic uncertainty, or a pathological fracture, curettage and grafting with or without osteosynthesis is usually the treatment of choice.

Keywords

Enchondroma · Benign cartilaginous neoplasm · Chondroma

Definition

Cartilaginous neoplasms are among the most common tumors of the appendicular skeleton and can involve almost any bone. Benign examples of these are enchondroma, osteochondroma, chondroblastoma, and chondromyxoid fibroma.

Enchondromas are the most common benign intraosseous form of cartilaginous neoplasms. They represent approximately 3% of all bone tumors and up to 15% of benign bone tumors. The vast majority are an intramedullary growth of

T. Zamora (✉)
Pontificia Universidad Católica de Chile, Santiago, Chile
e-mail: tzamora@med.puc.cl

hyaline cartilage, but a peripheral variant also exists around the bone surface (periosteal chondroma) [1, 2].

Syndromes with multiple enchondromas in the skeleton are infrequent, such as Ollier disease and Maffucci syndrome.

Clinical Presentation

Enchondromas are usually solitary tumors that are found incidentally, and therefore, their true incidence is likely to be higher than reported. Most of them are asymptomatic, and are found at any age, but usually from 15–40 years. In cases with multiple tumors and enchondromatosis the diagnosis is earlier in life, usually during the first decade, and they can present themselves with substantial deformity [3].

Small bones of the hands and feet are the most commonly affected bones, and that can occur in more than 50% of the cases, with long bones being next, such as the proximal humerus and distal femur. Axial skeleton involvement is rare in solitary enchondromas. In the hand, enchondromas can be diagnosed as a pathological fracture.

A frequent presentation is a young patient with an enchondroma in a long bone with a benign appearance, and a coexisting pathology in the contiguous joint that is causing symptoms (bursitis of the shoulder, for example). If symptoms and physical exam are also characteristic with this condition, and the cartilagenous lesion has a clear appearance of a benign process, the treatment should be addressed to manage the underlying condition and the cartilaginous tumor observed.

Imaging and Evaluation

Typically, enchondromas appear as central and metaphyseal lesions, with a well-delimitated border and central mineralization. Their appearance depends importantly on the amount of calcification, and they can range in size from

© Springer-Verlag London Ltd., part of Springer Nature 2021
J. Paulos and D. G. Poitout (eds.), *Bone Tumors*,
https://doi.org/10.1007/978-1-4471-7501-8_7

small punctuate to larger rings. They can also be described as having a popcorn-like appearance (Figs. 7.1 and 7.2). Endosteal scalloping can be observed on plain radiographs as well as in its low-grade malignant or atypical counterpart. In children, mineralization of the lesion might not be completed, and enchondromas can be confused with cystic lesions.

Even when the diagnosis in clearly benign lesions might seem simple, differentiating between an enchondroma and a more aggressive/malignant tumor, especially an atypical cartilaginous neoplasm, remains a diagnostic challenge, even for experienced specialists. A recent study published by our group showed that for 39 cartilaginous lesions, diagnosis and grading had only fair interobserver agreement (kappa = 0.44) between 10 experienced subspecialists, while treatment had only a poor intraobserver agreement (kappa = 0.21) [4]. Similar results have been found for radiologists and pathologists, showing us the complexity of this diagnosis [5, 6].

Various radiographic and clinical features can aid in the differentiation of a benign enchondroma from a chondrosarcoma [7, 8]. Murphey et al. [9] showed that for 187

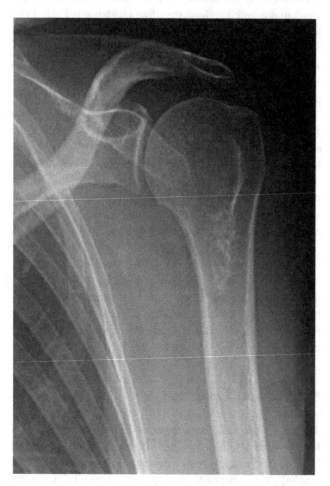

Fig. 7.1 Enchondroma of the left proximal humerus

cartilaginous neoplasms, cortical compromise more than 2/3 of cortical thickness, a neoplasm size >5 cm and the presence or absence of pain were the most prominent symptoms/signs for distinguishing between an enchondroma versus low-grade chondrosarcoma. Conversely, patient age, tumor location, and other variables did not influence the diagnosis. Studies by Ferrer-Santacreu [10, 11] showed that pain on palpation, cortical involvement, and bone scan uptake were essential factors in the diagnosis of low-grade chondrosarcoma as well.

CT and MRI can both be useful in the evaluation of these lesions. CT scan and axial reconstructions are useful to determine the presence of endosteal scalloping or cortical compromise. MRI can be helpful to evaluate soft tissue masses and edema in cases of impending fracture. Also, it can help demonstrate bone marrow replacement by the tumor and can guide surgical treatment if needed (Fig. 7.3).

18F-fluorodeoxyglucose positron emission tomography (18F FDG PET-CT) has been used to assess metabolic activity and to help differentiate between a benign enchondroma and a chondrosarcoma. A recent metanalysis of eight articles including 166 lesions, showed that maximum standardized uptake value (SUVmax) correlates with the histologic grade in intraosseous chondroid neoplasms, with low SUVmax being supportive of a benign tumor, while elevated SUVmax ≥ 4.4 being 99% specific for chondrosarcoma. A technetium-99 bone scan can also provide useful information. Radionuclide uptake within the lesion can be compared with an internal marker, such as the anterior superior iliac spine. Murphey et al. showed that 82% of chondrosarcomas in their series had lesion uptake higher than that of the anterior iliac crest.

Pathology and Genetics

Distinguishing between an enchondroma and a chondrosarcoma can be difficult even for trained histopathologists, and therefore, the final diagnosis has to be made by a multidisciplinary team in this clinical scenario more than ever. Samples from curettage are often fragmented, and they are composed of hyaline cartilage mixed with bone tissue (Fig. 7.4). Core needle biopsy might be prone to sampling error due to the heterogeneity that these tumors can have, with even high-grade chondrosarcoma having areas of benign hyaline cartilage. For this same reason, needle biopsy to differentiate between an enchondroma and a low-grade chondrosarcoma or an atypical cartilaginous neoplasm is not recommended as a considerable risk of error, and a non-representative sample can be found.

Enchondromas are composed of lobules of hyaline cartilage with low cellularity and atypia. The lobules are usually rimmed by bone, and small nodules of cartilage may be seen

Fig. 7.2 Distal femur AP and lateral X-ray on an 18-year-old male patient without any previous pain who had a knee contusion playing soccer; images show a central lesion with a cartilaginous matrix and calcifications

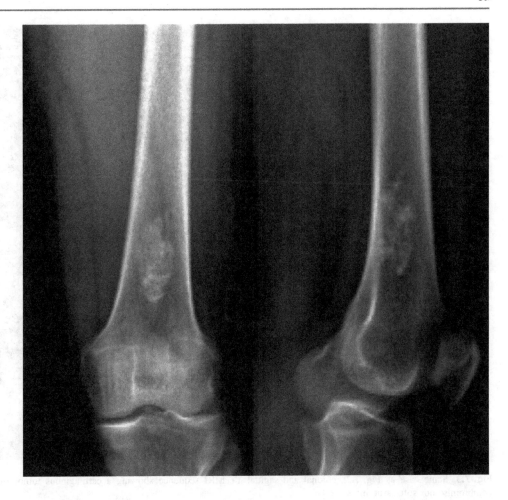

separated from the mass [2, 12]. As it was previously mentioned, that final histopathological diagnosis depends significantly from the clinical and radiographic appearance. For example, samples from the hand usually present more atypia and cellularity, but with clinical and radiographic manifestations of an enchondroma, they still maintain their benign status, while the same sample from the pelvis might be considered as a malignant variant. In general, binucleation, increased cellularity, atypia, bone permeation, and myxoid changes are indicative of malignancy [13, 14].

A few genetic abnormalities have been found in patients with multiple enchondromatosis with up to 8% of them demonstrating mutations in the gene encoding a Parathyroid hormone-like hormone (PTHLH) receptor (PTHR1) which is involved in enchondral bone formation. However, conflicting evidence exists regarding the real prevalence of these mutations [15, 16]. This being said, the exact cause of enchondromatosis is unknown. Recently, patients with solitary enchondromas as well as Ollier disease and Maffucci syndrome have been found to carry somatic mutations in isocitrate dehydrogenase-1 (IDH1) and 2 (IDH2) genes [17, 18]. This causes malfunction of the tricarboxylic acid cycle resulting in increased levels of the oncometabolite

D-2-hydroxyglutarate and a blockade of osteogenic differentiation during the formation of bone and instead cartilaginous tumor formation.

Treatment

As with most benign latent lesions, enchondromas that are asymptomatic can be treated non-operatively with observation alone. Single lesions with a characteristic radiographic appearance do not need to undergo a biopsy since follow up for more than 3–5 years without significant change has been usually considered to be enough for establishing an accurate diagnosis.

Indications for surgical treatment in an enchondroma are continuous symptoms; enlargement or radiographic changes during follow up to rule out a low-grade malignant variant; impending fracture or an actual fracture of the host bone. If surgical treatment is decided, curettage and bone grafting is usually the treatment of choice, with a low rate of recurrence if done adequately.

Several adjuvants for curettage have been described in order to reduce remaining microscopic foci of the tumor.

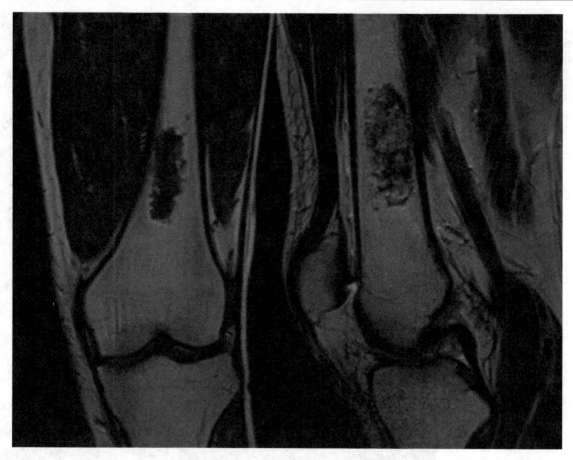

Fig. 7.3 Same case as Fig. 7.2:. coronal and sagittal T1 MRI sequence showing a cartilaginous tumor of 2 x 4 cm without any cortical compromise nor soft tissue mass

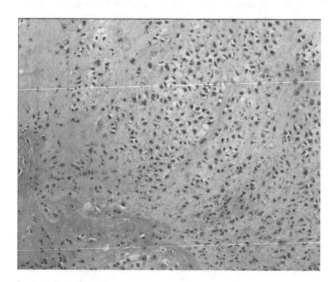

Fig. 7.4 Microscopic histology of enchondroma

Frequently used techniques are the use of thermal ablation with electrocautery and phenol, as well as cryotherapy. Grafting of the tumor can be done with either allo or autograft with excellent results. Other substitutes have been used to fill the cavitary defect after curettage beside bone graft. Filling the defect with methyl methacrylate is another alternative, especially if immediate stability is needed, with other benefits such as the adjuvant properties of thermal ablation and facilitating the postoperative evaluation of recurrence with better visualization of the bone-cement interface. Plate and screw fixation can be used as well if stability is needed on a weakened bone. Modification of activities and weight bear protection is usually recommended to prevent postoperative fractures after curettage, especially in the lower limb.

If a fracture occurs in a lesion suspected to be an enchondroma, treatment depends on the stability of the fracture, the localization of the lesion and the age of the patient. Young patients can usually be treated non-operatively, as fractures tend to heal as long as adequate stability and alignment are maintained. In cases where the lesion is close to the physis, surgical treatment should be delayed to prevent any damage to the growth plate of the bone. If the location of the fracture warrants acute stabilization, special attention should be paid to perform an adequate curettage and not contaminating other compartments. Fixation and osteosynthesis should be performed after curettage, and adjuvant therapy are performed, filling the defect with bone graft, substitutes, or cement.

Enchondromatosis

Several syndromes have been described in patients with multiple enchondromas, with recent classifications based on spinal involvement and genetic inheritance. The two most frequently described syndromes are Ollier disease and Maffucci syndrome, both non-hereditary and without spinal involvement [19, 20].

Ollier Disease is the most common subtype, with an estimated prevalence of 1/100.000. The lesions usually are distributed unilaterally, but bilateral distribution with lesions in the entire skeleton have been described as well (Fig. 7.4). Malignant transformation is significant, with a rate of 10–40%, being more frequent in long or flat bones, instead of the hands and feet. They also have a higher rate of other non-skeletal malignant tumors, like gliomas, ovarian juvenile granulosa cell tumors, and non-small cell lung cancer.

Maffucci syndrome is characterized by the presence of enchondromatosis with multiple haemangiomas of soft tissue or less commonly lymphangiomas. The disease develops in an important proportion before the first couple of years, and lesions are asymmetrically distributed. Both enchondromas and vascular lesions can transform to malignant tumors, with a higher risk of that happening than with Ollier disease. In the same way, a higher risk of developing intracranial malignancies is seen in these patients.

Similarly, other syndromes without spinal involvement, but with autosomal dominant inheritance have been described, such as Matachondromatosis and Genochondromatosis. Both of them are rare, the first one displaying a combination of multiple enchondromas along with osteochondroma-like lesions and the second one with characteristic chondroma in the clavicle or alteration of the flat bones of the hands or feet.

Syndromes with spinal involvement can be inherited or sporadic as well. Examples of this are Spondyloenchondrodysplasia, an autosomal recessive inherited disease with enchondromas of the appendicular skeleton combined with vertebral dysplasia. Other syndromes like Cheirospondyloenchondromatosis are characterized for marked hand and foot involvement, and Dysspondyloenchondromatosis that combines enchondromatosis with severe irregular vertebral lesions, including segmentation and severe kyphoscoliosis (Fig. 7.5).

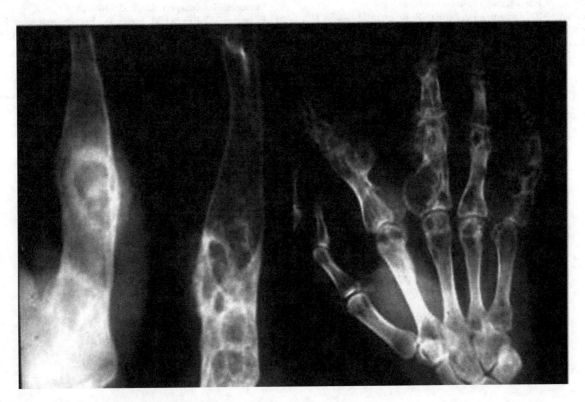

Fig. 7.5 35-year-old patient with enchondromatosis and hand lesions

References

1. Unni K, Inwards C. Dahlin's bone tumors: general aspects and data on 10,165 Cases, 6th edn. Baltimore, MD: Lippincott Williams & Wilkins; 2009.
2. Romeo S, Hogendoorn PC, Dei Tos AP. Benign cartilaginous tumors of bone: From morphology to somatic and germ-line genetics. Adv Anat Pathol. 2009;16(5):307–15.
3. Biermann J. Orthopaedic knowledge update: musculoskeletal tumors, vol. 3, 3rd edn. American Academy of Orthopaedic Surgeons; 2014.
4. Zamora T, Urrutia J, Schweitzer D, et al. Do orthopaedic oncologists agree on the diagnosis and treatment of cartilage tumors of the appendicular skeleton? Clin Orthop Relat Res. 2017;475:2176–86. https://doi.org/10.1007/s11999-017-5276-y.
5. Eefting D, Schrage YM, Geirnaerdt MJ, Le Cessie S, Taminiau AH, Bovee JV, Hogendoorn PC, EuroBoNeT consortium. Assessment of interobserver variability and histologic parameters to improve reliability in classification and grading of central cartilaginous tumors. Am J Surg Pathol. J. 2009; 33: 50–57.
6. Skeletal Lesions Interobserver Correlation among Expert Diagnosticians (SLICED) Study Group. Reliability of histopathologic and radiologic grading of cartilaginous neoplasms in long bones. J Bone Joint Surg Am. 2007; 89: 2113–2123.
7. Weiner SD. Enchondroma and chondrosarcoma of bone: clinical, radiologic, and histologic differentiation. Instr Course Lect. 2004;53:645–9.
8. Geirnaerdt MJ, Hermans J, Bloem JL, Kroon HM, Pope TL, Taminiau AH, Hogendoorn PC. Usefulness of radiography in differentiating enchondroma from central grade 1 chondrosarcoma. AJR Am J Roentgenol. 1997;169:1097–104.
9. Murphey MD, Flemming DJ, Boyea SR, Bojescul JA, Sweet DE, Temple HT. Enchondroma versus chondrosarcoma in the appendicular skeleton: differentiating features. RadioGraphics. 1998;18(5):1213-1237
10. Ferrer-Santacreu EM, Ortiz-Cruz EJ, Gonzalez-Lopez JM, Perez Fernandez E. Enchondroma versus low-grade chondrosarcoma in appendicular skeleton: clinical and radiological criteria. J Oncol. 2012;2012:437958
11. Ferrer-Santacreu EM, Ortiz-Cruz EJ, Diaz-Almiron M, Pozo Kreilinger JJ. Enchondroma versus chondrosarcoma in long bones of appendicular skeleton: clinical and radiological criteria-a follow-up. J Oncol. 2016;2016:8262079.
12. Bovée JV, Hogendoorn PC, Wunder JS, Alman BA. Cartilage tumours and bone development: molecular pathology and possible therapeutic targets. Nat Rev Cancer. 2010;10(7):481–8
13. Fletcher CD, Unni KK, Mertens F, editors. Pathology and genetics of tumours of soft tissue and bone. Lyon, France: IARC Press; 2002.
14. Schwartz HS, Zimmerman NB, Simon MA, Wroble RR, Millar EA, Bonfiglio M. The malignant potential of enchondromatosis. J Bone Joint Surg Am. 1987;69(2):269–74.
15. Hopyan S, et al. A mutant PTH/PTHrP type I receptor in enchondromatosis. Nat Genet. 2002;30:306–10.
16. Rozeman LB et al. Enchondromatosis (Ollier disease, Maffucci syndrome) is not caused by the PTHR1 mutation p.R150C. Hum Mutat. 2004; 24:466–473.
17. Pansuriya TC, van Eijk R, d'Adamo P, van Ruler MA, et al. Somatic mosaic IDH1 and IDH2 mutations are associated with enchondroma and spindle cell hemangioma in Ollier disease and Maffucci syndrome. Nat Genet. 2011; 43(12):1256–1261.
18. Amary MF, Damato S, Halai D, et al. Ollier disease and Maffucci syndrome are caused by somatic mosaic mutations of IDH1 and IDH2. Nat Genet. 2011; 43(12): 1262–1265.
19. Ranger A, Szymczak A. Do intracranial neoplasms differ in Ollier disease and maffucci syndrome? An in-depth analysis of the literature. Neurosurgery. 2009;65:1106–13.
20. Pansuriya TC, Kroon HM, Bovée JV. Enchondromatosis: Insights on the different subtypes. Int J Clin Exp Pathol. 2010;3(6):557–69.

Chondromyxoid Fibroma

8

Dominique G. Poitout

Abstract

The chondromyxoid fibroma is a rare beningn metaphyseal tumor that mainly affects children and adolescents. It is sometimes confused with enchondromas and condroblastomas, but it can be differentiated by histological analysis since it is composed of a mixture of chondroid, myxoid, and fibrous tissues. Clinically it can manifest with moderate pain and swelling in the case of large tumors. In the X-ray it appears as a lobulated, osteolyic lesion located eccentrically in the metaphysis of the bone. Surgical treatment is indicated in case of symptomatic lesions and at risk of pathological fracture, and consists of intralesional resection and filling the defect with bone graft.

Keywords

Chondromyxoid fibroma · Benign bone tumors

Etiology

This tumor occurs in children and adolescents; it is rare after 20 years of age [1]. Gender does not appear to be a significant etiologic factor.

The location of this tumor is always metaphyseal [2].

Gross Anatomy

Fibroma chondromyxoid appears as a rounded or oval mass, more or less irregular, whose major axis is parallel to the long axis of the bone. It is excentric, slimming or sometimes destroying the cortical in contact, but always remaining encapsulated [3].

Tumor tissue is yellowish white, brown in places (Fig. 8.1). Generally firm and grainy, it has roughly a cartilaginous appearance, but without the bluish appearance of the enchondroma in the microscopic anatomy [4]. Its polymorphism is a little confusing and explains the misinterpretation [5].

Topographically viewed, the appearance of the lesion is characterized by its lobulation, cell ranges being separated by connective and vascular tracts.

Microscopic anatomy: its polymorphism is a little confusing and explains the misinterpretation. Cells, are very dense and are encompassed within a myxoid ground substance. They are quite polymorphic, elongated, spindle-shaped or stellate. The cores are bulky chromophil. Some elements are multinucleated without abnormal mitosis, atypia or nucleolar chromatin [6, 7]. At the periphery of the cell areas, found in varying quantities, in connective tract support, are multinucleated giant cells, extravasated red blood cells, neutrophils, and macrophages loaded with hemosiderin. The basic substance which covers the whole is somewhat vacuolated and takes a bluish color when colored with hematoxylin. Myxoid, the nature of this substance, must be attributed to its aqueous composition rather than the presence of mucin, which is not demonstrated by specific dyes. In more advanced tumors, collagenation of the basic substance is more important. Note the presence in places where more or less developed hyaline substance flows. The chondroid aspect, the calcification foci are aging signs of the tumor [8].

Pathogenesis and Nosology

Although localized differently in relation to the growth plate, the chondroblastomas and chondro-myxoid fibroids seem to have a common origin [9, 10].

Clinical Study

Mild pain, but persistent, is the most common presenting sign; more rarely, in the case of large tumors, the swelling may be visible [11–13].

D. G. Poitout (✉)
Aix Marseille University, Marseille, France
e-mail: Dominique.poitout@live.fr

© Springer-Verlag London Ltd., part of Springer Nature 2021
J. Paulos and D. G. Poitout (eds.), *Bone Tumors*,
https://doi.org/10.1007/978-1-4471-7501-8_8

a b

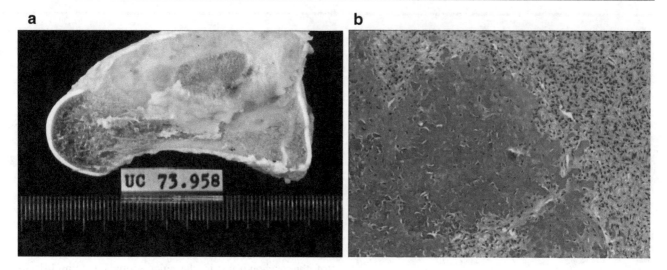

UC 73.958

Fig. 8.1 Chondromixoyd fibroma: **a** macroscopic aspect **b** histological aspect

Radiological Study

The image is metaphyseal, ovoid, rarely polycyclic. In the initial forms it is excentric, but may, subsequently, occupy the full width of the bone at the same time as it extends gradually toward the diaphysis (Fig. 8.2). It is surrounded by a border of more or less dense sclerosis; the cortical appears thinned, and may even disappear in some areas. The periosteum limiting the tumor can be the seat of a periosteal reaction giving a laminated and disturbing irregular appearance [14, 15].

Fig. 8.2 Rx chondromyxoid fibroma

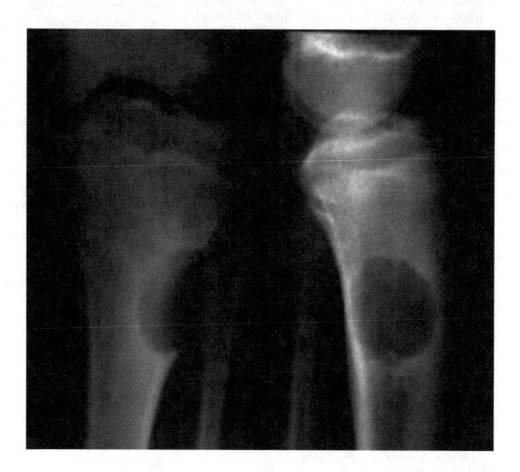

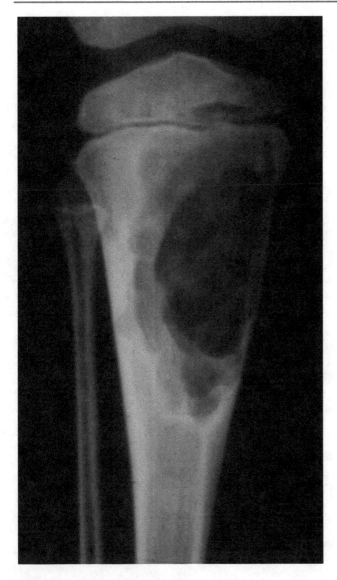

Fig. 8.3 Fibroma chondromixoid

Natural History

Malignant transformation is exceptional.

Bone lysis can lead to the occurrence of a pathological fracture.

Treatment

Surgical treatment should be strictly conservative. The block resection is unnecessary and exaggerated.The spongy tissue graft refill is the method of choice as evidenced by the excellent long-term results (Fig. 8.3).

References

1. Lersundi A, Mankin HJ, Mourikis A, Hornicek FJ. Chondromyxoid fibroma: a rarely encountered and puzzling tumor. Clin Orthop Relat Res. October 2005;439:171–5.
2. Sharma H, Jane MJ, Reid R. Chondromyxoid fibroma of the foot and ankle: 40 years' Scottish bone tumour registry experience. Int Orthop. 2006;30(3):205–9.
3. Dahlin DC, Wells AH, Henderson ED. Chondromyxoid fibroma of bone; report of two cases. J Bone Joint Surg Am 1953;35-A(4): 831–834.
4. Jaffe HL, Lichtenstein L. Chondromyxoid fibroma of bone; a distinctive benign tumor likely to be mistaken especially for chondrosarcoma. Arch Pathol (Chic). 1948;45(4):541–51.
5. Zustin J, Akpalo H, Gambarotti M, et al. Phenotypic diversity in chondromyxoid fibroma reveals differentiation pattern of tumor mimicking fetal cartilage canals development: An immunohisto-chemical study. Am J Pathol. 2010;177(3):1072–8.
6. Yasuda T, Nishio J, Sumegi J, et al. Aberrations of 6q13 mapped to the COL12A1 locus in chondromyxoid fibroma. Mod Pathol 2009;22(11):1499–1506.
7. Wu CT, Inwards CY, O'Laughlin S, Rock MG, Beabout JW, Unni KK. Chondromyxoid fibroma of bone: A clinicopathologic review of 278 cases. Hum Pathol. 1998;29(5):438–46.
8. Dahlin DC. Chondromyxoid fibroma of bone, with emphasis on its morphological relationship to benign chondroblastoma. Cancer. 1956;9(1):195–203.
9. Romeo S, Eyden B, Prins FA, Briaire-de Bruijn IH, Taminiau AH, Hogendoorn PC. TGF-beta1 drives partial myofibroblastic differentiation in chondromyxoid fibroma of bone. J Pathol. 2006;208 (1):26–34.
10. Park HR, Park YK, Jang KT, Unni KK. Expression of collagen type II, S100B, S100A2 and osteocalcin in chondroblastoma and chondromyxoid fibroma. Oncol Rep. 2002;9(5):1087–91.
11. Dürr HR, Lienemann A, Nerlich A, Stumpenhausen B, Refior HJ. Chondromyxoid fibroma of bone. Arch Orthop Trauma Surg. 2000;120(1–2):42–47.
12. Rahimi A, Beabout JW, Ivins JC, Dahlin DC. Chondromyxoid fibroma: a clinicopathologic study of 76 cases. Cancer. 1972;30 (3):726–36.
13. Armah HB, McGough RL, Goodman MA, et al. Chondromyxoid fibroma of rib with a novel chromosomal translocation: A report of four additional cases at unusual sites. Diagn Pathol. 2007;2:44.
14. Baker AC, Rezeanu L, O'Laughlin S, Unni K, Klein MJ, Siegal GP. Juxtacortical chondromyxoid fibroma of bone: a unique variant: a case study of 20 patients. Am J Surg Pathol. 2007;31(11):1662–1668.
15. Yamaguchi T, Dorfman HD. Radiographic and histologic patterns of calcification in chondromyxoid fibroma. Skeletal Radiol. 1998;27(10):559–64.
16. Unni KK, Inwards CY. Chondromyxoid fibroma. In: Unni KK, Inwards CY, editors. Dahlin's bone tumors, 6th edn. Philadelphia, PA: Wolters Kluwer, Lippincott Williams & Wilkins; 2010. p. 50–59.
17. Hasegawa T, Seki K, Yang P, et al. Differentiation and proliferative activity in benign and malignant cartilage tumors of bone. Hum Pathol. 1995;26(8):838–45.

Chondroblastoma

9

Franklin H. Sim

Abstract

Chondroblastoma is a benign primary bone tumor that represents less than 1% of all primary bone tumors [1]. It is frequently discovered in adolescents with a mean age of fifteen years. The symptomatology is very poor, usually characterized by pain related or not to trauma. Radiographically, chondroblastoma typically presents in the epiphysis of long bones of the extremities. It looks like a round or oval clarity occupying part of the epiphysis, bordered by a narrow edge of hypercondensation. The tumor is characterized histologically by the proliferation of chondroblasts along with areas of mature cartilage, giant cells, and occasionally, secondary aneurysmal bone cyst formation. Surgical management is the mainstay of treatment for chondroblastomas that threaten the physis or joint surface. Meticulous curettage, and bone-grafting or cementation are the gold standard of treatment.

Keywords

Chondroblastoma • Benign lesion • Bone tumor • Chondroblasts

Etiology

These tumors do not represent more than 1% of benign bone tumors. The average age is around 15 years, with a few extreme cases up to age 25, and more unusually a later age [2]. Sex seems to play no significant role.

The only etiological character value is almost always epiphyseal localization of the lesion encountered; most often at the lower end of the humerus or near the knee (Fig. 9.1).

F. H. Sim (✉)
Mayo Clinic, Rochester, MN 55905, USA
e-mail: sim.franklin@mayo.edu

© Springer-Verlag London Ltd., part of Springer Nature 2021
J. Paulos and D. G. Poitout (eds.), *Bone Tumors*,
https://doi.org/10.1007/978-1-4471-7501-8_9

Pathological Anatomy

Gross Anatomy

The study of resected lesions in their entirety makes the following findings: the diameter of the neoformation varies from 3 to 6 cm. The contours are regular yet without cleavable space with the normal cancellous bone which surrounds it.

The lesion is located in contact with the growth plate on which it seems to depend. Sometimes it invades the neighboring joint after cartilage erosion; the neighboring periosteum of the lesion is thickened and hyperemic, without any reaction forming subperiosteal bone. The tumor is dotted with yellowish areas of calcification, gray-blue areas (cartilage), red-brown areas (evidence of previous hemorrhage). The tumor is of elastic consistency, comprising, per space, stronger or more friable zones corresponding to calcification or hemorrhaic zones [3].

Microscopic Anatomy

The basic tissue is richly cellular and presents some analogy with that of giant cell tumors. The basis of these tumor cells is considered by most authors as a chondroblast: it is an egg cell, of medium height, with a wide core, round or oval, sometimes kidney-shaped. Its cytoplasm is highly acidic soils and border cells are clearly visible. There is little or no ground substance. Alternating with these cells are found, in varying numbers, multinucleated cells. They contain an average of five to 15 cores, rarely up to 50. Overall, it appears that these giant cells are smaller and less numerous than in giant cell tumors. These multinucleated cells are more abundant in contact with hemorrhagic foci, and cystic necrotic. There is also, in most chondroblastomas, sometimes extensive beaches of cartilaginous substance [3].

Fig. 9.1 Epidemiology chondroblastoma and frequent location

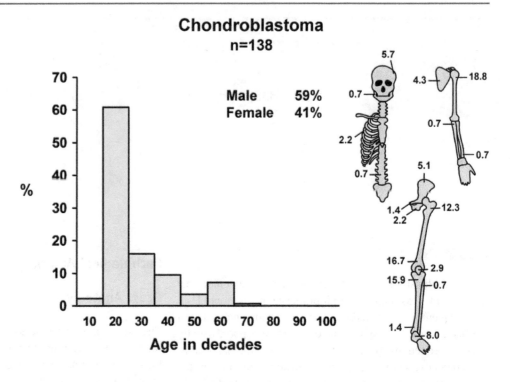

These can, in some cases, exceed in importance the cellular beaches. At the periphery of the tumor, we can note the presence of newly formed osteoid bone spans which penetrate the tumor and can be subdivided into lobes.Finally, if the level of a few cells contained images of mitosis, they are constantly normal, without any atypical unusual appearance [3] (Figs. 9.2, 9.3, and 9.4).

Clinical Study

The symptomatology is very poor. Some pain, more or less related to trauma, is sometimes the pretext for a radiological examination that discovers the injury. Do not expect to find any visible deformities because these tumors, usually of

Fig. 9.2 Chondroblastoma contains zones of chondroid matrix that are typically hypocellular when compared to the surrounding regions,as shown in this photomicrograph

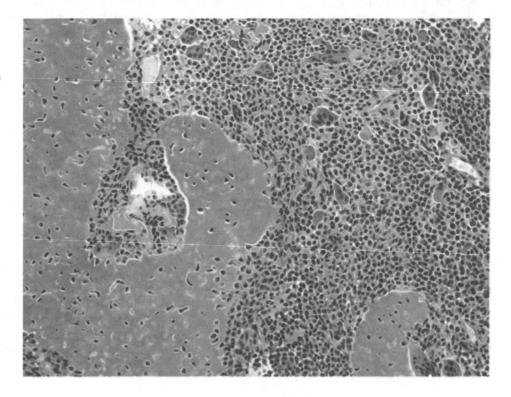

Fig. 9.3 At high magnification, chondroblastoma has a mononuclear cell with well-defined cytoplasmatic borders and rounded, well-stained nuclei with a typical longitudinal groove

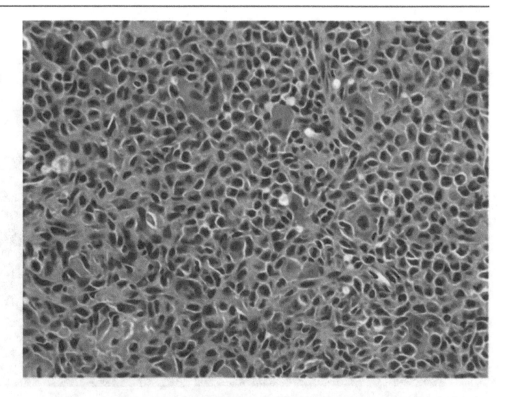

Fig. 9.4 Calcification is a typical feature that helps distinguish chondroblastoma and it may form a "chicken wire" pattern

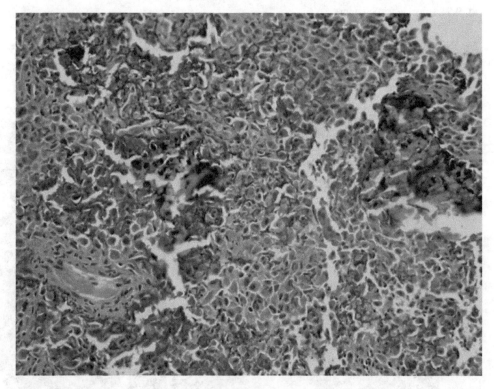

modest size, occur most often at deep epiphysis. In some cases suffering from the neighboring articulation draws attention to the type of functional impairment, or effusion.

The general condition is still well preserved and biological investigations are constantly negative [2].

Radiological Study

The location of the injury is almost always epiphyseal, metaphyseal exceptionally. It is in most cases at the upper epiphysis of the humerus, tibia, or femur. The image of the

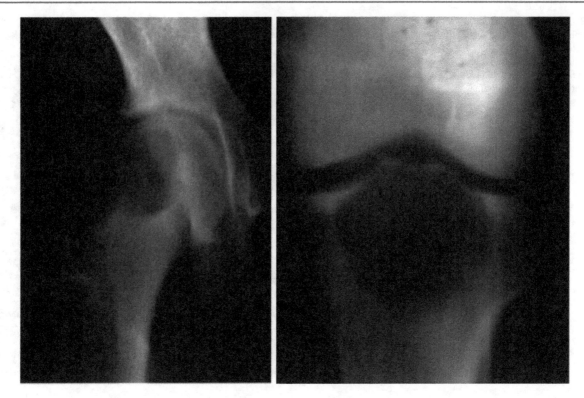

Fig. 9.5 X-ray chondroblastoma

lesion is represented by a round or oval clarity occupying part of the epiphysis, bordered by a narrow edge of

hypercondensation, corresponding to a reaction of an osteosclerosis area [4] (Figs. 9.5 and 9.6).

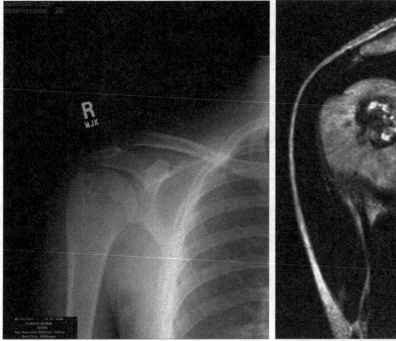
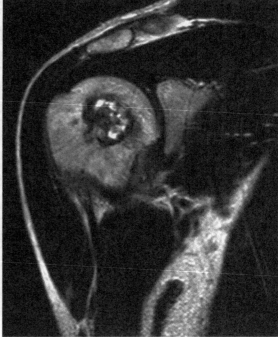

Fig. 9.6 Humeral head chondroblastoma; importance of advanced image on the diagnosis of chondroblastoma; radiograph of the right shoulder of a 17-year-old male who presented with a complaint of shoulder pain; the radiographic findings are subtle; coronal MRI clearly defines location at the epiphysis of the proximal humerus

Evolution

With discrete symptoms,and slow extension, it is rare that this injury is the seat of very remarkable evolutionary phenomena.

Treatment

It must be strictly conservative; the Jam recess is the method of choice and gives good results.

Surgical Treatment of Chondroblastoma

After a cortical window is opened the tumor is exposed as demonstrated in Fig. 9.7. The specimen is sent to frozen section analysis to confirm the diagnosis of chondroblastoma.

After complete curettage and use of a high speed burr a cavity is created. In this case the cavity was filled with phenol and later neutralized by alcohol as adjuvant.

Figure 9.8 shows the final aspect after cancellous allograft is applied and impacted [5].

-Surgical treatment of chondroblastoma:

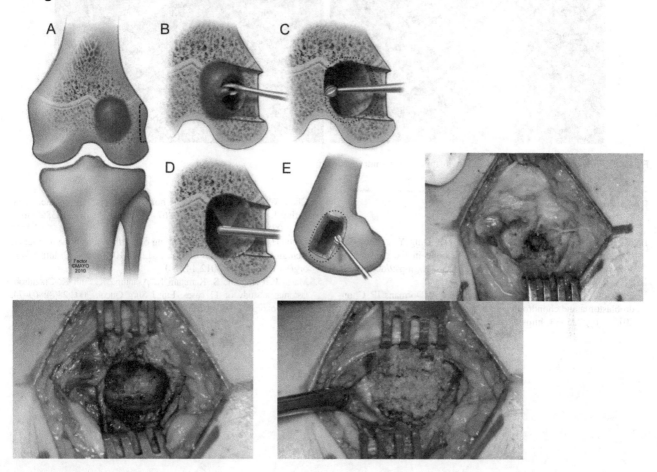

Fig. 9.7 Surgical treatment of chondroblastoma: **A** cortical window is opened; **B** tumor exposed and then resected; **C** fullfilment of bone defect with cancellous allograft

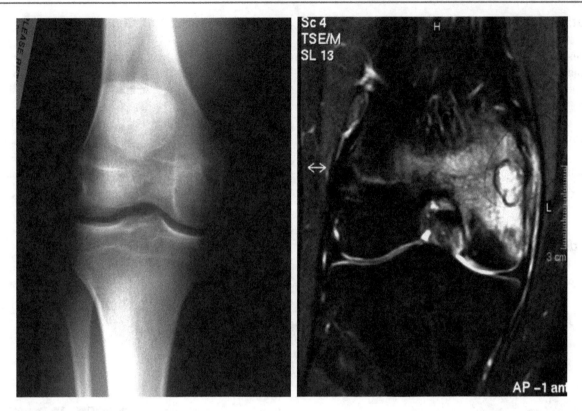

Fig. 9.8 Final aspect after cortical window treatment of chondroblastoma

References

1. Xu H, Nugent D, Monforte HL, Binitie OT, Ding Y, Letson GD, Cheong D, Niu X. Chondroblastoma of bone in the extremities. J Bone Joint Surg Am. 2015;97(11):925–31. https://doi.org/10.2106/jbjs.n.00992.
2. De Mattos CBR, Angsanuntsukh C, Arkader A, Dormans JP. Chondroblastoma and chondromyxoid fibroma. J Am Acad Orthop Surg. 2013;21(4):225–33. https://doi.org/10.5435/JAAOS-21-04-225.
3. Chen W, DiFrancesco LM. Chondroblastoma: an update. Arch Pathol Lab Med. 2017;141(6):867–71. https://doi.org/10.5858/arpa.2016-0281-RS.
4. Douis H, Saifuddin A. The imaging of cartilaginous bone tumours I: Benign lesions. Skeletal Radiol. 2012;41(10):1195–212. https://doi.org/10.1007/s00256-012-1427-0.
5. Masui F, Ushigome S, Kamitani K, Asanuma K, Fujii K. Chondroblastoma: a study of 11 cases. Eur J Surg Oncol. 2002;28(8):869–74. https://doi.org/10.1053/ejso.2002.1276.

Chondrosarcoma

10

Jaime Paulos

Abstract

Chondrosarcoma is a malign bone tumor forming cartilage. It occurs in adults, mostly during the fourth to sixth decades of life forming a big tumoral mass. Frequent locations are the femur, pelvis, and ribs. Different grades have different prognoses including clinical and biomolecular features. The treatment requires wide surgical resection and reconstruction.

Keywords

Chondrosarcoma • Malign bne tumor • Pelvis and limb reconstruction

Definition

Chondrosarcoma is a malign tumor characterized by the formation of cartilageneous tissue without presence of osteoid tissue.

The clinical, and therapeutic features of chondrosarcoma are a significant challenge for the surgeon. Most cases appear in adults during the fourth, fifth, and sixth decades of life in both genders (Fig. 10.1). Chondrosarcomas are rare in children or adolescents.

The tumor frequently grows slowly, with little pain, and with the appearance of a tumoral mass. These clinical features induce the patient to seek medical attention relatively late (Fig. 10.2).

The most frequent localizations for this tumor are: the pelvis, femur, proximal humerus and ribs [1].

There are many forms of chondrosarcomas (CS) described below:

- primary chondrosarcoma
- secondary chondrosarcoma: from an osteochondroma or osteochondromatosis or secondary to an en chondroma (Ollier, Mafucci).
- yuxtacortical chondrosarcoma
- mesenchymal chondrosarcoma
- clear cells chondrosarcoma
- dedifferenciated CS
- soft tissue CS
- craneal base CS

Malignancy

In general, malignancy can be classified as:

- low grade malignancy or grade 1
- intermediate grade malignancy or grade 2
- high grade malignancy or grade 3.

However, histopathological grade on a chondrosarcoma doesn't always correlate with its clinical course and prognosis. For example, a low grade chondrosarcoma located in the pelvis can have an aggresive behavior, while a higher grade chondrosarcoma in a phalanx can result in an indolent course, with a better overall prognosis. [2] (Fig. 10.3).

Parameters that influence the prognosis of a patient with a chondrosarcoma are: age, location, size, histological grade, speed of growth, soft tissue compromise, and the existence of metastasis. All these factors can guide the physician to a more exact prognosis.

In young adults high grade CS can frequently exhibit an agressive behavior, with progressive and rapid growth, culminating in metastasis. However, low grade CS tends to grow slowly.

Chondroid tumors located in axial bones such as the pelvis, ribs, scapula, and proximal femur and humerus tend to have an aggresive behaviour and worse overall prognosis

J. Paulos (✉)
Pontificia Universidad Católica de Chile, Santiago, Chile
e-mail: paulos.jaime@gmail.com

© Springer-Verlag London Ltd., part of Springer Nature 2021
J. Paulos and D. G. Poitout (eds.), *Bone Tumors*,
https://doi.org/10.1007/978-1-4471-7501-8_10

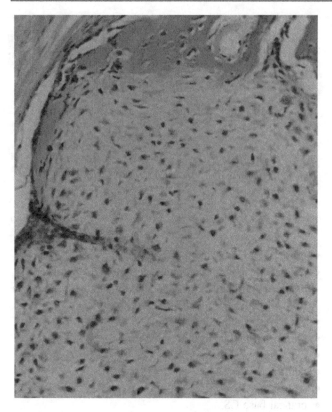

Fig. 10.1 Histopathology of chondrosarcoma

[3, 4] (Fig. 10.4). Similarly, rapid growth tumors, with an extensive soft tissue mass or metastasis generally exhibit a poor prognosis.

On the other hand, chondroid tumors located in appendicular bones, especially in the hands and feet, usually have a better prognosis (Figs. 10.5 and 10.6).

Most CSs result in metastasis at a very late stage, reaching a large size. They also have a tendency to local recurrence after resection, even in the biopsy tract.

Imaging

A typical raduiographic image of CS shows a tumor with irregular calcifications, circular limits, cortical invasion, and ill defined margins with a wide zone of transition.

In long bones they are mostly located on the metaphysis and sometimes on the shaft. There is usually little or no periosteal reaction.

The computed tomography (CT) and magnetic resonance imaging (MRI) will evaluate the cortical and soft tissue invasion, along with the endomedular progression and adyacent neurovascular structures [5].

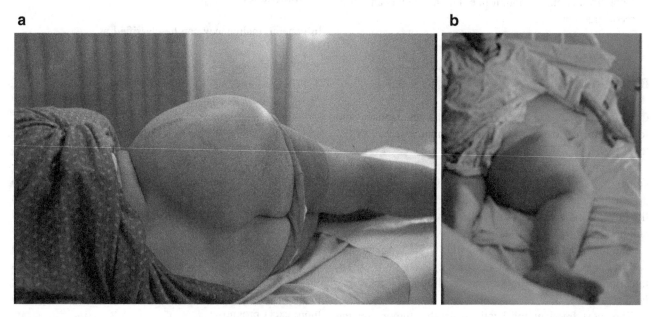

Fig. 10.2 Clinical aspects of chondrosarcoma: **a** iliac chondrosarcoma; **b** femur chondrosarcoma

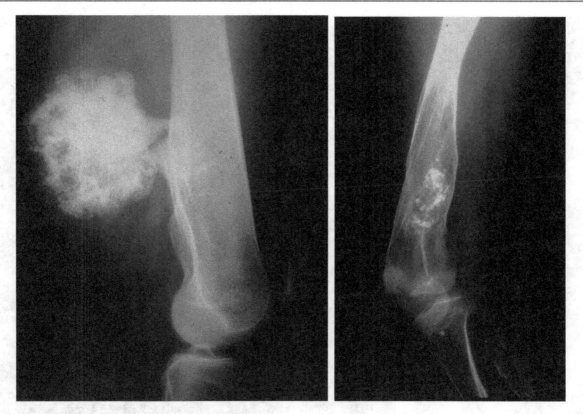

Fig. 10.3 Examples of radiological aspects of chondrosarcoma

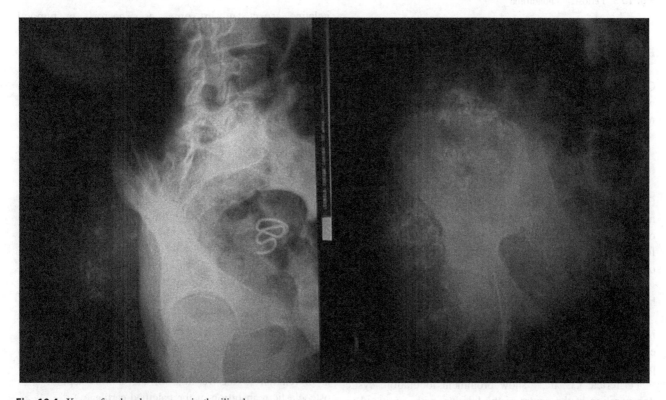

Fig. 10.4 X-ray of a chondrosarcoma in the iliac bone

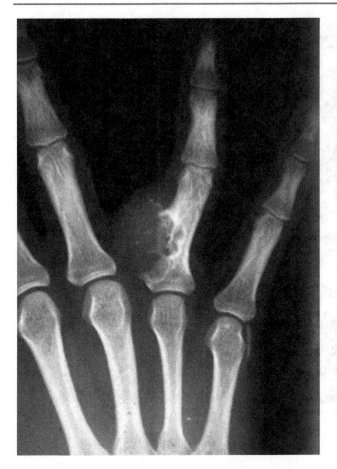

Fig. 10.5 Periosteal chondroma

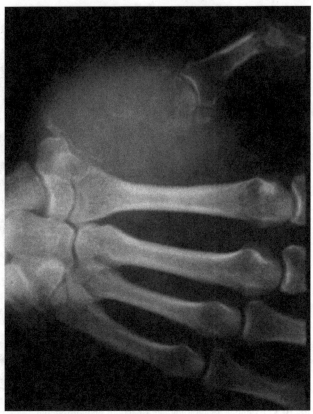

Fig. 10.6 Chondrosarcoma (very rare in the hand)

Pathology

Chondrosarcoma is a sarcoma with tumoral cells asociated with a cartilagineous matrix; the formation of bone is only reactive or through endochondral ossification.

Macroscopy

CS can reach a large size of about 10–20 cms or more. The most extensive ones are found in flat bones. They are formed of solid tissue, lobulated in the periphery and in well differentiated cases. Some zones can have yellow calcifications or a focus of endochondral calcification. In cases of high grade malignancy it is possible to find mixoid areas with hemorrhagic features and necrosis.

Central chondrosarcomas: these show festoneted endostal borders, focal destruction or thickening of the cortex. The extension through the soft tissues around it is limited with a pseudocapsule or new periosteal bone formation.

Periferical CS: these show prominent lobulation, cystic degeneration in the center of the lobules, with a mucoid or gelatine aspect and in some cases necrosis or tumoral liquefaction.

Histopathology

It is important to say that the pathologist can evaluate the cellular components only in not calcified areas.

The nuclei of the tumoral chodrocites are sometimes bigger with nucleolus and they can be mono-, bi- or multi-nucleated. They have nuclear pleiomorphism and nuclear hyperchcromasia. They can have intracitoplasmatic vacuolas, looking like ring cells that can be confused with metastasis of an adenocarcinoma of ring cells.

The tumoral chondrocites have a distribution in groups of differents sizes and irregular form separated by fibrous tissue. The matrix is chondroid or myxoid (in this case the cells are fused or star-like). The cellularity is higher in the periphery of the lobules where there is more chance to find mitosis. The fusiform tumoral cells in the periphery can be near the fibrous septum. Around the lobules it is possible to find calcifications, or reactive bone with osteoblasts. The enchondral ossification is in relation to the vascular of the fibrous septum with osteoclastic reabsortion of the calcified cartilage.

The tumor grows inside the trabecular bone and it is possible to see necrotic bone partially reabsorbed by the tumoral mass, which is characteristic of a malignant lesion. The surrounding bone is in remodelation.

Grades of Chondrosarcoma

The grades of chondrosarcome are made by evaluating the cellularity intercellular matrix, the number of binucleated cells, their size, form and mitosis. The mixoid stroma is related to a worse clinical prognosis. Cellularity shows the main difference between low or high grade chondrosarcoma. The nuclear size is the best index for prognosis, and the number of mitoses is not related to the clinical behaviour.

- Grade 1
  - these make up 26–50% of all chondrosarcomas
  - the cellularity is augmented in relation to chondromas
  - chondrocites are small, with a dense nucleus a little bigger, and irregular or elongated
  - few chondrocites are binucleated
  - lobules are mostly chondroides, very few or none exhibit mixoid changes
  - there is sometimes extensive calcification
  - no mitosis.
- Grade 2
  - these make up 30–60% of all chondrosarcomas
  - there is higher cellularity in the periphery of the lobules.
  - larger nucleus and hyperchromatics
  - there is frequently more than a cell in one lacune
  - chondrocytes can be binucleated
  - there is less calcification
  - mixoid stroma appears around long necrotics areas
  - fewer mitoses
- Grade 3
  - these make up 8–25% of all chondrosarcomas
  - cellularity is augmented
  - nuclei are pleomorphic and vesicoulous, 5–10 times larger
  - there can be fusiform cells, many of them are binucleated
  - tumoral chondrocites are disposed in cordons or irregulars groups
  - giants multinucleated tumoral cells can be found
  - there is mitotic activity
  - predominant mixoid stroma over chondroid
  - necrosis can be extensive
  - calcification is rare or absent.

Differential Diagnosis

The most common clinical scenario is the need to differentiate a Chondroma versus a low-grade Chondrosarcoma (or atypical cartilageous neoplasm in case of a tumor of the appendicular skeleton) [6].

Chondroma

Chondroma is completely or partially wrapped by lamellar mature calcifications; the loboules are separated with bone marrow. They show less cellularity and a smaller nucleus size. Mixoid areas are rare, except in chondromatosis. There is no necrosis.

Chondrosarcoma

Chondrosarcomas have a permeative growth, infiltrating the intertrabecular spaces; necrotic bone can be found; or destroyed bone enveloped by lobes of cartilage which are separated by fibrous tissue. They have more cellularity and a bigger nucleus. The stroma can be mixoid and focal or extensive necrosis can be found.

It is not always possible for the pathologist to find clear characteristics and the diagnosis can be less precise,such as cartilageneous lesion of uncertain malignant potential or cartilageneous borderline neoplasia. In these cases the pathologist must also evaluate the histological aspect in front of the clinical and radiological background of the case.

Others differential diagnoses are:

- mixoid chondrosarcomas versus chondromixoid fibroma
- high grade versus dedifferentiated chondrosarcoma
- chondrosarcomas versus chondroblastic osteosarcoma.

Assessment of Chondrosarcomas

Chondrosarcomas have been evaluated in different ways with the aim of assisting in the diagnosis. Nowadays most diagnoses analyze the biochemical features with cytopathology, histochemistry [7], flow citometry and electronic microscopy, immunohistochemistry and molecular biology [8], because they help to best differentiate between benign and malignant cartilaginous lesions:

- Immunohistochemistry. KI-67 Antigen (Scotlandi et al. 1995)

- Nuclear antigen present in all active phases of the cellular cycle.
- There is significant difference in the number of positive nuclei when comparing chondrosarcomas of different grades.
- P53 Antigen (Oshiro et al. 1998)
- These antigens are the protein of the gene located in the chromosome 17p13 and its role is to control cellular proliferation keeping DNA fidelity.
- High grade tumors over-express p53 antigen, while low grade chondrosarcomas and benign tumors do not.
- Protooncogen c-erb-B2 (Wrba et al. 1989)
- Growth factor, member of tirosine kinase receptors family.
- It is found in chondrosarcomas and not in benign cartilaginous tumors.
- Its impact on the prognosis is not well established.
- Catepsina B y Plasminogen activating Urokinase (Haeckel et al. 2000)
- Proteases which dregradate stromal elements.
- When overexpressed, correlates with higher local recurrence and metastasis. (Hirakoa et al. 2002)
- Cylcin dependent kinase inhibitor. If present it correlates with a better prognosis.
- Tenascina (Koukoulis et al. 1991)
- Extracellular matrix glycoprotein transiently expressed during embryionary development. It has been found in the tumoral lobe periphery or in high grade chondrosarcoma matrix.
- Collagen (Ueda et al. 1990). The different types of collagen distribution demonstrate tumoral cell maturity.
- S-100 (Weis et al. 1986) Intense (+) in low grade tumors, weak or negative in high grade tumours.
- Vimentina (+). Desmina, actina (+ and −).

Molecular Biology

- There is a considerable genetic heterogenecity within chondrosarcomas. Between genetic alterations we found:
- numeric anomalies: chromosomes 5, 7, 8 and 18
  structural anomalies: chromosomes 1, 12 and 15
- Structural anomalies have been found in region 12q13–15. Collagen type II gen, a major component of normal cartilage, is localized in this same region. The same thing happens for mesenchymal neoplase. (Clinical Oncology genetic factors 2000).
- Chondrosarcomas and osteosarcomas studies have shown genetic alterations in 8q24.1 region (EXT1) which supports the hypothesis that EXT1 loss mutation (a tumor

suppressor gene) is important for these tumors' pathogenesis.
- There is evidence that aberrations in region 6q13–21 correlates with local aggressive behavior of cartilagenous tumors (Sawyer et al. 1997). In extra-osseus mixoid condrosarcomes it has been described that a tumor specific translocation t(9;22) (q22:q12) is a reorder of EWS gene in 22q12 with a new gene in the region 9q22 called TEC.
- These findings are not present in osseus mixoid chondrosarcoma (Sjorgen et al 1999; Olveira et al. 2000).
- Genetic changes in p53 could be an important predictor for the aggressive behavior of chondrosarcomas.
- Genetic changes in p16 are very important in high grade chondrosarcomas but not in low grade.
- Fluorescent in-situ hybridization (FISH) and genotipification have been used to determine the cellular line of an specific abnormal clone in dedifferentiated chondrosarcomas.

These are just some of the numerous genetic changes describe in the literature. In the future there will be a technique which will help us to differentiate the diagnosis of cartilagenous lesions, to know the origin of this neoplasy, and its cure.

Chondrosarcoma Variants

I: Periosteal Chondrosarcoma

This corresponds to 1–2% of chondrosarcomas and they are found mostly in the fourth decade of life. It is localized in the methaphysis or metadiaphisys of the femur, humerus, pelvis, metatarsals and hands.

The macroscopic aspect looks like chondrosarcoma, but from the histological point of view they are Grade I or II with areas of calcification of endochondral ossification.

II: Mesenchymal Chondrosarcomas

These correspond to 2% of chondrosarcomas and are found usually in the second or third decade of life. They are located in the femur, craniofacial bones, the pelvis ribs, ribs and extraosseus at the epiphysis, diaphysis or periostal.

The macroscopic aspect is a firm or soft mass, grey or reddish with cartilage, hemorrhage, necrosis, cysts and calcifications.

From the histological point of view they combine components of indifferentiated cells with a variable amount of well differentiated cartilagenous areas.

III: Clear Cell Chondrosarcomas

These correspond to less than 2% of chondrosacomas and are found mostly in the third and fourth decade of life, being located in the proximal femur, proximal humerus and tibia (epiphys).

Macroscopically they do not look like a typical chondroid tissue. Histologically most of the tumoral cells have a clear and huge cytoplasm with an hyperchromatic and central nucleus or a vacuolated nucleus with a prominent nucleolus. Some cells are binucleated, but mitosis is rare. There are typical areas of grade II chondrosarcoma in 50% of cases. They can be confused with metastasis of other clear cells tumors.

IV: Osseus Mixoid Chondrosarcoma

This is a rare variant. Histologically it has formed on round cells with very few cytoplasms, in chordons or nests with a hyperchromatic nucleus and the occasional nucleolus. There is no mitotic activity.

Treatment

The treatment for this tumor is surgical resection with a wide margin [9, 10].

These tumors are resistant to both chemotherapy and radiotherapy. Radiotherapy is used as palliative treatment in tumors that cannot be reached by surgery (spine, sacral, skull).

In undifferentiated chondrosarcoma, chemotherapy might be of benefit.

Surgical reconstruction will depend on tumor location. Some clinical cases are described as examples of treatment:

Case 1

See Fig. 10.7. A 28-year-old man who consults for right shoulder and arm pain. Physical examination reveals a hard tumor that can be easily palpated in the arm. The imaging study shows: a tumor that invades the cortex and calcifications inside the lesion. Biopsy: grade II chondrosarcoma. Treatment: En block resection and autograft reconstruction using the patient's fibula as an autograft.

Case 2

See A.. 10.8. A 49-year-old male, a radiological assessment for a hip contusion accidentally reveals: metaphyseal lesion of proximal femur with ill definded margins with a chondroid aspect.

Percutaneous biopsy: chondrosarcoma.

Treatment

Block resection and mega-prosthetic hip reconstruction.

Follow-up at ten years: there is no evidence of local or distant recurrence, and he walks with minimal limping.

Case 3

See Figs. 10.9 and 10.10. This patient was 60 years old, with moderate hip pain whose X-ray study shows a periacetabular lesion, well localized as well in the MRI. Core needle biopsy under CT scan shows a grade 1 chondrosarcoma. The clinical decision was curettage and filling with impacted morcelized bone allograft. The patient is controlled every six months and after four years he has pain again and the X-ray and MRI showed a periacetabular lesion in I and IIA zones (according to Sim's classification). A biopsy reveals a high grade chondrosarcoma.

Surgical Treatment

Given the extension to the periacetabular Sim zones I, IIA and permeative through zone 3 the surgical option proposed was an hemipelvectomy and reconstruction with massive hemipelvic allograft with hip endoprosthesis.

Follow up: After eight years post-op the patient continues to walk and there is no evidence of recurrence.

Pelvic Chondrosarcoma

The pelvis is the second more frequent location between chondrosarcomas and for that deserves special consideration (Fig. 10.11). Surgical treatment is mandatory because chemotherapy and radiotherapy have no therapeutic good results and also this location is predictive of poor outcomes. Surgical treatment is challenging for the surgeon because of the regional anatomy, vascular, nervous and visceral tissues, significant tumoral size and higher complication rates.

The resection needs wide margins and therefore big bone resection respecting and conserving the surrounding structures. And also reconstructive surgery to obtain a functional limb needs complex elements like massive allograft or graft combined with prosthesis or massive endoprosthesis (Fig. 10.10).

Condroid lesions in the pelvis have a high risk of malignant transformation.

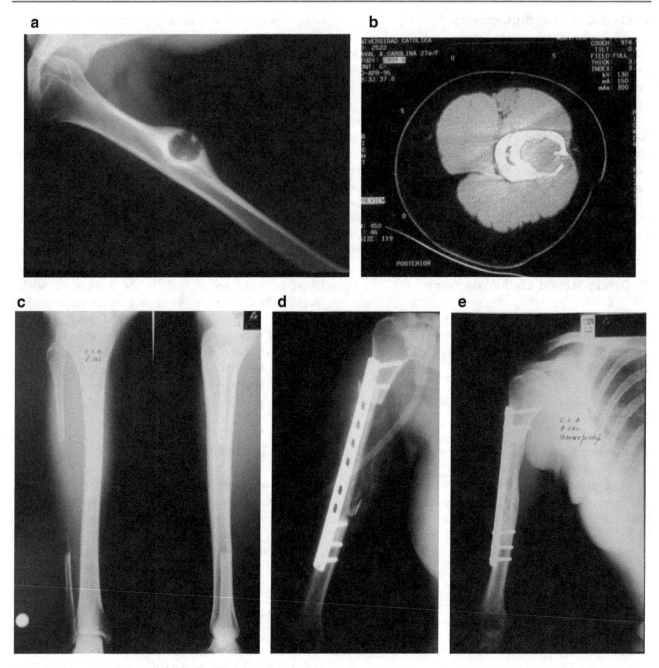

Fig. 10.7 Images of clinical Case 1: **a** and **b**; preoperative study, the tumor invades the cortex and calcifications are observed within the lesion; **c** fíbula autograft harvest; **d** and **e** post-operative images showing progressive consolidation

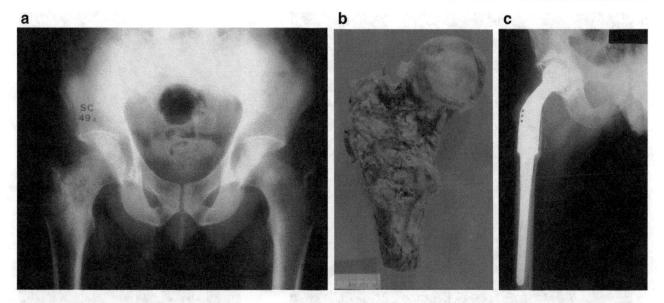

Fig. 10.8 Images of clinical Case 2: **a** pre-operative radiography; **b** resected bone, intraoperative piece; **c** post-operative radiography

Surgical resection and reconstruction is a complex issue, involving complex surgical procedures and high morbidity. But is possible to obtain good results conserving the limb with a very good long term function. Pelvic sarcomas affecting the sacrum that will need sacral roots resection might result in severe impairment of vesicorectal and lower extremities function, and therefore, this should be considered when the sacrum is affected.

Pelvic reconstruction can be made with a massive allograft or massive prosthesis (pelvic and hip prosthesis). Cases with pelvic reconstruction can present up to 50% of complications requiring allograft or endoprosthesis extraction or infection. To perform a limb salvage surgery involves a judicious evaluation of oncologic and psicologic factors, with the possibilities of functional and anatomic restauration of the remaining limb even if no reconstruction is performed (Fig. 10.10).

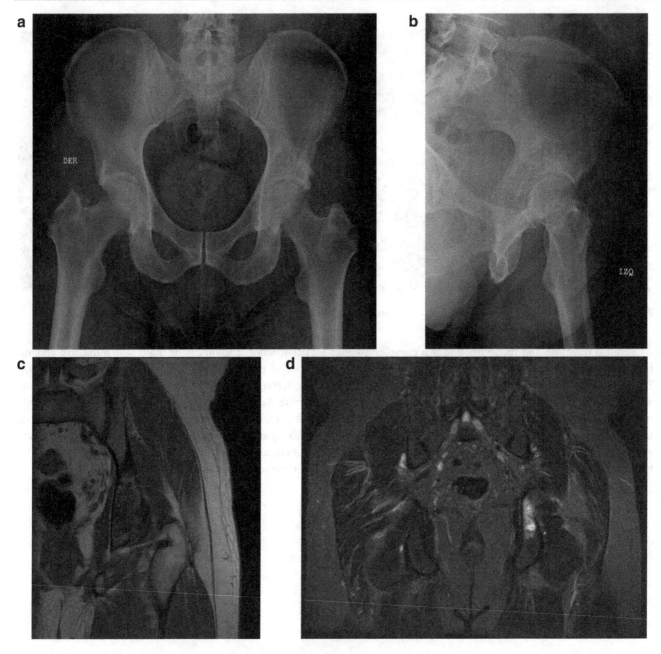

Fig. 10.9 Pre-operative images in clinical Case 3: **a** and **b** X-ray; **c** and **d** MRI

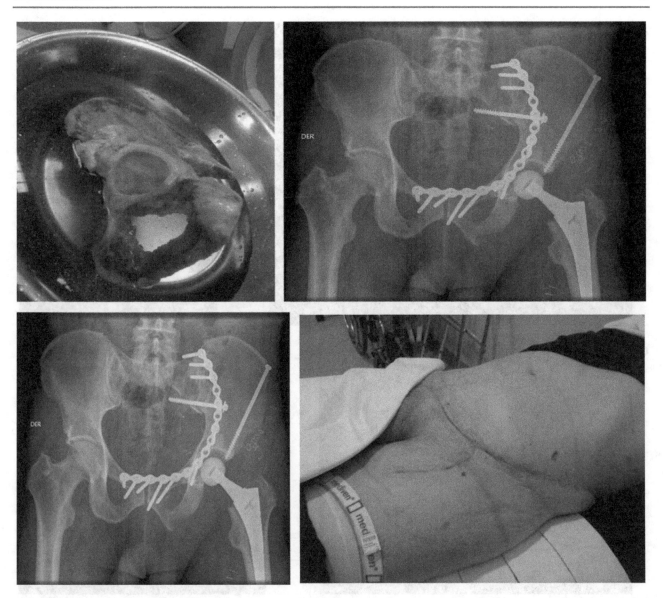

Fig. 10.10 Operative images of clinical Case 3: **a** bone bank allograft; **b** post-op X-ray; and **c** iliofemoral incision

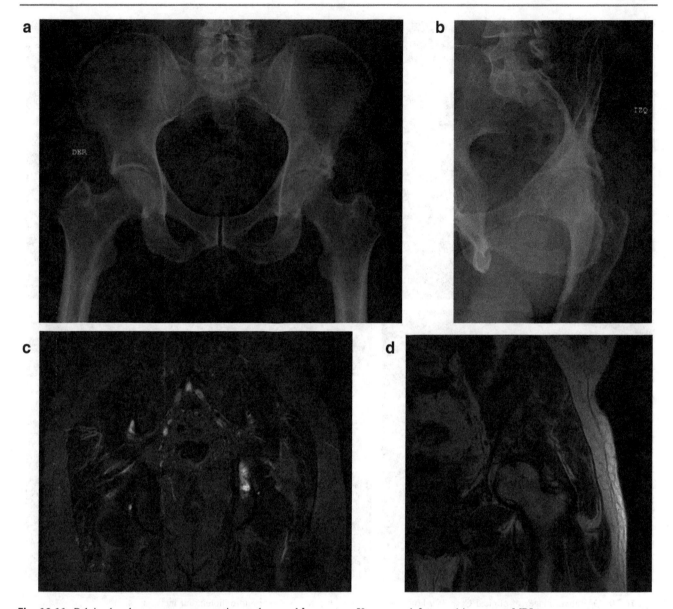

Fig. 10.11 Pelvic chondrosarcoma, pre-operative study: **a** and **b** aspect on X-ray; **c** and **d** coronal images on MRI

References

1. Leddy LR et al. Chondrosarcoma of bone. Cancer Treat Res. 2014.
2. Atalay İB, Yılmaz S, Şimşek MA, Ekşioğlu MF, Güngör BŞ. Chondrosarcomas of the phalanges of the hand. Eklem Hastalik Cerrahisi. 2018;29(1):34–9. https://doi.org/10.5606/ehc.2018. 58876 PMID:29526157.
3. Bani MA, Gargouri F, Mansouri N, Bouziani A, Msakni I. Secondary chondrosarcoma arising in solitary sacro-iliac osteo- chondroma: a case report. Tunis Med. 2017;95(5):386–7.
4. Richard L, McCoughIII MD. Chondrosarcoma of bone OKU 3, chapter 17.
5. Fritz B, Müller DA, Sutter R, Wurnig MC, Wagner MW, Pfirrmann CWA, Fischer MA. Magnetic resonance imaging-based grading of cartilaginous bone tumors: added value of quantitative texture analysis. Invest Radiol. 2018. https://doi. org/10.1097/RLI.0000000000000486.
6. Mulligan ME. How to diagnose enchondroma: bone infarct, and chondrosarcoma. Curr Probl Diagn Radiol. 2018:S0363-0188 (18)30047-1. https://doi.org/10.1067/j.cpradiol.2018.04.002.
7. Terek RM. Recent advances in the basic science of chondrosar- coma. Orthop Clin North Am. 2006;37(1):9–14.
8. Jeong W, Kim HJ. Biomarkers of chondrosarcoma. J Clin Pathol. 2018. pii: jclinpath-2018-205071. https://doi.org/10.1136/ jclinpath-2018-205071.
9. Bus MPA, Campanacci DA, Albergo JI, Leithner A, Van De Sande MAJ, Gaston CL, Sander Dijkstra PD et al. Prognostic factors and outcome of surgical treatment in 162 patients. J Bone Joint Surg Am. 2018; 100(4):316–325 https://doi.org/10.2106/ JBJS.17.00105
10. Donati D, Colangeli S, Colangeli M, Di Bella C, Bertoni F. Surgical treatment of grade I central chondrosarcoma. Clin Orthop Relat Res. 2010;468(2):581–9.

Giant Cell Tumors

Dominique G. Poitout

Abstract

Giant cell tumors are benign bone tumors, representing 5% of primary bone tumors with variable biological aggressiveness and controversial treatment. It more commonly occurs between the third and fourth decades of life and affects preferably the epiphysis of long bones, most of them with an eccentric lytic lesion around the knee.

Keywords

Bone neoplasms · Giant cell tumor of bone · Campanacci staging · Neoplasm recurrence · Curetage · Adjuvant therapy · Denosumab

Introduction

The giant cell tumor represents 5% of the primary bone tumors with variable biological aggressiveness and controversial treatment. There is a low prevalence in females between the third and fourth decades of life and affects preferably the epiphysis of long bones, most of them around the knee (Szendroi, 2004). According to Campanacci grades 1 and 2 represent 52% of the total of GCT and grade 3 represents 48%. There was no correlation between this classification and recurrence. There was a better correlation between the aggressiveness of the treatment and the appearance of recurrence [1].

Histopathology

Giant cell tumors were first described in 1818 by Sir Astley Cooper who denominated it as "fungi medular exostosis" [2]. Nowadays it has a very well defined clinical, radiological and histopathological identity. Its local aggressiveness was described by Nelaton and its potential malignancy by Virchow [3, 4].

The WHO has defined this tumor as an aggressive tumor, very well vascularized, formed by ovoids or fusiform cells with an association of multiple giants cells of osteoclastic type, uniformly distributed in the tumoral tissue (Fig. 11.1).

The pathogenesis is still not very well known [5], but its origin may derive from the mono cells of the local stroma or the bone marrow [6].

The typical giant cell of this tumor is not different to those found in other bone lesions where these giant cells appear similar to chondroblastomas, pigmented villonodular synovitis, the brown tumor of hyperparathyroidism, reparative granuloma of giants cells and Paget [3].

The expression of a receptor activator of nuclear factor kappa–B ligand (RANKL) has been found in osteoclast-like macrophages. This is the basis of the use of RANKL inhibition for medical management which interferes with osteoclastic stimulation.

Jaffe et al. tried to establish a histological gradient with a prognostic correlation for this tumor; however, this gradient was not correlated with treatment and long term prognosis, so it was finally discarded [7].

Clinical Features

Age, location and X-ray imaging are the clues for the clinical diagnosis. Local pain and swelling in the affected joint appears slowly over weeks or months. Pathological fractures can occur.

D. G. Poitout (✉)
Aix Marseille University, Marseille, France
e-mail: Dominique.poitout@live.fr

© Springer-Verlag London Ltd., part of Springer Nature 2021
J. Paulos and D. G. Poitout (eds.), *Bone Tumors*,
https://doi.org/10.1007/978-1-4471-7501-8_11

Fig. 11.1 Histologic aspect of giant cell tumors

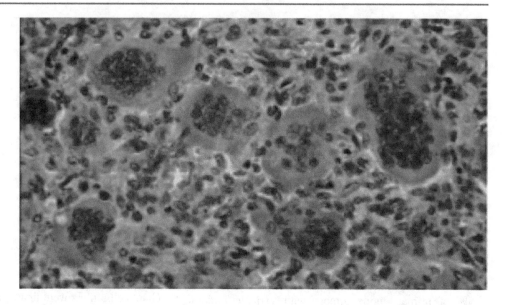

The GCT is developed in a mature skeleton: 70% appearing in people between 20 and 40 years old [8], with a slightly higher female-to-male ratio (60% females). Its occurrence in children is rare [9]. Less than 2% of cases are found under 10 years of age, and only 10% over 55 years of age.

GCTs are usually located in the epiphysis of the long bones; 55% are developed around the epiphysis of the knee, most commonly found in the distal femur [10], proximal tibia and distal radius. An intermediate frequency is found in the proximal femur, proximal fibula (Fig. 11.2) and distal tibia.

In the axial spine, GCT is most often located in the sacrum. GCT is found infrequently in the vertebral body of the mobile spine and rarely in the posterior elements [11, 12]. It is not found in the clavicle or breastbone and few cases are seen in the scapula, hands or feet [5]. Metachronous and multicentric GCTs of bone are even less common [13].

Imaging

Radiologically the GCT is located in the epiphyseal-metaphyseal zone of the long bones, like a osteolytic and excentric lesion. Sometimes there is a fine trabeculated image like soap bubbles [14]. It is a very destructive local bone tumor (Fig. 11.3).

Campanacci developed a radiological classification in 3 grades [1, 15]:

- **Grade 1**: osteolytic tumor with very well-defined edges in a halo of mature bone with an intact or thinned cortex but not deformed;
- **Grade 2**: well-defined edges without an opaque halo and thin limits and more expansive;
- **Grade 3**: badly defined edges suggesting quick growth and invasion of soft tissues and without bone limits.

Around 50% of the cases are found in grade 1 or 2.

Enneking, using radiological, scintigraphic, angiographic, TC and pathologic parameters classified benign tumors as latent, active and aggressive [16].

MRI in grade 2 or 3 cases is useful to evaluate soft tissue compromise revealing an aggressive behavior. T1-weighted MRI demonstrates a low to intermediate signal, mostly homogenous but in T2 sequences showing heterogeneity, due to hemosiderin producing a lower signal and the high water content a high signal. Gadolinium-enhanced images confirm a solid lesion.

Bone scintigraphy with technetium can be useful in looking for other multifocal lesions, showing multiple increased radiotracer uptake helping with the differential diagnosis with hyperparathyroidism whose histology has multinucleated cells.

Lung metastasis has been described even in benign GCT in about 2% of cases [11, 15]. The malignancy can be primary, secondary (post-radiation) or evolutive [17]. Recurrence cases have a greater chance of GCT metastasis. Metastasis can show a benign GCT tumor like in the initial location.

Treatment

Several treatments have been proposed [18]: curettage [19, 20], curettage and bone grafting [21], cryotherapy post-curettage, phenol or cauterization post-curettage, radiation, embolization, bone cement [22], hydrogen peroxide, argon beam coagulation [23], resection and massive allograft [24] and prosthetic reconstruction.

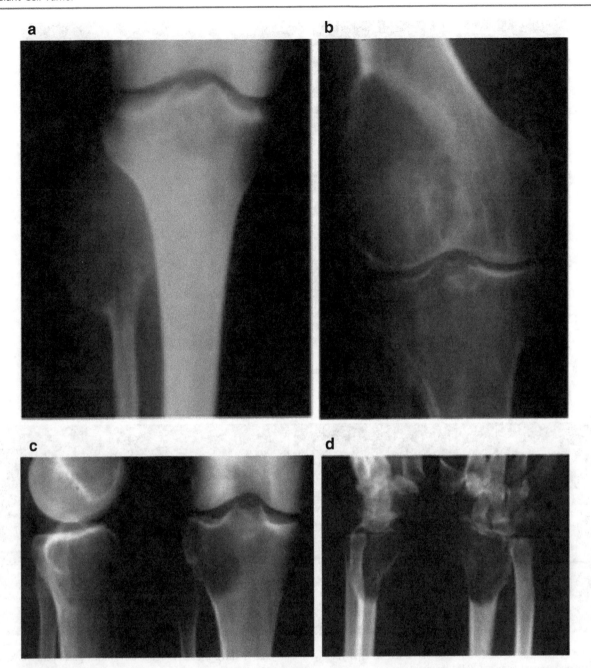

Fig. 11.2 Giant cell tumor located on the epiphysis of long bones: **a** proximal epiphyseal fibula; **b** proximal tibia; **c** and **d** distal epiphyseal femur and distal radius

Most authors recommend curettage or intralesional resection and cryotherapy, phenol or cementing adjuvant therapy (Fig. 11.4)

Curettage must be performed with additional adjuvant therapy, otherwise recurrence is very high (30% or higher).

After a tidy suitable curettage has been performed, a high-speed burr to remove the tumor can be used, but seems insufficient. Cryotherapy with liquid nitrogen poured directly into the tumor cavity reduces the chance of recurrence, but is difficult to manage, with a risk of necrosis of tissuues around

the area, so that this technique must be managed by expert hands. Other chemical products have been used, like phenol, but it is a toxic agent, and also ethanol and hydrogen peroxide. Thermal techniques using cementing with PMM (Fig. 11.5) or cauterization from argon beam coagulation have demonstrated better results.

Bone grafting makes the identification of recurrences difficult. The remodeling associated with bone graft integration can lead to difficulties in image interpretation when looking for local recurrences (Fig. 11.6).

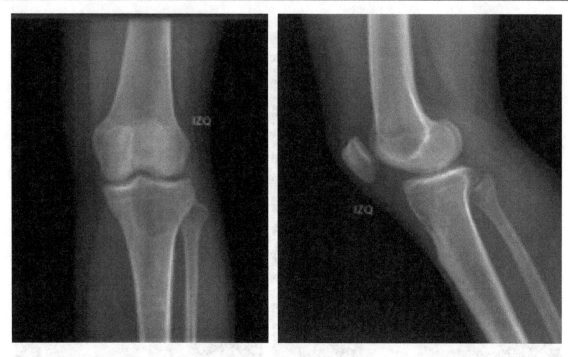

Fig. 11.3 X-ray of giant cell tumor epiphyseal proximal tibia grade 1

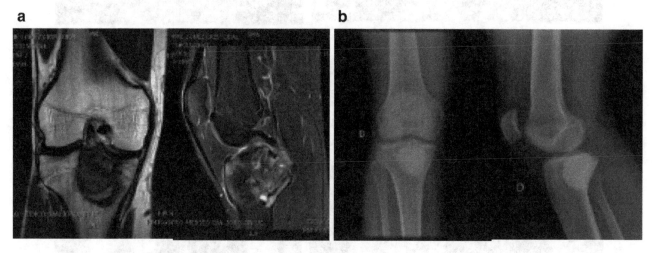

Fig. 11.4 Treatment of GCT, curettage and filled with polymethylmethacrylate (PMM): **a** and **b** preoperative MRI, post-operative X-ray of curettage and cement adjuvant PMM therapy

Bone tumoral resection can be indicated in aggressive Campanacci grade 3 GCT and replacement with allograft. The wrist is a good example of this procedure with an arthrodesis (Fig. 11.7).

Amputation has been necessary in some cases in advanced recurrences.

Radiotherapy is not recommended except when there are no available surgical locations, there is danger of secondary malignization or secondary radioirritation of surrounding tissues. Embolization to reduce the volume of the tumor and with difficult anatomical locations can be useful [25, 26].

Medical management has been used in GCT with biphosfonates (pamidronate, zoledronate) but in recently years with denosumab, a human monoclonal antibody and a RANKL inhibitor [25, 27]. Very good results have been reported decreasing the tumoral mass and the potential agressivity [28–30]. Denosumab is used monthly; the optimal duration of therapy is not yet determined but reports indicate that after stopping the medication the tumor becomes activate again. So surgical treatment continues to be the treatment of choice.

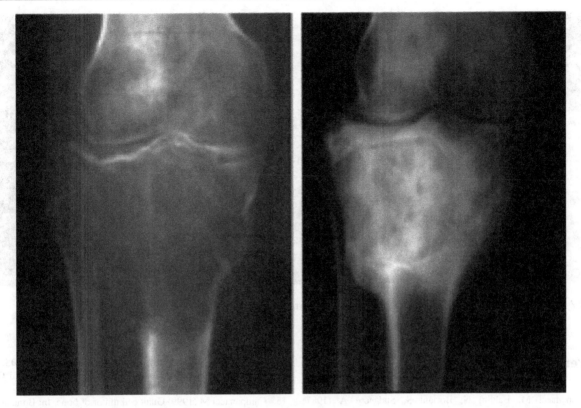

Fig. 11.5 GCT treated with curettage and filled with PMM; 9 years follow-up

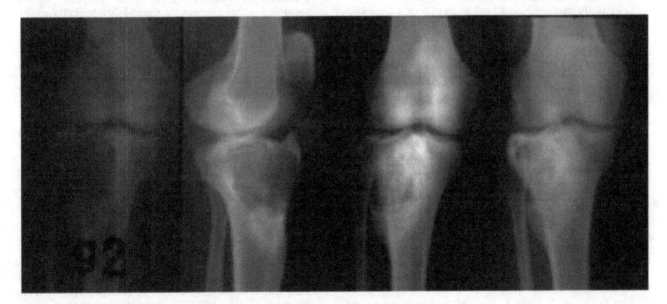

Fig. 11.6 GCT grade 2 treated with curettage and bone graft impaction

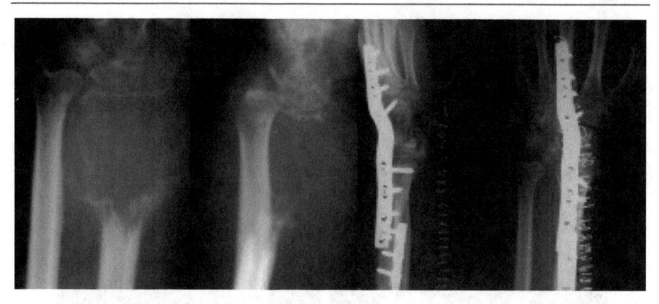

Fig. 11.7 Distal radius GCT, grade 3, bone resection, allograft and wrist arthrodesis

References

1. Campanacci M, Baldini N, Boriani S, Sudanese A (1987) Giant-cell tumor of bone. J Bone Joint Surg Am 69(1):106–114.
2. Cooper A, Travers B (1818) Surgical Essays Part 1. Cox and Son.
3. Coley B (1960) Giant cell tumor (osteoclastoma). In: Neoplasms of bone and related conditions, 2nd ed. p. 196–235.
4. Coley B, Higinbotham N. Giant cell tumor of bone. J Bone Joint Surg Am. 1938;20(4):870–84.
5. Prince H. Giant cell tumor of the os calcis. J Orthop Surg. 1916;2–14(11):641–53.
6. Schajowicz F. Giant cell tumors of bone (osteoclastoma): a pathological and histochemical study. J Bone Joint Surg Am. 1961;43(1):1–29.
7. Jaffe HL (1953) Giant-cell tumour (osteoclastoma) of bone: its pathologic delimitation and the inherent clinical implications. Ann R Coll Surg Engl 13(6):343–355. https://pubmed.ncbi.nlm.nih.gov/13114840.
8. Lichtenstein L (1951) Giant-cell tumor of bone; current status of problems in diagnosis and treatment. J Bone Joint Surg Am 33(1):143–150.
9. Picci P, Manfrini M, Zucchi V, Gherlinzoni F, Rock M, Bertoni F, Neff JR (1983) Giant-cell tumor of bone in skeletally immature patients. J Bone Joint Surg Am 65(4):486–490.
10. Szendroi M (2004) Giant-cell tumour of bone. J Bone Joint Surg Br. 86(1):5–12.
11. Donthineni R, Boriani L, Ofluoglu O, Bandiera S (2009) Metastatic behaviour of giant cell tumour of the spine:497–501. https://doi.org/10.1007/s00264-008-0560-9.
12. Scott D, Pedlow F, Hecht A, Hornicek F. Primary benign and malignantant extradural spine tumors. In: Frymoyer J, Wiesel S, editors. The adult and pediatric spine, 3rd edn. Lippincott Williams and Wilkins; 2003.
13. Hoch B, Inwards C, Sundaram M, Rosenberg AE (2006) Multicentric giant cell tumor of bone: clinicopathologic analysis of thirty cases. J Bone Joint Surg Am 88(9):1998–2008. https://doi.org/10.2106/JBJS.E.01111.
14. Raskin KA, Schwab JH, Mankin HJ, Springfield DS, Hornicek FJ. Giant cell tumor of bone abstract. J Am Acad Orthop Surg. 2013;21:118–26.
15. Campanacci M (1999) Giant cell tumor of bone. In: Bone and soft tissue tumors, 2nd ed. Springer Verlag, p. 99–132.
16. Enneking W (1983) Musculoskeletal tumor surgery, 1st ed. Churchill Livingstone.
17. Domovitov SV, Healey JH (2010) Primary malignant giant-cell tumor of bone has high survival rate:694–701. https://doi.org/10.1245/s10434-009-0803-z.
18. Johnson EWJ, Dahlin DC (1959) Treatment of giant-cell tumor of bone. J Bone Joint Surg Am 41(5):895–904.
19. Meyerding H. Treatment of benign giant cell tumors. J Bone Joint Surg Am. 1936;18(4):823–41.
20. Miller G, Bettelli G, Fabbri N, Capanna R. Curettage of giant cell tumor of bone. La Chirurgia Degli Organi Di Movimento. 1990;75 (1 Suppl.):203.
21. McDonald DJ, Sim FH, McLeod RA, Dahlin DC (1986) Giant-cell tumor of bone. J Bone Joint Surg Am 68(2):235–242.
22. O'Donnell RJ, Springfield DS, Motwani HK, Ready JE, Gebhardt MC, Mankin HJ (1994) Recurrence of giant-cell tumors of the long bones after curettage and packing with cement. J Bone Joint Surg Am 76(12):1827–1833. https://doi.org/10.2106/00004623-199412000-00009.
23. Lewis VO, Wei A, Mendoza T, Primus F, Peabody T, Simon MA. Argon beam coagulation as an adjuvant for local control of giant cell tumor. Clin Orthop Relat Res. 2007;454:192–7. https://doi.org/10.1097/01.blo.0000238784.98606.d4.
24. Mankin HJ, Hornicek FJ. Treatment of giant cell tumors with allograft transplants: a 30-year study. Clin Orthop Relat Res. 2005;439:144–50. https://doi.org/10.1097/01.blo.0000174684.85250.b5.
25. Chawla S, Henshaw R, Seeger L, et al. Safety and efficacy of denosumab for adults and skeletally mature adolescents with giant cell tumour of bone: Interim analysis of an open-label, parallel-group, phase 2 study. Lancet Oncol. 2013;14(9):901–8.
26. Onishi H, Kaya M, Wada T, Nagoya S, Sasak IM, Yamashita T. Giant cell tumor of the sacrum treated with selective arterial embolization. Int J Clin Oncol. 2010; 15(4): 416–419.

27. Thomas D, Henshaw R, Skubitz K, et al. Denosumab in patients with giant-cell tumour of bone: an open label, phase 2 study. Lancet Oncol. 2010;11(3):275–80.

28. Karras NA, Polgreen LE, Ogilvie C, Manivel JC, Skubitz KM, Lipsitz E. Denosumab treatment of metastatic giant-cell tumor of bone in a 10-year-old girl. J Clin Oncol. 2013;31(12):e200–2.

29. Branstetter DG, Nelson SD, Manivel JC, et al. Denosumab induces tumor reduction and bone formation in patients with giant-cell tumor of bone. Clin Cancer Res. 2012;18(16):4415–24.

30. Sung HW, Kuo DP, Shu WP, Chai YB, Liu CC, Li SM. Giant-cell tumor of bone: analysis of two hundred and eight cases in Chinese patients. J Bone Joint Surg Am. 1982; 64(5):755–761.

31. Stewart M, Richardson T. Giant cell tumor of bone. J Bone Joint Surg Am. 1952;34(2):372–86.

Ewing's Sarcoma

Jean Camille Mattei and Dominique G. Poitout

Abstract

Ewing's sarcoma is a malignant bone tumor histologically formed by round blue cells and is among the most aggressive tumors found in children. Its incidence is low and all bones can be affected. Local pain and swelling are common signs of presentation. There are sometimes inflammatory signs such as fever and a macroscopic aspect looking like pus, thus mimicking infectious presentation. The presence of metastasis is high at the moment of the diagnosis. Imaging can be characteristic with soft tissue involvement, which can be massive. Histology and cytogenetics make the final diagnosis. Treatment must be performed by a team of specialists dedicated to sarcoma management. Multidrugs chemotherapy, sometimes radiotherapy and surgery are indicated for the systemic and local control of the disease. The expected survival rate is around 70% at five years of age when the patient is properly treated.

Keywords

Ewing's sarcoma • Malign bone tumours • Cytogenetic • Chemotherapy • Radiotherapy • Reconstructive surgery

Introduction

Ewing's sarcoma is a primary malign bone tumour derived from bone marrow mesenchymal stem cells, belonging to a group of neoplasms characterized by round blue cells.

Diagnosis relies on the detection of a translocation involving the EWSR1 gene, located on chromosome 22 band q12 (usually t(11;22) (q24;q12), for 85–90% of cases), though this mandatory feature can be associated with diverse genetical aberrations [1]. Ewing's family of tumors include the classic Ewing's sarcoma (bone tumor), the Askin tumor (chest wall) and the Primitive Neuro Ectodermal Tumors (PNET).

As to the location, less than a third of Ewing's sarcoma occurs in soft tissues, whereas PNET occur equally in the bone and soft tissue and is five times less common than Ewing's sarcoma.

The incidence of Ewing's sarcomas is of one case/million people in the US, which has remained unchanged over the last decades, with ethnic variabilities (more common in Caucasians than African Americans [2]). Ewing's sarcoma is a tumor of the first and second decade with a peak incidence between eight and 15 years. It rarely occurs in children before five years of age or in adults older than 30 years. Most patients are teenagers and a majority are males (60% [3]).

It is absolutely crucial that the whole management of Ewing's sarcoma is performed in an expert centre dedicated to bone and soft tissue tumours and the patient is evaluated and treated by specialists from the appropriate discipline (e.g., surgeons, radiologists, radiation oncologists, pathologists, medical oncologists), as early as possible.

Diagnosis

Clinical presentation: the most common locations are in diaphysis and meta-diaphysis of long bones, pelvis and ribs but can affect any bone.

Bone disease repartition is as follows [3]:

- lower extremity (40%)
- pelvis (25%)
- chest wall (15%)
- upper extremity (10%)
- spine (5%)
- hand and foot (3%)
- skull (2%)

J. C. Mattei · D. G. Poitout (✉)
Aix Marseille University, Marseille, France
e-mail: dominique.poitout@live.fr

© Springer-Verlag London Ltd., part of Springer Nature 2021
J. Paulos and D. G. Poitout (eds.), *Bone Tumors*,
https://doi.org/10.1007/978-1-4471-7501-8_12

For extraosseous diseases [4]:

- trunk (32%)
- extremity (26%)
- hHead and neck (18%)
- retroperitoneum (16%)
- pther sites (9%)

Pain is the most common symptom and pathological fracture may be a mode of revelation.

Swelling is often present at diagnosis especially at the bone surface, being tense, elastic, often painful and quickly increasing in volume as Ewing's sarcoma remains a high-grade aggressive tumour. Local inflammation signs may be present and Ewing's sarcomas can also mimic an infection, sometimes with high fever, weight loss and myalgia, but should not lead to misdiagnosis of the pathology.

Median time from symptoms to diagnosis is around two to five months, with longer times in deep localizations (e.g., the pelvis) and does not seem to be linked with poorer oncological outcomes [5].

Metastases can be present at diagnosis in 25% of cases [6], of various locations: skeleton (all bones can be affected); lungs and pleura; and less frequently to the liver, heart, kidney, pancreas, the thyroid gland, and central nervous system. Lymph node metastases are rare.

Imaging

In addition to a physical examination and the patient's medical history, diagnostic evaluation relies on:

X-Rays

The most common aspect is ill-limited osteolysis. The **cortex** is first thinned and then destroyed by the evolutionary process. **Periosteal reaction** is a major sign and might present with the classic image of an onion bulb (small bone superposed sheets parallel to the shaft). **Endostal osteogenic periosteal reaction** is possible, but not as clear or important as in neoplastic osteogenesis osteosarcoma. There may be osteosclerosis with increased bone density. But the usual presentation is purely lytic with no matrix. Specific attention to X-ray analysis is crucial as signs of Ewing's sarcoma can be very subtle in the initial stages of the disease. The growth plate and epiphysis may be respected by the tumor process for a long time.

The **soft tissue involvement** can present as opacity, or as muscle being pushed aside by the tumor. It is often major considering the aggressiveness of those neoplasms.

Computed Tomography (CT/CAT Scan)

Periosteal reaction lamellar organization and lysis are better defined. At the epiphyseal level, tumor extension is usually not well-defined.

The **tumor extension** is a bit clearer than on X-rays and a **gadolinium** injection allows better definition of its extent; most importantly, it helps with clarifying vascular vicinity/ involvement.

Magnetic Resonnance Imaging (MRI)

This is mandatory in the diagnosis and local staging of Ewing's sarcoma. It specifies the bone extension of the tumor (T1 sequences) and soft tissue involvement (T2, with T1 help in the analysis of critical anatomical structures involvement as nerves and vessels). Full bone has to be in the field to detect skip metastases.

Blood Tests

The **sedimentation rate and/or PCR** is often increased. Sometimes **anemia** and mild leukocytosis are present.

An increase in **serum LDH** is common in Ewing's sarcoma, while it is not found in some differential diagnoses such as osteomyelitis.

They are usually not useful for the diagnosis.

Biopsy

A surgical or image-guided biopsy is mandatory for the diagnosis of Ewing's sarcoma, taking as much tissue as possible from the tumor, favoring its soft tissue component to avoid decalcification, which takes time and might delay diagnosis and therefore the treatment. An appropriate imaging (MRI) has to be performed first, to assess the most cellular part of the tumor and target it with the biopsy (avoiding necrotic areas). It is of an utmost importance that the biopsy path is performed or decided by the surgeon who will resect the tumor.

The biopsy should be taken as often as possible in the soft tissues to avoid pathological fracture risk [7] and to accelerate the diagnosis (if the biopsy is bone only, the examination by the pathologists necessitates a decalcification first, which also limits the possibility to perform genetics tests on the sample). It is important to send fresh tissue in the laboratory for cytogenetics and molecular profiling.

If a needle biopsy is performed, the specialized radiologist has to ensure that the biopsy path complies with the surgeon's opinion. It is far more comfortable for the patient (no anaesthesia, no hospitalization) and has the same diagnostic performance [8] but limits the opportunity to perform research on small-sized samples. If a needle biopsy is performed, its tract has to be tattoed by the radiologist to remove the scar, as for a surgical case.

The biopsy assessment should include:

- a standard histological examination
- immunocytochemistry study
- a cytogenetic examination carried out on a fresh and sterile fragment

Macroscopic Aspect

Ewing's sarcoma is a grey soft, translucent, encephaloid tumor. Some hemorrhagic necrotic areas can be observed, sometimes with a milky/ liquid/ purulent appearance (similar to osteomyelitis). There is bone destruction and often already a significant spread of the tumor in the adjacent tissues.

Microscopic Aspect

Cellularity is high with small, oval or polyhedral cells arranged in checkerboard or lobules separated by thin or absent connective septa. Nuclei are round or oval, intensely colored, chromatin is finely punctuated and the nucleolus is small, mitoses are rare with pale, sparse, vacuolated cytoplasm (Fig. 12.1).

Sometimes these cells are grouped around a vessel or small necrotic focus, forming a pseudorosette, different from the rosette of neuroblastoma. Neoplastic tissue propagates along Haversian canals.

The presence of glycogen in the cytoplasm of these cells can give a special pink coloring periodic acid Schift (PAS); this may allow clinicians to differentiate Ewing's sarcoma from malignant lymphoma, or bone metastases of neuroblastoma, because the cytoplasm of those cells contains no glycogen.

Specific immunodetection can recognize a possible lymphoid lineage if there is still a doubt on lymphoma.

Immuno-Histochemistry

The **NSE (Neuron Specific Enolase)** often shows an intracytoplasmic marking, but without specificity as for **HNK (Human Natural Killer)** but Kovar et al. highlighted both in Ewing's sarcoma and in PNETs (Primitive Neuro Ectodermal Tumors) the overexpression of the **MIC2** gene [9].

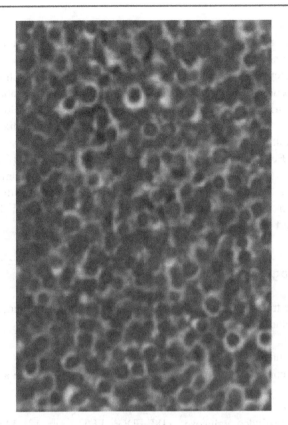

Fig. 12.1 Histology of Ewing's sarcoma

The presence of this gene confirms the neuroectodermal origin of Ewing's sarcoma and clinically allows diagnosis of these tumors in 90% of cases. *MIC2* positivity is not unique to Ewing's sarcoma, and positivity by immunochemistry is found in several other tumors, including synovial sarcoma, non-Hodgkin lymphoma, and gastrointestinal stromal tumors.

Cytogenetics

The detection of a translocation involving the *EWSR1* gene on chromosome 22 band q12 and any one of a number of partner chromosomes is the key feature in the diagnosis of Ewing's sarcoma [1].

The most frequent anomaly found in Ewing's sarcoma is the translocation **t(11; 22) (q24; q12)**, found in 90% of cases. This anomaly was described for the first time in 1983 by Turc-Carel et al. [10] and corresponds to an exchange of reciprocal translocations between chromosome 11 and chromosome 22, at the level of 11q24 and 22q12 bands. Translocations variants are described but all involve chromosomes 22 at the q12 band,

The highlight of this translocation is a major diagnostic interest. Indeed, histologically differential diagnosis of small round cell tumors such as rhabdomyosarcoma and neuroblastoma, and bone lymphoma can be difficult. The presence of the translocation t [11, 22] is used to confirm the diagnosis of Ewing's sarcoma. These translocations are detectable with both reverse transcriptase-polymerase chain reaction (RT-PCR) and fluorescence in situ hybridization (FISH) in formalin-fixed paraffin-embedded tissue. However, RT-PCR is less sensitive in formalin-fixed paraffin-embedded than frozen tissue [11].

Besides these consistent aberrations involving the *EWSR1* gene at 22q12, additional numerical and structural aberrations have been observed in Ewing's sarcoma, including gains of chromosomes, translocation and deletions on the short arm of chromosome 6.

Staging

Pre-treatment staging studies for Ewing's sarcoma should include:

- magnetic resonance imaging (MRI)
- computed tomography (CT) scan of the primary site and chest
- ositron emission tomography using fluorine F 18-fludeoxyglucose (18F-FDG PET) or 18F-FDG PET-CT
- bone scan
- bone marrow aspiration/biopsy.

When diagnosis is confirmed, **CT and MRI** are both equivalent in terms of staging and might also help the radiation oncologist in the determination of volumes [12]. The chest CT is meant to detect pulmonary metastases, which is the most common secondary location in Ewing's Sarcoma.

18F-FDG PET or 18F-FDG PET-CT have demonstrated high sensitivity and specificity in Ewing's sarcoma and may provide additional information that alters therapy planning. 18F-FDG PET has a very high correlation with the bone scan and tends to progressively replace the bone scan for the initial extent of disease evaluation [13]. 18F-FDG PET-CT has also been assessed as more accurate than 18F-FDG PET alone in Ewing's sarcoma [14].

Bone marrow aspiration or biopsy have been in the standard of care for several years in Ewing's sarcoma. However, these tests were negative in every case where bone scan and/or the PET scan and lung CT did not show secondary localizations in several studies [15]. Furthermore, isolated bone marrow involvement (i.e., without any other metastatic sites) is exceptional and the need for such tests is now in question since bone marrow involvement would not change the type of treatment [16].

At the end of local and general work-up the tumor is defined as localized when no spread beyond the primary site is detected. If regional lymph node involvement is suspected, pathologic confirmation is indicated, though such a condition is exceptional in Ewing's Sarcoma.

Treatment

Ewing's sarcoma without treatment has a mortality rate near to 100%.

The optimal treatment of patients with localized Ewing's sarcoma includes a combined treatment: systemic (chemotherapy) and local (surgery and/or radiation therapy) [17]. Patients usually receive chemotherapy before local-control treatment (neoadyuvant and multidrug protocols). Adjuvant therapies are then guided by the results of surgery (surgical margins and oncologic response to chemo). Metastases often respond well to pre-operative chemotherapy, but control is unfortunately partial [18]. Lung localization of metastasis is considered as of a better prognosis than patients with other type of secondary disease (bone, liver, bone marrow) and dedicated local treatment of oligometastatic diseases (especially in bone and lungs locations) is becoming a subject of interest in local control and survival [19].

One should also not forget that Ewing's sarcoma most often arises in young patients and that lots of health workers will be involved in global care (primary care physicians, hematologists, rehabilitation specialists, pediatric nurse specialists, social workers, child-life professionals, psychologists, school support, etc.). Chemotherapy regimens are also as aggressive as the disease, and fertility management will also have to be considered.

Chemotherapy

Currently, the standard of care is based first on chemotherapy, followed by a conservative surgery when it is possible. Indications of radiotherapy depend for most teams on the response to the initial chemotherapy and the quality of surgical resection. Before the advent of chemotherapy, the prognosis of localized Ewing's sarcoma was dark, with a mortality rate at five years of over 90% due to pulmonary metastasis and/or bone-marrow metastasis.

Several protocols of chemotherapy have been used, beginning in the 1980s with VACA (vincristine, actinomicina, cyclophosphamide, adriamicina) looking for better results. Research with chemotherapy is ongoing.

Chemotherapy in Ewing's sarcoma is always based on four drugs (vincristine, doxorubicin, ifosfamide, and etoposide). Most protocols also use cyclophosphamide, and some teams may add dactinomycin. Cyclophosphamide doses and intensity however vary among different protocols.

To simplify, US protocols [20] tend to alternate vincristine, cyclophosphamide, and doxorubicin with ifosfamide/etoposide, while European [21] centers usually combine vincristine, doxorubicin, and an alkylating agent with or without etoposide in a single treatment cycle. For all protocols, the duration neoadjuvant chemotherapy ranges from six months to one year.

For patients with a high risk of relapse with conventional treatments, certain centers have utilized high-dose chemotherapy with hematopoietic stem cell transplant (HSCT) as a consolidation treatment, to improve the outcome [22]. In the Euro Ewing's trial, improved outcomes with such treatment have been observed for patients with a poor response to initial therapy [23].

Local Treatment

Sarcoma local management always tries to optimize local control while limiting morbidity and optimizing function, when feasible.

Local control remains controversial and it does not replace prospective randomized trial that has compared surgery with radiotherapy versus radiotherapy alone, especially in primitive pelvic tumors. But in general, resection is recommended in cases of small localized tumors or if the team thinks that surgery is curative. In very young patients, surgery should be preferred when feasible because radiation therapy is a significant cause of morbidity.

Surgery remains the gold standard for local control. However, radiation therapy remains a reasonable and effective option when morbidity is considered as too severe by orthopaedic oncologists (impact on function, cosmetics, especially in certain localizations such as the pelvis or spine). Besides, when complete surgical resection with pathologically negative margins cannot be obtained, post-operative radiation therapy is indicated. A multidisciplinary discussion between expert radiation oncologists and the surgeon needs to determine the best treatment options for local control for a given case, when surgery is not the simplest way to obtain a satisfying local control. A combined approach is also an option when a marginal resection (close to the tumor/R1 margins) is expected, with neo-adjuvant radiotherapy followed by surgery. The timing of local therapy is crucial, as the overall survival rate is better for patients who were taken in charge earlier.

There is basically no questioning of surgery versus radiation therapy as the few studies that exist are based by selection criteria (with apparent superiority of surgery in local control and survival) and are retrospective.

Some studies using propensity scoring may conclude to the equivalency of radiation, surgery and combined treatment in pelvic localizations.

However, Euro Ewing's trial showed improved survival with combined radiation therapy and surgery in pelvic localization. In non-sacral tumors, combined local treatment was associated with a lower recurrence rate compared with surgery alone. Even when surgery was wide (R0 margins) and with good histologic response to chemo, combined treatment did seem to achieve better overall survival rates (87% vs. 51% at five years). Furthermore, patients who did not undergo complete removal of the affected bone, patients with a poor histologic response to induction chemotherapy and patients who did not receive additional radiation therapy had a higher risk of death. Finally, for patients who undergo resection with microscopic residual disease, a radiation therapy dose is indicated.

In summary, surgery is adapted for suitable patients, but radiation therapy remains a standard of care for patients with unresectable disease when functional or cosmetic issues are at stake when considering surgery. Adjuvant radiation therapy should also be considered in case of close or inadequate margins.

Also, when local staging suggests that surgical margins will be close or positive, pre-operative radiation therapy may allow tumor shrinkage with clear surgical margins and limit recurrence risk [24].

Surgery

Resection

Surgery remain the standard of care for local control. Limb salvage wide excisions or amputations have the same results especially for extremity sarcomas. Amputation was historically considered the gold standard in the treatment of extremity sarcomas but started to be questioned through a randomized trial comparing patients undergoing amputation with patients operated with limb-salvage wide excision and adjuvant radiation. Amputation had an impact on local recurrence, but no difference in the overall survival rate or disease-specific survival rate was observed between the two groups. Progressively, limb-sparing surgery was then preferred to amputation for the majority of patients with extremity sarcoma [25] and for that reason, amputation is rarely employed in the management of extremity sarcomas in modern series from referral centers.

Initially, limb-sparing consisted in the resection of an entire muscular body containing a sarcoma. It is now recognized that a 1 cm margin circumferentially is adequate in most cases to achieve negative margins and minimize the risk of local recurrence. In cases of soft tissue sarcomas, histologic subtypes with infiltrative borders should however benefit from wider margins and/or specific radiation therapy considerations (Myxofibrosarcomas or UPS).

However, even when a standard 1 cm margin is planned, safe margins are sometimes limited by neurovascular bundles. If the bundle is just pushed aside without being encased in the tumor, the sarcoma can be removed with the bundle sheath to achieve negative margin. Usually this is performed by exposing the bundle in a safe zone and protecting it as the tumor is progressively retracted from the surgical bed. Microscopic positive margin following complete resection close to a bundle does not necessarily result in local recurrence, so resection of an adjacent artery or nerve to obtain an R0 versus R1 resection is not indicated in the context of a primary lesion [26].

When the tumor cannot be separated from those critical structures to obtain R1 margins (especially in cases of local recurrence when the tumor was initially close to a bundle), the vascular bundle is sacrificed, which might necessitate vascular reconstruction too. Bypass indication is usually carefully assessed by vascular surgeons and depends on the location and the length of sacrificed vessel(s). For example, there is usually no need of vascular reconstruction if the deep femoral vessels are encased, but resection of an Ewing's sarcoma of the knee involving the superficial femoral bundle will lead to vascular reconstruction if limb salvage is considered. There are still debates regarding venous bypass, which depends on the level of the resection (e.g., the external iliac will usually be reconstructed, whereas the superficial femoral will not, especially if the saphenous and/or deep femoral are kept intact). In the event of significant swelling, compression and elevation will temporize symptoms until collateral vessels develop. Regarding nerves, resection of perineal or sciatic are usually well managed with orthoses but the patient must be warned about the risk of unrecognized injuries due to foot anaesthesia, as the foot will indeed have to be examined on a regular basis, just like a diabetic foot [27]. Femoral nerve resection leads to more frequent complications with long-term joint damage and falls related to the impossibility of locking the knee. These falls are responsible for a higher rate of fractures after limb-preserving procedures and should be prevented with knee bracing like the Zimmer splint or articulated knee splints [28]. Resection of one of three of the major upper extremity nerves usually preserves opposition in the hand and a fair function.

If a wide resection implies the resection of major nerves with complex vascular bypass reconstruction, many teams might favor amputation because of high rates of complications and failures, combined with the risk of resulting in poor functional outcomes. In such cases, especially in the lower limbs, amputation might be preferred.

Reconstruction

Resection of tumors in bones such as the fibula, patella, scapula, or radius/ulna, is often successful without reconstruction (and in pelvic localizations which are subject to intense debates). In weight-bearing locations, biomechanics must be restored as best as possible to optimize function and limit the morbidity of oncological surgery. Many reconstructive options are at a surgeon's disposal: allograft, allograft-prosthetic composite, endoprosthesis (including expandable prostheses), biological reconstructions and extracorporeal irradiated autografts. New technologies will have an impact on decreasing complication rates, implant design/fixation/function and operative techniques.

(1) **Allograft reconstruction**: This might allow for: bone stock restoration, sparing of uninvolved joints (intercalary techniques), and anatomical reattachment of tendons [29], which is needed to restore good function to the joint. However, a weight-bearing protection is needed until healing, with a risk of osteoarthritis in osteoarticular grafts, disease transmission (exceptional) or graft rejection (very rare too). They are also known for high rates of complications (nonunion, fracture, and infection) [29, 30], as almost 20% of procedures could fail, with more than 50% of patients requiring additional surgery [31, 32]. The various types of reconstruction have different behaviors: intercalary allografts have fair long-term functional outcomes in more than 80% of patients [31, 33] and excellent limb survival rates (>90%) [31],

Osteoarticular reconstruction studies report variable outcomes (60% of satisfying results (30)) with interesting results by Poitout and al. [35] who found that cartilage preserved in DMSO was functional, without significant joint destruction, with with living chondrocytes, several years after implantation.

In a recent intercalary allograft reconstruction assessment (30), more than 75% of patients had >1 complications, mostly non-union (40%). Risk factors for failure and complications were age > 18 years, allograft length > 15 cm, intramedullary nail-only fixation, and diaphyseal localization. Those findings were consistent with the literature [34, 35] as there is general consensus regarding age, length, lack of rigid fixation, and diaphyseal location as risk factors for complications after such procedures.

Those pitfalls (graft fracture, non-union and infection) may be due to the avascular nature of some parts of the allograft [36, 37]. For that reason, Campanna et al. developed in the 1980s a technique using massive allograft combined with vascularized fibula autograft incorporated in the allograft canal and reported a significant improvement in fracture risk and union rate at a long-term follow-up [38]. However, Houdek et al. [37] were unable to confirm those results, finding high fracture and low union rates, comparable to those of classic allograft reconstruction; but the proportion of patients achieving limb preservation was high (94%) with good functional results in >90% of cases and an acceptable complication rate (30%). This technique may represent an improvement in surgical outcomes of allograft reconstruction, though technically demanding and time-consuming, and the future will most probably see some breakthrough as our understanding of the technique's failure mechanisms and bone healing is growing every day.

(2) **Composite allograft-prosthetic reconstructions**: Chondrocytes cannot survive cryo-presentation procedures and for that reason, osteo-articular allografts are challenging and subject to failure because of instability due to non-anatomical graft fixation, resulting in fast cartilage destruction [39]. Composite allograft-prosthetic reconstructions (CAPR) are supposed to combine joint plasty of a standard prosthesis with the bone stock and soft tissues attachments of an allograft [40].

Several studies have shown that CAPR might provide better stability than massive replacements, most probably because of muscles and capsule reattachments for joint stabilization [41] so that constraints are transferred as in a classic arthroplasty rather than directly to the junction between the endoprosthesis and the bone [40].

Though usually performed in the lower extremities, this technique is also useful in reverse shoulder arthroplasties (Fig. 12.2) [42]. As for allograft-only reconstructions, weight-bearing must be postponed until bone healing, usually delayed by chemotherapy in Ewing's sarcoma. This must be considered when discussing reconstruction options with the patient as non-union remains the most common complication (>20%) in these procedures [43].

According to Poitout et al. [44], the reconstruction has to be done with massive allografts or allografts surrounding massive metallic prostheses. The integration of massive deep-frozen allografts is enhanced when the fixation of the graft is even, with a perfect contact between the allografts and the recipient bone. Infectious issues are equivalent to those obtained with massive prostheses and the risk of fracture is decreased when the allografted bone is well protected by a stem or a plate.

(3) **Endoprosthetic reconstruction** (Figs. 12.2, 12.3 and 12.4): This is the most widespread reconstruction method in the adult population thanks to their

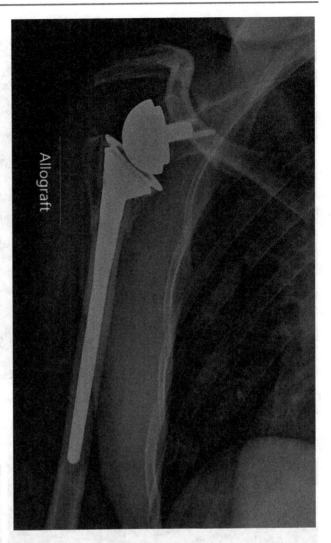

Fig. 12.2 Reverse shoulder arthroplasty after proximal humerus resection for Ewing's sarcoma; composite reconstruction with long stem cemented prosthesis with rotator-cuff reattachment on the allograft portion

immediate availability and to the early weight-bearing possibilities of modern implants [45]. They also provide a fair implant survival rate at almost 80% in the lower extremities and 90% in the upper limbs [46, 47], and a very high limb preservation rate (>90%); but the counterparty of such results are the high revision rates (>30%) [48], essentially due to mechanical failures and infection, then recurrence [49].

When comparing CAPR with endoprosthetic reconstruction in the proximal femur, complication rates were similar, with 10% aseptic loosening in massive replacements and 10% non-union in CAPR. Function scores and survival rates were not different, though abductor strength was higher in CAPR [50].

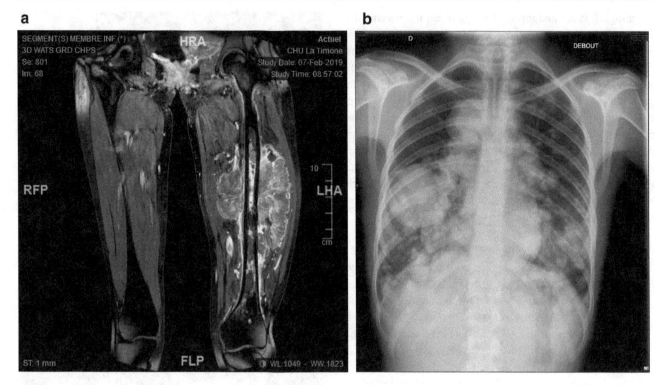

Fig. 12.3 a, b: femoral/thigh Ewing's sarcoma before chemotherapy: **a** involvement of several compartments of the thigh; **b** chest X-rays: multiple metastases

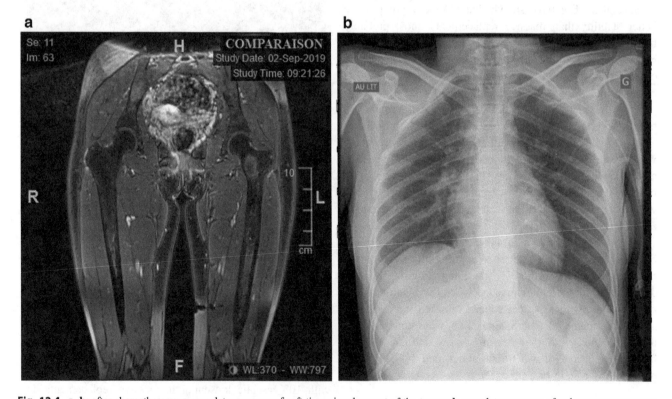

Fig. 12.4 a, b: after chemotherapy: **a** complete response of soft-tissue involvement of the tumor; **b** complete response of pulmonary metastases

Distal femoral massive replacements have poorer outcomes due to the complexity of the knee joint compare to the coxo-femoral location, which was illustrated in studies comparing CAPR with massive implants. Whereas biomechanics were mostly preserved in CAPR, endoprosthetic replacements showed abnormal kinetics [51] in the knee with strength loss and abnormal gait pattern when medialis and intermedius had to be resected for tumor consideration [52]. These findings suggest that recreating normal joint kinematics and soft tissue reattachment in metal implants remains challenging, however remaining popular among orthopedic oncologic surgeons. This also has to be put into perspective with several ongoing debates regarding which implant (custom versus modular), fixation (cemented or not) and hinge type to use in distal femoral replacements [53]. It seems that all these parameters should be addressed depending on the patient profile, which relies on randomized and homogenous studies that are complex to build in rare pathologies such as sarcomas (Figs. 12.3a, b, 12.4a, b, and 12.5a, b).

(4) **Extra-corporeal irradiation and autograft** [54]: some authors have used extra-corporeal irradiation of a resected bone tumor segment with re-implantation, that may facilitate reconstruction of defects with an inexpensive, anatomically identical graft that restores bone stock, theoretically limiting the risk of disease transmission and graft rejection. The technique uses rotational markers to optimize alignment at reimplantation, soft tissue stripping from the bone, with wrapping in sterile-antibiotic loaded gauzes during administration of a single 50-Gy dose of radiation. Endo-medullar

reaming with bone cement in the canal completes the procedure before the specimen reimplantation and internal fixation. The osteotomy site is united primarily in 88% of cases, higher than for cadaveric allograft fixation, with a 13.0% infection rate and comparable recurrence rate as in other techniques [33]. Fractures could be as high as 20% [55] and adjunction of vascularized fibula autograft might mitigate this risk, with almost 90% good or excellent functional outcomes [56].

(5) **Reconstruction options in children:** (a) biological reconstruction: Paediatrics orthopaedic oncology surgeons tend to limit the use of prostheses due to ultimate implant failure probability in children. Considering that physis might also be preserved, several techniques are used to prefer segmental bone resection with joint sparing to a massive prosthetic replacement.

Autogenous bone grafts are used commonly to reconstruct bone voids or to induce bone healing and the iliac crest remains a widespread autograft in orthopedic oncology and especially in children. Alternative sites include the proximal tibia, the distal radius, the distal tibia, and the greater trochanter [57]. Cortical bone grafts might be used in structural defects in which immediate mechanical stability is required for healing [57] whereas cancellous bone grafts provide higher rates of remodeling and incorporation while of a limited mechanical strength. Cortico-cancellous bone grafts offer the advantages of both cortical and cancellous bone while vascularized bone grafts offer the best incorporation and healing due to vascular pedicles and are indicated for large bone defects. Pedicled or free vascularized fibula grafts are among the most used grafts in orthopedic oncology and

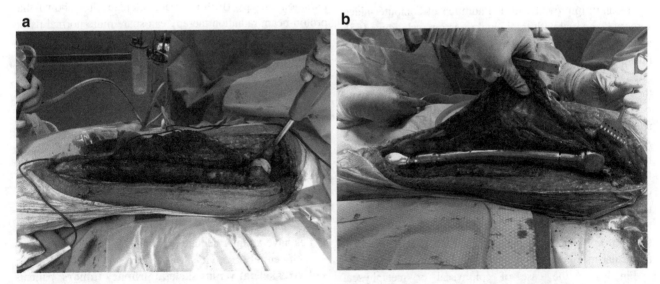

Fig. 12.5 **a**, **b**. Femur: Ewing's sarcoma, surgical treatment; **a** progressive resection of total femur considering MRI findings, leaving layer of vastus intermedius as margin on the bone; **b** intra-operative view of total femoral reconstruction

might be used in various sites such as the humerus, ulna, or radius. Furthermore, they are also an option for growth plate reconstruction (with proximal fibula for example) [58].

(b) *Expandable prostheses*: these remain an option in pediatrics with mitigation of length discrepancy thanks to various systems allowing the expansion of the prothesis over the year, accompanying the child's growth. They offer fair outcomes and limit the morbidity of donor sites in case of autograft harvesting. However, revision is inevitable and can be quite challenging when the patient becomes an adult [59].

What comes next?
Rates of aseptic mechanical loosening are expected to rise as young survivors of sarcoma will unfortunately see their implant or reconstruction fail. One strategy is to optimize fixation devices. Compress prosthesis [60], designed to apply compression at the bone-implant interface, resulting in hypertrophic bone growth (Wolff's Law [61]) and the use of a hydroxy-apatite collar at the bone-prosthesis junction [53] are two different ways which might limit aseptic loosening rates, with interesting long-term results.

Follow-up on operated patients relies on the reliability of recurrence detection techniques, often limited by implant-related artifacts, and radiolucent implants minimizing the artifact on MRI or CT scans might improve cross-sectional imaging surveillance during oncological follow-up [62] with interesting biomechanical profiles [63].

Optimizing resection safety, efficiency and margins is high on the stakes in orthopedic oncology. Navigation technology is widely used for spine and trauma surgery, and arthroplasty improves the precision and reproducibility of hardware placement [64]. In orthopedic oncology, for example, studies have shown that in intralesional resection rates of pelvic tumors the accuracy of planned osteotomies significantly improved with the addition of computer-aided surgery compared with traditional resection techniques [65]; and Cho et al. [66] suggested a decrease in local recurrence rates as a result of improved margin status.

In the same vein, pre-operative MRI and CATs scan allow the engineering of 3D-printed custom cutting jigs, with patient-specific instrumentation to achieve patient-matching reconstruction of bone defects and hardware placement [67]. Advanced pre-operative computer-aided planning would also help two surgical teams to work simultaneously, one performing the resection and the other creating an allograft identical to the resection specimen to be used for reconstruction [68]. A similar technique can be applied to custom-made metallic implants, in which the implant manufacturer and surgeon work on the same pre-operative plan to create a trabecular-metal implant that precisely matches the resection.

Finally, in the case of epiphyseal or metaphyseal long-bone sarcomas, navigation or custom cutting jigs would optimize and allow periarticular resection to preserve the whole or partial epiphysis, with a defect reconstructed by a 3D-printed implant or custom-osteotomized allograft [69]. Those techniques could be especially valuable in Ewing's sarcomas challenging localizations such as the pelvis.

Radiation Therapy

Ewing's sarcoma is considered as a radiosensitive tumor and can be treated with adequate management and doses of radiation, which, however, include radiation pitfalls and complications.

When no resection is scheduled, radiation therapy is generally administered in fractionated doses of 55.8 Gy total to the initial tumor volume [70]. For patients with residual disease after surgery, the Intergroup Ewing's Sarcoma recommended 45 Gy to the original disease site plus a 10.8 Gy boost for patients with gross residual disease, and 45 Gy plus a 5.4 Gy boost for patients with microscopic residual disease [71]. No radiation therapy was recommended for those who have no evidence of microscopic residual disease after surgical resection [72].

We should not not forget that radiation therapy is delivered to young patients and might be associated with a long follow-up with the development of subsequent neoplasms. A retrospective study found that patients who received 60 Gy or more were at risk of secondary malignancy in 20% of cases, compared to 5% when between 48 and 60 Gy was administered, and 0% for those who received less than 48 Gy [73].

For that reason, a radiation therapy regimen is at the center of many studies which try to limit radiation fields and/or doses and/or number of sessions. A comparison of proton-beam radiation therapy with intensity-modulated radiation therapy (IMRT) treatment plans has shown that proton-beam radiation therapy can spare more normal tissue than IMRT [74]. However, the small number of samples and short follow-up limit the extent of these conclusions, especially in terms of local-recurrence risk, which might be higher when reducing the doses.

Prognosis Factors

Pre-treatment Factors

- **Site of tumor**: distal extremities have a better prognosis. Patients with Ewing's sarcoma in the proximal extremities have an intermediate prognosis, followed by patients with central or pelvic sites [75].
- **Extraskeletal versus skeletal primary tumors**: patients with extraskeletal primary tumors had a statistically

significant better prognosis than patients with skeletal primary tumors [76].

- **Tumor size or volume** is an important prognostic. Cut-offs of a volume of 100 ml or 200 ml and/or single dimension greater than 8 cm define larger tumors, which also tend to occur in unfavorable sites [77].
- **Age**: infants and younger patients have a better prognosis than patients >15 years of age [78].
- **Sex**: girls have a better prognosis [75].
- **Serum LDH**: increased serum LDH levels before treatment are associated with inferior prognosis, also correlated with large primary tumors and/or metastatic disease [79].
- **Metastases**: the single most powerful predictor of outcome. Metastases confined to the lungs show better outcomes [80] and their numbers does not seem to have an impact though patients with unilateral lung involvement do better than bilateral localizations [81]. Metastasis to bone only seem to have a better outcome than patients with metastases to both bone and lung [18] and lymph node involvement is associated with inferior overall outcomes [82].
- **Pathologic fracture**: seems to be associated with inferior event-free survival (EFS) and OS [83].
- **Previous treatment for cancer**: 5-year OS for patients with secondary Ewing's sarcoma was of 45% compared to 65% in patients with primary Ewing's sarcoma in a study [84].
- **Standard cytogenetics**: complex karyotype and chromosome numbers could signify a worse prognosis [85].
- **Circulating tumor DNA in peripheral blood** seems to be associated with inferior 3-year EFS rates and OS rates [86].
- **Detectable fusion transcripts in morphologically normal marrow**: fusion transcript detection in marrow or peripheral blood was associated with an increased risk of relapse [87].
- **Other biological factors**: overexpression of the p53 protein, Ki67 expression, and loss of 16q may be adverse prognostic factors [88]. High expression of microsomal glutathione S-transferase (associated with resistance to doxorubicin), is associated with poorer outcomes [89].

The following are *not* considered to be adverse prognostic factors for Ewing's sarcoma:

- Histopathology: the degree of neural differentiation is not a prognostic factor in Ewing's sarcoma [90].
- Molecular pathology: the *EWSR1-ETS* translocation breakpoint site is not an adverse prognostic factor [91]

Post-treatment Factors

- Patients with **minimal or no residual viable tumor** after presurgical chemotherapy have a better EFS than do patients with larger amounts of viable tumor [92].
- **Female sex and younger age predict a good histologic response to pre-operative therapy** [93].
- **Decreased PET uptake** after chemotherapy correlated with good histologic response and better outcome [94].
- Patients with **poor response to presurgical chemotherapy** have an increased risk for local recurrence [95].
- **Adverse risk factors for local recurrence** [96]: pelvic localization, marginal/intralesional resection. But the addition of radiation therapy was associated with improved outcome.
- **Adverse risk factors for pulmonary metastasis** [96]: less than 90% necrosis, previous pulmonary metastasis
- **Adverse risk factors for death** [96]: pulmonary metastasis, bone or other metastasis, less than 90% necrosis and early local recurrence (0–24 months).

Summary of Treatments According to Specific Situations

Localized Disease

Most patients are expected to have an occult metastatic spread even if the disease appears to be localized on the initial work-up. For that reason, the usual course of treatment is multidrug chemotherapy then local treatment (surgery and/or radiation) then adjuvant chemotherapy. Such treatment allows for an overall survival of 70% at five years, all localizations included [20].

Metastatic Sarcoma

As previously exposed, metastases are detected in 25% of cases upon diagnosis [6], with poor prognosis. Current therapies achieve approximately 30% of a five-year overall survival rate [18], slightly better (40%) when only lungs are involved and with whole lung radiation therapy [81]. The prognosis is even poorer when there is secondary bone or visceral disease [97].

The usual treatments includes chemotherapy, alternating vincristine, doxorubicin, cyclophosphamide, and ifosfamide/etoposide combined with adequate local-control measures applied to both primary and metastatic sites. Complete or partial responses may be achieved but the overall cure rate is 20% [80]. Surgery and radiation therapy for metastatic sites may improve overall outcome in patients with extrapulmonary metastases [19, 98]. Other therapies might be used such as high-dose chemo with stem cell support, melphalan or irinotecan with inconstant outcomes.

Recurring Ewing's Sarcoma

Approximately 80% of recurring sarcomas will recur within two years after the initial diagnosis [99] though late recurrence (>five years) represent more than 10% of cases [100]. The overall prognosis is poor; with a five-year survival rate after recurrence of 10–15% [17]. A shorter recurrence time and distant recurrence from the original site are among adverse prognosis factors.

Combinations of chemotherapy (cyclophosphamide and topotecan or irinotecan and temozolomide with or without vincristine) can be considered [101]. Radiation therapy to bone lesions can be used as a palliative option, however radical resection may improve outcome [99]. Lung metastases which were not previously irradiated may be considered for whole-lung irradiation and lung residual disease may be surgically removed [102]. High doses chemo with stem cell support, monoclonal antibody therapy (e.g., IGF1R) and immunotherapy (e.g., anti HER2 or anti CD99) may offer some partial and objective responses in specific cases, but it is too early to pinpoint their exact indication.

References

1. Delattre O, Zucman J, Melot T, Garau XS, Zucker JM, Lenoir GM et al. The Ewing family of tumors: a subgroup of small-round-cell tumors defined by specific chimeric transcripts. N Engl J Med. 1994; 331(5):294–299.
2. Beck R, Monument MJ, Watkins WS, Smith R, Boucher KM, Schiffman JD, et al. EWS/FLI-responsive GGAA microsatellites exhibit polymorphic differences between European and African populations. Cancer Genet. 2012;205(6):304–12.
3. Jiang S, Wang G, Chen J, Dong Y. Comparison of clinical features and outcomes in patients with extraskeletal vs skeletal Ewing sarcoma: an SEER database analysis of 3,178 cases. Cancer Manag Res. 2018;10:6227–36.
4. Raney RB, Asmar L, Newton WA, Bagwell C, Breneman JC, Crist W, et al. Ewing sarcoma of soft tissues in childhood: a report from the Intergroup Rhabdomyosarcoma Study, 1972 to 1991. J Clin Oncol Off J Am Soc Clin Oncol. 1997;15(2):574–82.
5. Brasme JF, Chalumeau M, Oberlin O, Valteau-Couanet D, Gaspar N. Time to diagnosis of Ewing tumors in children and adolescents is not associated with metastasis or survival: a prospective multicenter study of 436 patients. J Clin Oncol Off J Am Soc Clin Oncol. 2014; 32(18):1935–1940.
6. Esiashvili N, Goodman M, Marcus RB. Changes in incidence and survival of Ewing sarcoma patients over the past 3 decades: surveillance epidemiology and end results data. J Pediatr Hematol Oncol. 2008;30(6):425–30.
7. Fuchs B, Valenzuela RG, Sim FH. Pathologic fracture as a complication in the treatment of Ewing sarcoma. Clin Orthop. 2003;415:25–30.
8. Hoffer FA, Gianturco LE, Fletcher JA, Grier HE. Percutaneous biopsy of peripheral primitive neuroectodermal tumors and Ewing sarcomas for cytogenetic analysis. AJR Am J Roentgenol. 1994;162(5):1141–2.
9. Kovar H, Dworzak M, Strehl S, Schnell E, Ambros IM, Ambros PF, et al. Overexpression of the pseudoautosomal gene MIC2 in Ewing sarcoma and peripheral primitive neuroectodermal tumor. Oncogene. 1990;5(7):1067–70.
10. Turc-Carel C, Philip I, Berger MP, Philip T, Lenoir G. Chromosomal translocation (11; 22) in cell lines of Ewing sarcoma. Comptes Rendus Seances Acad Sci Ser III Sci Vie. 1983;296 (23):1101–3.
11. Bridge RS, Rajaram V, Dehner LP, Pfeifer JD, Perry A. Molecular diagnosis of Ewing sarcoma/primitive neuroectodermal tumor in routinely processed tissue: a comparison of two FISH strategies and RT-PCR in malignant round cell tumors. Mod Pathol Off J U S Can Acad Pathol Inc. 2006; 19(1):1–8.
12. Meyer JS, Nadel HR, Marina N, Womer RB, Brown KLB, Eary JF et al. Imaging guidelines for children with Ewing sarcoma and osteosarcoma: a report from the Children's oncology group bone tumor committee. Pediatr Blood Cancer. 2008; 51 (2):163–170.
13. Ulaner GA, Magnan H, Healey JH, Weber WA, Meyers PA. Is methylene diphosphonate bone scan necessary for initial staging of Ewing sarcoma if 18F-FDG PET/CT is performed? AJR Am J Roentgenol. 2014;202(4):859–67.
14. Treglia G, Salsano M, Stefanelli A, Mattoli MV, Giordano A, Bonomo L. Diagnostic accuracy of ^{18}F-FDG-PET and PET/CT in patients with Ewing sarcoma family tumors: a systematic review and a meta-analysis. Skeletal Radiol. 2012; 41(3):249–256.
15. Kopp LM, Hu C, Rozo B, White-Collins A, Huh WW, Yarborough A, et al. Utility of bone marrow aspiration and biopsy in initial staging of Ewing sarcoma. Pediatr Blood Cancer. 2015;62 (1):12–5.
16. Cesari M, Righi A, Colangeli M, Gambarotti M, Spinnato P, Ferraro A, et al. Bone marrow biopsy in the initial staging of Ewing sarcoma: Experience from a single institution. Pediatr Blood Cancer. 2019;66(6):e27653.
17. Bacci G, Longhi A, Briccoli A, Bertoni F, Versari M, Picci P. The role of surgical margins in treatment of Ewing sarcoma family tumors: experience of a single institution with 512 patients treated with adjuvant and neoadjuvant chemotherapy. Int J Radiat Oncol Biol Phys. 2006; 65(3):766–772.
18. Ladenstein R, Pötschger U, Le Deley MC, Whelan J, Paulussen M, Oberlin O, et al. Primary disseminated multifocal Ewing sarcoma: results of the Euro-EWING 99 trial. J Clin Oncol Off J Am Soc Clin Oncol. 2010; 28(20):3284–3291.
19. Haeusler J, Ranft A, Boelling T, Gosheger G, Braun-Munzinger G, Vieth V, et al. The value of local treatment in patients with primary, disseminated, multifocal Ewing sarcoma (PDMES). Cancer. 2010;116(2):443–450.
20. Grier HE, Krailo MD, Tarbell NJ, Link MP, Fryer CJH, Pritchard DJ et al. Addition of ifosfamide and etoposide to standard chemotherapy for Ewing sarcoma and primitive neuroectodermal tumor of bone. N Engl J Med. 2003; 348(8):694–701.
21. Juergens C, Weston C, Lewis I, Whelan J, Paulussen M, Oberlin O et al. Safety assessment of intensive induction with

vincristine, ifosfamide, doxorubicin, and etoposide (VIDE) in the treatment of Ewing tumors in the EURO-Ewing 99 clinical trial. Pediatr Blood Cancer. 2006; 47(1):22–29.

22. Loschi S, Dufour C, Oberlin O, Goma G, Valteau-Couanet D, Gaspar N. Tandem high-dose chemotherapy strategy as first-line treatment of primary disseminated multifocal Ewing sarcomas in children, adolescents and young adults. Bone Marrow Transplant. 2015;50(8):1083–8.

23. Whelan J, Le Deley MC, Dirksen U, Le Teuff G, Brennan B, Gaspar N et al. High-dose chemotherapy and blood autologous stem-cell rescue compared with standard chemotherapy in localized high-risk ewing sarcoma: results of euro-EwinG 99 and Ewing-2008. J Clin Oncol Off J Am Soc Clin Oncol. 2018; JCO2018782516.

24. Wagner TD, Kobayashi W, Dean S, Goldberg SI, Kirsch DG, Suit HD, et al. Combination short-course pre-operative irradiation, surgical resection, and reduced-field high-dose post-operative irradiation in the treatment of tumors involving the bone. Int J Radiat Oncol Biol Phys. 2009; 73(1):259–266.

25. Rosenberg SA, Tepper J, Glatstein E, Costa J, Baker A, Brennan M, et al. The treatment of soft-tissue sarcomas of the extremities: prospective randomized evaluations of (1) limb-sparing surgery plus radiation therapy compared with amputation and (2) the role of adjuvant chemotherapy. Ann Surg. 1982;196(3):305–15.

26. Crago AM, Brennan MF. Principles in management of soft tissue sarcoma. Adv Surg. 2015;49(1):107–12.

27. Brooks AD, Gold JS, Graham D, Boland P, Lewis JJ, Brennan MF, et al. Resection of the sciatic, peroneal, or tibial nerves: assessment of functional status. Ann Surg Oncol. 2002;9(1):41–7.

28. Jones KB, Ferguson PC, Deheshi B, Riad S, Griffin A, Bell RS, et al. Complete femoral nerve resection with soft tissue sarcoma: functional outcomes. Ann Surg Oncol. 2010;17(2):401–6.

29. Fox EJ, Hau MA, Gebhardt MC, Hornicek FJ, Tomford WW, Mankin HJ. Long-term followup of proximal femoral allografts. Clin Orthop. 2002;397:106–13.

30. Bus MPA, Dijkstra PDS, van de Sande MAJ, Taminiau AHM, Schreuder HWB, Jutte PC, et al. Intercalary allograft reconstructions following resection of primary bone tumors: a nationwide multicenter study. J Bone Joint Surg Am. 2014; 96(4):e26.

31. Aponte-Tinao L, Ayerza MA, Muscolo DL, Farfalli GL. Survival, recurrence, and function after epiphyseal preservation and allograft reconstruction in osteosarcoma of the knee. Clin Orthop. 2015;473(5):1789–96.

32. Sorger JI, Hornicek FJ, Zavatta M, Menzner JP, Gebhardt MC, Tomford WW, et al. Allograft fractures revisited. Clin Orthop. 2001;382:66–74.

33. Ortiz-Cruz E, Gebhardt MC, Jennings LC, Springfield DS, Mankin HJ. The results of transplantation of intercalary allografts after resection of tumors: A long-term follow-up study. J Bone Joint Surg Am. 1997; 79(1):97–106.

34. Aponte-Tinao L, Farfalli GL, Ritacco LE, Ayerza MA, Muscolo DL. Intercalary femur allografts are an acceptable alternative after tumor resection. Clin Orthop. 2012;470(3):728–34.

35. Frisoni T, Cevolani L, Giorgini A, Dozza B, Donati DM. Factors affecting outcome of massive intercalary bone allografts in the treatment of tumours of the femur. J Bone Joint Surg Br. 2012;94 (6):836–41.

36. Berrey BH, Lord CF, Gebhardt MC, Mankin HJ. Fractures of allografts: frequency, treatment, and end-results. J Bone Joint Surg Am. 1990; 72(6):825–833.

37. Houdek MT, Wagner ER, Stans AA, Shin AY, Bishop AT, Sim FH, et al. What is the outcome of allograft and intramedullary free fibula (capanna technique) in pediatric and adolescent patients with bone tumors? Clin Orthop. 2016;474(3):660–8.

38. Capanna R, Campanacci DA, Belot N, Beltrami G, Manfrini M, Innocenti M, et al. A new reconstructive technique for intercalary defects of long bones: the association of massive allograft with vascularized fibular autograft. Long-term results and comparison with alternative techniques. Orthop Clin North Am. 2007; 38 (1):51–60, vi.

39. Aponte-Tinao LA, Ritacco LE, Albergo JI, Ayerza MA, Muscolo DL, Farfalli GL. The principles and applications of fresh frozen allografts to bone and joint reconstruction. Orthop Clin North Am. 2014;45(2):257–69.

40. Gitelis S, Piasecki P. Allograft prosthetic composite arthroplasty for osteosarcoma and other aggressive bone tumors. Clin Orthop. 1991;270:197–201.

41. Benedetti MG, Bonatti E, Malfitano C, Donati D. Comparison of allograft-prosthetic composite reconstruction and modular prosthetic replacement in proximal femur bone tumors: functional assessment by gait analysis in 20 patients. Acta Orthop. 2013;84 (2):218–23.

42. King JJ, Nystrom LM, Reimer NB, Gibbs CP, Scarborough MT, Wright TW. Allograft-prosthetic composite reverse total shoulder arthroplasty for reconstruction of proximal humerus tumor resections. J Shoulder Elbow Surg. 2016;25(1):45–54.

43. Hejna MJ, Gitelis S. Allograft prosthetic composite replacement for bone tumors. Semin Surg Oncol. 1997;13(1):18–24.

44. Poitout D, Nouaille de Gorce E, Tropiano P, Volpi R, Merger A. Long-term outcome of large bone and osteochondral allografts. Bull Acad Natl Med. 2008;192(5):895–910; discussion 910–911.

45. Racano A, Pazionis T, Farrokhyar F, Deheshi B, Ghert M. High infection rate outcomes in long-bone tumor surgery with endoprosthetic reconstruction in adults: a systematic review. Clin Orthop. 2013;471(6):2017–27.

46. Gosheger G, Gebert C, Ahrens H, Streitbuerger A, Winkelmann W, Hardes J. Endoprosthetic reconstruction in 250 patients with sarcoma. Clin Orthop. 2006;450:164–71.

47. Ahlmann ER, Menendez LR, Kermani C, Gotha H. Survivorship and clinical outcome of modular endoprosthetic reconstruction for neoplastic disease of the lower limb. J Bone Joint Surg Br. 2006;88(6):790–5.

48. Houdek MT, Wagner ER, Wilke BK, Wyles CC, Taunton MJ, Sim FH. Long term outcomes of cemented endoprosthetic reconstruction for periarticular tumors of the distal femur. Knee. 2016;23(1):167–72.

49. Jeys LM, Kulkarni A, Grimer RJ, Carter SR, Tillman RM, Abudu A. Endoprosthetic reconstruction for the treatment of musculoskeletal tumors of the appendicular skeleton and pelvis. J Bone Joint Surg Am. 2008;90(6):1265–71.

50. Farid Y, Lin PP, Lewis VO, Yasko AW. Endoprosthetic and allograft-prosthetic composite reconstruction of the proximal femur for bone neoplasms. Clin Orthop. 2006;442:223–39.

51. AlGheshyan F, Eltoukhy M, Zakaria K, Temple HT, Asfour S. Comparison of gait parameters in distal femoral replacement using a metallic endoprosthesis versus allograft reconstruction. J Orthop. 2015;12(Suppl 1):S25–30.

52. Benedetti MG, Catani F, Donati D, Simoncini L, Giannini S. Muscle performance about the knee joint in patients who had distal femoral replacement after resection of a bone tumor: an objective study with use of gait analysis. J Bone Joint Surg Am. 2000; 82(11):1619–1625.

53. Mattei JC, Chapat B, Ferembach B, Le Nail LR, Crenn V, Bizzozero P et al. Fixed-hinge cemented modular implants: An effective reconstruction technique following primary distal femoral bone tumor resection: a 136-case multicenter series. Orthop Traumatol Surg Res OTSR. 2020.

54. Puri A, Gulia A, Jambhekar N, Laskar S. The outcome of the treatment of diaphyseal primary bone sarcoma by resection,

irradiation and re-implantation of the host bone: extracorporeal irradiation as an option for reconstruction in diaphyseal bone sarcomas. J Bone Joint Surg Am. 2012;94(7):982–8.

55. Currey JD, Foreman J, Laketić I, Mitchell J, Pegg DE, Reilly GC. Effects of ionizing radiation on the mechanical properties of human bone. J Orthop Res Off Publ Orthop Res Soc. 1997;15(1):111–7.

56. Krieg AH, Davidson AW, Stalley PD. Intercalary femoral reconstruction with extracorporeal irradiated autogenous bone graft in limb-salvage surgery. J Bone Joint Surg Am. 2007;89(3):366–71.

57. Myeroff C, Archdeacon M. Autogenous bone graft: donor sites and techniques. J Bone Joint Surg Am. 2011; 93(23):2227–2236.

58. Kunz P, Bernd L. Methods of biological reconstruction for bone sarcoma: indications and limits. Recent Results Cancer Res Fortschritte Krebsforsch Progres Dans Rech Sur Cancer. 2009;179:113–40.

59. Savvidou OD, Kaspiris A, Dimopoulos L, Georgopoulos G, Goumenos SD, Papadakis V, et al. Functional and surgical outcomes after endoprosthetic reconstruction with expandable prostheses in children: a systematic review. Orthopedics. 2019; 42(4):184–190.

60. Zimel MN, Farfalli GL, Zindman AM, Riedel ER, Morris CD, Boland PJ, et al. Revision distal femoral arthroplasty with the compress(®) prosthesis has a low rate of mechanical failure at 10 Years. Clin Orthop. 2016;474(2):528–36.

61. Cristofolini L, Bini S, Toni A. In vitro testing of a novel limb salvage prosthesis for the distal femur. Clin Biomech Bristol Avon. 1998;13(8):608–15.

62. Zimel MN, Hwang S, Riedel ER, Healey JH. Carbon fiber intramedullary nails reduce artifact in post-operative advanced imaging. Skeletal Radiol. 2015;44(9):1317–25.

63. Steinberg EL, Rath E, Shlaifer A, Chechik O, Maman E, Salai M. Carbon fiber reinforced PEEK Optima: a composite material biomechanical properties and wear/debris characteristics of CF-PEEK composites for orthopedic trauma implants. J Mech Behav Biomed Mater. 2013;17:221–8.

64. Richter M, Cakir B, Schmidt R. Cervical pedicle screws: conventional versus computer-assisted placement of cannulated screws. Spine. 2005; 30(20):2280–2287.

65. Jeys L, Matharu GS, Nandra RS, Grimer RJ Can computer navigation-assisted surgery reduce the risk of an intralesional margin and reduce the rate of local recurrence in patients with a tumor of the pelvis or sacrum? Bone Jt J. 2013; 95-B(10): 1417–1424.

66. Cho HS, Oh JH, Han I, Kim HS. The outcomes of navigation-assisted bone tumor surgery: minimum three-year follow-up. J Bone Joint Surg Am. 2012;94(10):1414–20.

67. Wong KC, Kumta SM, Sze KY, Wong CM. Use of a patient-specific CAD/CAM surgical jig in extremity bone tumor resection and custom prosthetic reconstruction. Comput Aided Surg Off J Int Soc Comput Aided Surg. 2012;17(6):284–93.

68. Docquier PL, Paul L, Cartiaux O, Delloye C, Banse X. Computer-assisted resection and reconstruction of pelvic tumor sarcoma. Sarcoma. 2010; 125–162.

69. Muscolo DL, Ayerza MA, Aponte-Tinao LA, Ranalletta M. Partial epiphyseal preservation and intercalary allograft reconstruction in high-grade metaphyseal osteosarcoma of the knee. J Bone Joint Surg Am. 2005; 87 Suppl 1(Pt 2):226–236.

70. Krasin MJ, Rodriguez-Galindo C, Billups CA, Davidoff AM, Neel MD, Merchant TE et al. Definitive irradiation in multidisciplinary management of localized Ewing sarcoma family of tumors in pediatric patients: outcome and prognostic factors. Int J Radiat Oncol Biol Phys. 2004; 60(3):830–838.

71. Yock TI, Krailo M, Fryer CJ, Donaldson SS, Miser JS, Chen Z et al. Local control in pelvic Ewing sarcoma: analysis from INT-0091: a report from the Children's Oncology Group. J Clin Oncol Off J Am Soc Clin Oncol. 2006; 24(24):3838–3843.

72. Granowetter L, Womer R, Devidas M, Krailo M, Wang C, Bernstein M et al. Dose-intensified compared with standard chemotherapy for nonmetastatic Ewing sarcoma family of tumors: a Children's Oncology Group Study. J Clin Oncol Off J Am Soc Clin Oncol. 2009; 27(15):2536–2541.

73. Kuttesch JF, Wexler LH, Marcus RB, Fairclough D, Weaver-McClure L, White M, et al. Second malignancies after Ewing sarcoma: radiation dose-dependency of secondary sarcomas. J Clin Oncol Off J Am Soc Clin Oncol. 1996;14(10):2818–25.

74. Rombi, B., DeLaney, T.F., MacDonald, S.M., Huang, M.S., Ebb, D.H., Liebsch, N.J., et al. Proton radiotherapy for pediatric Ewing sarcoma: initial clinical outcomes. Int J Radiat Oncol Biol Phys. March 1, 2012; 82(3): 1142–1148.

75. Karski EE, McIlvaine E, Segal MR, Krailo M, Grier HE, Granowetter L, et al. Identification of Discrete Prognostic Groups in Ewing Sarcoma. Pediatr Blood Cancer. 2016;63(1):47–53.

76. Cash T, McIlvaine E, Krailo MD, Lessnick SL, Lawlor ER, Laack N, et al. Comparison of clinical features and outcomes in patients with extraskeletal versus skeletal localized Ewing sarcoma: A report from the Children's Oncology Group. Pediatr Blood Cancer. 2016;63(10):1771–9.

77. Ahrens, S,. Hoffmann, C., Jabar, S., Braun-Munzinger, G., Paulussen, M., Dunst, J., et al. Evaluation of prognostic factors in a tumor volume-adapted treatment strategy for localized Ewing sarcoma of bone: the CESS 86 experience. Cooperative Ewing Sarcoma Study. Med Pediatr Oncol. March 1999; 32(3): 186–195.

78. Ahmed SK, Randall RL, DuBois SG, Harmsen WS, Krailo M, Marcus KJ, et al. Identification of Patients With Localized Ewing Sarcoma at Higher Risk for Local Failure: A Report From the Children's Oncology Group. Int J Radiat Oncol Biol Phys. 2017; 99(5):1286–1294.

79. Bacci G, Longhi A, Ferrari S, Mercuri M, Versari M, Bertoni F. Prognostic factors in non-metastatic Ewing sarcoma tumor of bone: an analysis of 579 patients treated at a single institution with adjuvant or neoadjuvant chemotherapy between 1972 and 1998. Acta Oncol Stockh Swed. 2006;45(4):469–75.

80. Miser JS, Krailo MD, Tarbell NJ, Link MP, Fryer CJH, Pritchard DJ et al. Treatment of metastatic Ewing sarcoma or primitive neuroectodermal tumor of bone: evaluation of combination ifosfamide and etoposide: a Children's Cancer Group and Pediatric Oncology Group study. J Clin Oncol Off J Am Soc Clin Oncol. 2004; 22(14):2873–2876.

81. Paulussen M, Ahrens S, Craft AW, Dunst J, Fröhlich B, Jabar S, et al. Ewing tumors with primary lung metastases: survival analysis of 114 (European Intergroup) Cooperative Ewing Sarcoma Studies patients. J Clin Oncol Off J Am Soc Clin Oncol. 1998;16(9):3044–52.

82. Applebaum MA, Goldsby R, Neuhaus J, DuBois SG. Clinical features and outcomes in patients with Ewing sarcoma and regional lymph node involvement. Pediatr Blood Cancer. 2012;59(4):617–20.

83. Schlegel M, Zeumer M, Prodinger PM, Woertler K, Steinborn M, von Eisenhart-Rothe R, et al. Impact of pathological fractures on the prognosis of primary malignant bone sarcoma in children and adults: a single-center retrospective study of 205 patients. Oncology. 2018;94(6):354–62.

84. Applebaum MA, Goldsby R, Neuhaus J, DuBois SG. Clinical features and outcomes in patients with secondary Ewing sarcoma. Pediatr Blood Cancer. 2013;60(4):611–5.

85. Roberts P, Burchill SA, Brownhill S, Cullinane CJ, Johnston C, Griffiths MJ, et al. Ploidy and karyotype complexity are powerful prognostic indicators in the Ewing sarcoma family of tumors: a study by the United Kingdom cancer cytogenetics and the children's cancer and Leukaemia Group. Genes Chromosomes Cancer. 2008;47(3):207–20.

86. Shulman DS, Klega K, Imamovic-Tuco A, Clapp A, Nag A, Thorner AR, et al. Detection of circulating tumor DNA is associated with inferior outcomes in Ewing sarcoma and osteosarcoma: a report from the Children's Oncology Group. Br J Cancer. 2018;119(5):615–21.

87. Schleiermacher G, Peter M, Oberlin O, Philip T, Rubie H, Mechinaud F et al. Increased risk of systemic relapses associated with bone marrow micrometastasis and circulating tumor cells in localized Ewing tumor. J Clin Oncol Off J Am Soc Clin Oncol. 2003; 21(1):85–91.

88. Ozaki T, Paulussen M, Poremba C, Brinkschmidt C, Rerin J, Ahrens S, et al. Genetic imbalances revealed by comparative genomic hybridization in Ewing tumors. Genes Chromosomes Cancer. 2001;32(2):164–71.

89. Scotlandi K, Remondini D, Castellani G, Manara MC, Nardi F, Cantiani L et al. Overcoming resistance to conventional drugs in Ewing sarcoma and identification of molecular predictors of outcome. J Clin Oncol Off J Am Soc Clin Oncol. 2009; 27 (13):2209–2216.

90. Luksch R, Sampietro G, Collini P, Boracchi P, Massimino M, Lombardi F, et al. Prognostic value of clinicopathologic characteristics including neuroectodermal differentiation in osseous Ewing sarcoma family of tumors in children. Tumori. 1999;85 (2):101–7.

91. Le Deley MC, Delattre O, Schaefer KL, Burchill SA, Koehler G, Hogendoorn PCW et al. Impact of EWS-ETS fusion type on disease progression in Ewing sarcoma/peripheral primitive neuroectodermal tumor: prospective results from the cooperative Euro-E.W.I.N.G. 99 trial. J Clin Oncol Off J Am Soc Clin Oncol. 2010; 28(12):1982–1988.

92. Oberlin O, Deley MC, Bui BN, Gentet JC, Philip T, Terrier P, et al. Prognostic factors in localized Ewing tumors and peripheral neuroectodermal tumors: the third study of the French Society of Paediatric Oncology (EW88 study). Br J Cancer. 2001; 85 (11):1646–1654.

93. Ferrari S, Bertoni F, Palmerini E, Errani C, Bacchini P, Pignotti E, et al. Predictive factors of histologic response to primary chemotherapy in patients with Ewing sarcoma. J Pediatr Hematol Oncol. 2007;29(6):364–8.

94. Palmerini E, Colangeli M, Nanni C, Fanti S, Marchesi E, Paioli A, et al. The role of FDG PET/CT in patients treated with neoadjuvant chemotherapy for localized bone sarcomas. Eur J Nucl Med Mol Imaging. 2017;44(2):215–23.

95. Lin PP, Jaffe N, Herzog CE, Costelloe CM, Deavers MT, Kelly JS, et al. Chemotherapy response is an important predictor of local recurrence in Ewing sarcoma. Cancer. 2007; 109(3):603–611.

96. Bosma SE, Rueten-Budde AJ, Lancia C, Ranft A, Dirksen U, Krol AD, et al. Individual risk evaluation for local recurrence and distant metastasis in Ewing sarcoma: a multistate model for Ewing sarcoma. Pediatr Blood Cancer. 2019;66(11):e27943.

97. Paulussen M, Ahrens S, Burdach S, Craft A, Dockhorn-Dworniczak B, Dunst J, et al. Primary metastatic (stage IV) Ewing tumor: survival analysis of 171 patients from the EICESS studies: European Intergroup Cooperative Ewing Sarcoma Studies. Ann Oncol Off J Eur Soc Med Oncol. 1998; 9 (3):275–281.

98. Casey DL, Wexler LH, Meyers PA, Magnan H, Chou AJ, Wolden SL. Radiation for bone metastases in Ewing sarcoma and rhabdomyosarcoma. Pediatr Blood Cancer. 2015;62(3):445–9.

99. Stahl M, Ranft A, Paulussen M, Bölling T, Vieth V, Bielack S, et al. Risk of recurrence and survival after relapse in patients with Ewing sarcoma. Pediatr Blood Cancer. 2011;57(4):549–53.

100. Wasilewski-Masker K, Liu Q, Yasui Y, Leisenring W, Meacham LR, Hammond S et al. Late recurrence in pediatric cancer: a report from the Childhood Cancer Survivor Study. J Natl Cancer Inst 2009; 101(24):1709–1720.

101. Raciborska A, Bilska K, Drabko K, Chaber R, Pogorzala M, Wyrobek E, et al. Vincristine, irinotecan, and temozolomide in patients with relapsed and refractory Ewing sarcoma. Pediatr Blood Cancer. 2013;60(10):1621–5.

102. Scobioala S, Ranft A, Wolters H, Jabar S, Paulussen M, Timmermann B et al. Impact of whole lung irradiation on survival outcome in patients with lung relapsed ewing sarcoma. Int J Radiat Oncol Biol Phys. 2018; 102(3):584–592.

Hemangioma

13

Jaime Paulos

Abstract

Hemangioma is a benign bone tumor forming blood vessels. It is found in vertebral bodies and cranial bones, many times as an incidental finding having a typical radiological aspect. The treatment requires observation, and in those cases with increased risk of pathological fractures, surgery is needed.

Keywords

Vascular bone tumors • Benign bone tumors

Hemangioma is a benign intraosseous tumor with formation of blood vessels. Hemangiomas are mostly found in the soft tissues while the intraosseous location is found mostly in the vertebral bodies and the craniofacial bones. In a smaller number of cases, they can be found in the ribs, pelvis, scapula, and in long bones such as the humerus, femur and tibia [1].

Clinical Presentation

Most vertebral hemangiomas are asymptomatic; they are found in an X-ray study of the spine taken because of some other medical reason. They may also occured as a pathologic fracture or pain.

Imaging

In the vertebral bodies, it is typical the formation of vertical bone striations with lytic lesions among them, giving a honeycomb appearance [2]. The bone scan is positive, being warm or hot (Fig. 13.1).

J. Paulos (✉)
Pontificia Universidad Católica de Chile, Santiago, Chile
e-mail: paulos.jaime@gmail.com

© Springer-Verlag London Ltd., part of Springer Nature 2021
J. Paulos and D. G. Poitout (eds.), *Bone Tumors*,
https://doi.org/10.1007/978-1-4471-7501-8_13

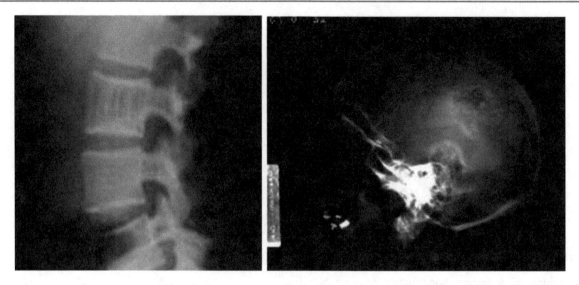

Fig. 13.1 Vertebral and cranial hemangioma

Fig. 13.2 Histology of
an hemangioma

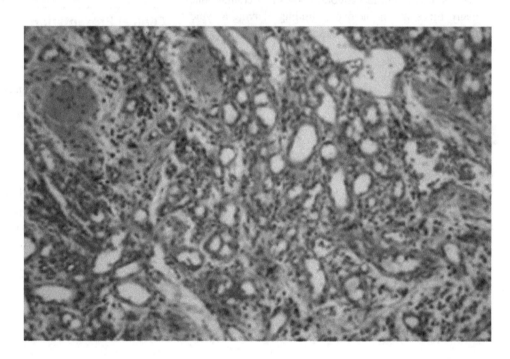

Histology shows cavernous lesions with thin walled blood lesions (Fig. 13.2).

Treatment

When the patient is asymptomatic and there is no risk of fracture, only observation is indicated.

Curettage and bone filling are indicated in symptomatic cases. For inaccessible surgical cases, a low dose of radiation can be indicated (25 to 40 Gy) [2].

References

1. Rigopoulou A, Saifuddin A. Intraosseous hemangioma of the appendicular skeleton: Imaging features of 15 cases, and a review of the literature. Skeletal Radiol. 2012;41(12):1525–36.
2. Miszczyk L, Tukiendorf A. Radiotherapy of painful vertebral hemangiomas: The single center retrospective analysis of 137 cases. Int J Radiat Oncol Biol Phys. 2012;82(2):e173–80.

Hemangiosarcoma or Angiosarcoma

Eduardo Botello

Abstract

These are rare malignant bone tumors of the lining of blood vessels. Locally they have an aggressive behavior whith local enlargement and can spread out very quickly. Treatment is based on wide or radical surgical resection.

Keywords

Vascular tumor • Malign bone tumor

Hemangiosarcomas or angiosarcomas are rare malign bone tumors arising of the angioblastic endothelial cells. Locally they have an aggressive behavior with local enlargement and can spread out via hematogenous and/or lymphatic metastasis. They grow locally over some months resulting in metastases. Usually the prognosis is bad with an overall survival rate of 20% at 5 years. The aetiology is unkown, and some cases appear secondarily in sites of prior radiation [1].

Imaging

Imaging reveals a lytic lesion without a reactive bone and areas of cortical destruction. MRI shows an expansive mass, destroying bone, and with soft tissue invasion (Fig. 14.1).

Clinical features shows a sensitive local mass appearing in few weeks or months. These mostly affect the long bones (femur) and spine and occur in adults (men 40–70 years old).

Histology

The pathology shows endothelial cells with highly atypical features and necrosis. Also an angiocentric growth expanding the vessel wall, obliterating the lumen and spreading centrifugally into surrounding tissue (Fig. 14.2).

Microscopic view: arranged in single files, cords and small nests, typically lacking well-formed vascular channels, with only immature, intracytoplasmic lumina. Mitotic activity is present with less histological differentiation [2, 3].

Treatment

Wide or radical surgical resection is indicated. The role of chemotherapy and radiation therapy can be used for these tumors but their role is not well established.

E. Botello (✉)
Pontificia Universidad Católica de Chile, Santiago, Chile
e-mail: ebotello@med.puc.cl

© Springer-Verlag London Ltd., part of Springer Nature 2021
J. Paulos and D. G. Poitout (eds.), *Bone Tumors*,
https://doi.org/10.1007/978-1-4471-7501-8_14

Fig. 14.1 MRI of angiosarcoma proximal femur

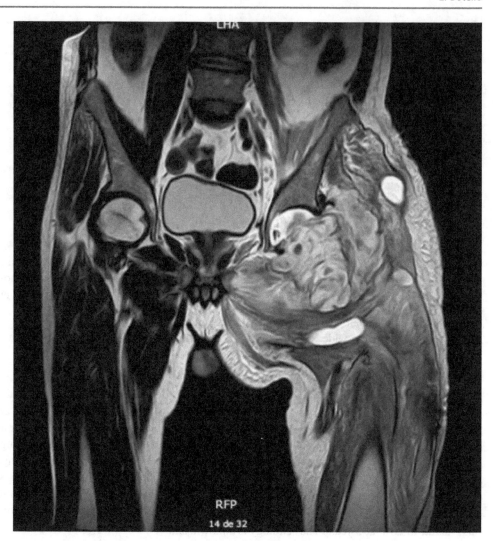

Fig. 14.2 Histology of a malign angiosarcoma

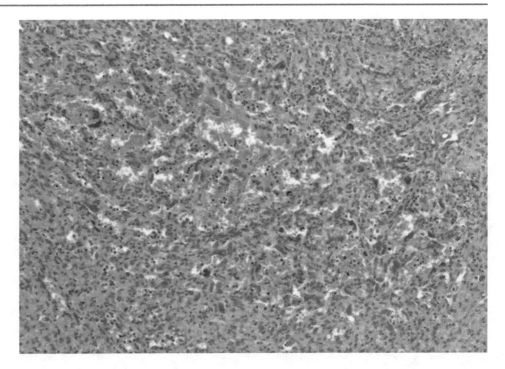

References

1. Chen KT, Hoffman KD, Hendricks EJ. Angiosarcoma following therepeutic irradiation. Cancer 44: 2044–2048.
2. Roessner A, Boehling T. Angiosarcoma. In Fletcher CDM, Unni KK, Mertens F, editors. Pathology and genetics of tumors of soft tissue and bone: world health organization classification of tumors. Lyon, France: IARC Press; 2002. p. 322–3. http://www.iarc.fr/en/publications/pdfs-online/pat-gen/bb5/BB5.pdf   Accessed August 1, 2012.
3. Deyrup AT, Tighiouart M, Montag AG, Weiss SW. Epithelioid hemangioendothelioma of soft tissue: A proposal for risk stratification based on 49 cases. Am J Surg Pathol 2008; 32(6):924–927.

Hemangiopericitoma

15

Jaime Paulos

Abstract

Hemangiopericitoma is an uncommon tumor, born from the pericytes of blood vessel walls. This origin is disputed and considered to have a fibrous origin. The treatment needs a wide resection combined with radiotherapy or chemotherapy.

Keyword

Malignant vascular bone tumor

Hemangiopericitoma is a malignant tumor derivating from the pericytes, found in the surrounding thin-walled vessels. Actually, it is classified as a solitary fibrous tumor because its origin is fibrous and not pericytic [1]. It is a rare bone tumor and can be found in any bone, mostly in the pelvis, proximal femur, vertebrae or humerus. Most cases are presented in adults, which have have few cases in different casuistics. Even though it has a slow growth. It produces metastases.

Imaging

Most cases are lytic and have no specific radiographic appearance; sometimes, they can have a honeycomb appearance.

Histology

The gross features show a firm, red bloody mass.

The tumor is hypercellular composed of round to oval cells with thin walled blood vessels in the tumor. The channels of the vascular ramification are described like "deer antlers."

A silver stain highlights the reticulin sheath surrounding each cell and confirms that tumor cells are outside the vascular spaces. The fact that tumor cells do not stain positive for actin suggests that the perycites may have some other cellular origin [2].

Treatment

Block resection is indicated with a wide margin. Amputation can be necessary. Radiotherapy and multiple drug chemotherapy may be employed.

References

1. Crawford EA, Slotcavage RL, King JJ, Lackman RD, Ogilvie CM. Ethanol sclerotherapy reduces pain in symptomatic musculoskeletal hemangiomas. Clin Orthop Relat Res. 2009;467(11):2955–61.
2. Brouchet A, Amoretti N, Penel N, Héritier S, Thariat J. Tumeurs vasculaires primitives osseuses 08/08/12[14-799]. https://doi.org/10.1016/s0246-0521(12)59302-2.

J. Paulos (✉)
Pontificia Universidad Católica de Chile, Santiago, Chile
e-mail: paulos.jaime@gmail.com

© Springer-Verlag London Ltd., part of Springer Nature 2021
J. Paulos and D. G. Poitout (eds.), *Bone Tumors*,
https://doi.org/10.1007/978-1-4471-7501-8_15

Desmoid Fibroma

16

Antonieta Solar

Abstract

Desmoid fibroma is an infrequent benign bone tumor but can have an aggressive behavior. It derives from fibroblastic cells producing collagen. Repeated recidives can change to a malignant form like a fibrosarcoma. It can be considered between a benign fibroma to a fibrosarcoma. Local recurrence has been reported in up to 40% of cases.

Keywords

Desmoplastic fibroma · Fibroblasts

Imaging

Desmoid fibroma looks like a benign osteolytic local lesion in the femur, tibia, pelvis or jaw [1].

Macroscopic Pathology

Desmoid fibroma ranges in size from 2.5 to 10 cm, although larger lesions have been described. It is a grayish white, dense, rubbery and firm mass; the cut surface has a whorled or fasciculated appearance. A complete excision is usually easy to peel away from the bone. Occasionally minor cystic areas are found. The endosteal cortical surface frequently shows focal destruction [2].

Microscopic Pathology

Desmoplastic fibroma is a hypocellular, spindle cell tumor associated to various amounts of collagen. The cells are fusiform or stellate, organized in sheets or in haphazardly interlacing fascicles, have a monotonous appearance, slender and elongated, sometimes an oval nucleus, with vesicular chromatin pattern and inconspicuous small round nucleoli. Some nuclei may be large or hyperchromatic, but the cells typically lack pleiomorphism or other bizarre features. Mitotic figures are rare. The amount of cellularity is variable, and some areas may be relatively hypercellular. nonetheless, striking hypercellularity should not be found in desmoplastic fibroma. Expanded, thinned wall, vascular spaces are a frequent finding. The collagen appears fibrillar and wavy or hyalinized; keloid-like collagen is not often seen. In a few tumors the stroma has a myxoid appearance [2]. Sometimes the occurrence of desmin has also been reported. Additionally, vimentin, MIB-1, and bcl 2 react with some of the desmoplastic fibroma cells.

Microscopic Differential Diagnosis

Histologically the differential diagnosis of desmoplastic fibroma includes fibrous dysplasia, low-grade fibrosarcoma and central low-grade osteosarcoma. Fibrous dysplasia can have large areas of spindle cell proliferation without bone formation, which may be erroneously diagnosed as

A. Solar (✉)
Pontificia Universidad Católica de Chile, Santiago, Chile
e-mail: asolar@med.puc.cl

© Springer-Verlag London Ltd., part of Springer Nature 2021
J. Paulos and D. G. Poitout (eds.), *Bone Tumors*,
https://doi.org/10.1007/978-1-4471-7501-8_16

desmoplastic fibroma. In spite of this, the typical roentgenographic features and sufficient sampling, including areas with the classic "alphabetic" shaped bone trabecules, should eliminate this histological error. Discriminating between desmoplastic fibroma and low-grade fibrosarcoma is the most difficult differential diagnosis, although the clinical course is similar. A low grade fibrosarcoma may show a "herringbone" pattern and usually shows at least slight pleiomorphism and hyperchromasia. Any osteoid or bone formation by the tumor eliminates the possibility of desmoplastic fibroma and supports the diagnosis of a central low-grade osteosarcoma.

References

1. Zhang F, Ni B, Zhao L et al. Desmoplastic fibroma of the cervical spine: case report and review of the literature. Spine (Phila Pa 1976) 2010; 35(14):E667–E671, 88.
2. Taconis WK, Schütte HE, Van der Heul RO. Desmoplastic fibroma of bone: a report of skeletal 18 cases. Radiol. 1994;23(4):283–8.

Fibrosarcoma

17

Antonieta Solar

Abstract

Fibrosarcoma is a malignant bone tumor that grows rapidly; it looks like an osteosarcoma with no forming osteoid tissue.

Keywords

Fibrosacoma • Malign bone sarcoma

Fibrosarcoma is a malignant tumor deriving from fibroblasts. It is a rare bone tumor more frequently found in the soft tissues [1–3].

Osseous fibrosarcoma is presented across all age ranges, being more frequent in adults within the fourth to sixth decades. The distal femur and proximal tibia are the most frequent locations.The ratio of male:female is not revelant.

As with other malign bone tumors its clinical presentation begins with dull pain and local swelling which can be palpated like a mass. Symptoms appear in weeks or a few months.

Imaging

Fibrosarcoma has a metaphyseal or diaphyseal location like a osteolytic, poorly marginated lesion (distal femur more frequent), destroying the cortical without periostic reaction or sclerosis, and can show invasion of soft tissues. There is a risk of pathological fracture.

Macroscopic Pathology

About two-thirds of fibrosarcomas measure 9 cm or less and the rest 10 cm or more at their largest dimension. The gross appearance of these tumors depends on their grade; low grade tumors are usually grayish to white, firm and rubbery, with a whorled cut surface or they can be soft and friable, with a evidently permeative pattern in high grade tumors, which may show areas of necrosis, hemorrhage, cystic degeneration or rarely, myxoid areas. Most tumors destroy the cortex.

Microscopic Pathology

Fibrosarcomas consists of interlacing fascicles of spindle cells arranged in a "herringbone" pattern in the majority of cases [4]. The nuclei are elongated and thin, with a fine or granular chromatin often with nucleoli and tapered ends. The cytoplasm is usually indistinguishable. The amount of collagen varies, ranging from slight to massive in well-differentiated fibrosarcomas. The tumor has a permeative growth pattern, leaving entrapped pre existent bone trabeculae in the lesion. Rarely, the tumor may be markedly myxoid or consist of small cells suggestive of Ewing's sarcoma. The grade of fibrosarcomas correlates well with the prognosis, hence the importance of grading these tumors. The four-grade Broders' system has been widely use, although some authors prefer to use a two- or three-grade system, both methods depending upon the production. The cells are fusiform with slight pleiomorphism, if any. The nuclei are ovoid or slender, some can be plump, with fine chromatin and little hyperchromasia. Nucleoli are inconspicuous and small. The mitotic count is low. High grade or poorly differentiated (Broders' III and IV) fibrosarcomas are exceedingly cellular and have scarce or no collagen production. The cells are spindle shaped and plump with moderated pleiomorphism; some cells are multinucleated; the nuclei are very dense, have fine and coarse irregular clumps of chromatin with hyperchromasia. Nucleoli can be small or large, but inconsistent; the mitotic count is overtly high. Foci of necrosis, hemorrhage or myxoid stroma are common.

A. Solar (✉)
Pontificia Universidad Católica de Chile, Santiago, Chile
e-mail: asolar@med.puc.cl

© Springer-Verlag London Ltd., part of Springer Nature 2021
J. Paulos and D. G. Poitout (eds.), *Bone Tumors*,
https://doi.org/10.1007/978-1-4471-7501-8_17

Special Techniques: Fibrosarcoma cells are strongly positive for vimentin and focally positive with smooth muscle actin.

Microscopic Differential Diagnosis

Well-differentiated fibrosarcoma differential diagnosis includes fibrous dysplasia and desmoplastic fibroma. The cells of fibrous dysplasia are usually plump, while fibrosarcoma cells are slender. No mineralized matrix should be found in fibrosarcoma, while the finding of "alphabet" appearing metaplastic bone formation confirms the diagnosis of fibrous dysplasia. Trying to distinguish between well-differentiated fibrosarcoma and desmoplastic fibroma is very complicated. Fibrosarcoma should have at least in some areas nuclear pleiomorphism, slight mitotic activity and a "herringbone" pattern. Poorly differentiated fibrosarcoma differential diagnosis includes fibroblastic osteosarcoma, malignant fibrous histiocytoma, spindle cell or sarcomatoid carcinoma and spindle cell melanoma. The identification of the osteoid matrix supports the diagnosis of osteosarcoma. A storiform pattern, epitheliod cells and evident cellular pleiomorphism favor malignant fibrous histiocitoma, obvious pleiomorphism is not a distinguishing quality of the fibrosarcoma cells. Spindled carcinoma cells or melanoma cells are usually distinguished by a good clinical history and immunohistochemical techniques for epithelial markers or melanocitic markers, respectively.

Treatment

Pre-operative chemotherapy similar to osteosarcoma can be indicated plus wide resection if posible with a wide surgical margin or amputation [5, 6].

Radiotherapy is indicated for surgically inaccessible tumors.

References

1. Kleihues P, Cavenee WK, editors. Classification of Tumors. Lyon, France: IARC Press;2002, p. 289–290.
2. Kahn LB, Vigorita V. Fibrosarcoma of Bone. In Fletcher CDM, Unni KK, Mertens F, editors. Pathology and genetics of tumors of soft tissue and bone. World Health Organization: www.iarc.fr/en/publications/pdfs-online/pat-gen/bb5/BB5.pdf. Accessed August 1, 2012.
3. Pritchard DJ, Soule EH, Taylor WF, Ivins JC. Fibrosarcoma clinicopathologic and statistical study of 199 tumors of the soft tissues of the extremities and trunk. Cancer. 1974;33:888–97.
4. Larsson SE, Lorentzon R, Boquist L. Fibrosarcoma of bone: Swedish Cancer Registry from 1958 to 1968. J Bone Joint Surg. 1976; 58B: 412–417.
5. Scott SM, Reiman HM, Pritchard DJ, Ilstrup DM Soft tissue fibrosarcoma: a clinicopathologic study of 132 cases. Cancer 1989; 64; 925–931.
6. Bahrami A, Folpe AL. Adult-type fibrosarcoma: A reevaluation of 163 putative cases diagnosed at a single institution over a 48-year period. Am J Surg Pathol. 2010;34:1504–13.
7. Ropars M, Heurtin T, Odri GA. Autres sacomes osseux: fibrosarcomes, sarcomes pleomorphes indifirencies de haut grade et leiomyosarcomes. EM consulte, Tumeurs: 25/07/19 [14–185], https://doi.org/10.1016/s1286-935x(19)42727-5.

Lipoma

18

Antonieta Solar

Abstract

Lipomas are benign bone tumors formed by fat tissue. They are usually a bone local tumor. MRI shows that a typical signal for fat is useful for diagnosis. Curettage is the definitive treatment.

Keywords

Benign bone tumor • Lipoma

Lipoma is a very frequent lesion in soft tissues but a rare intraosseous benign bone tumor formed by mature fat cells.

They can be found in various bones such as the femur, tibia, pelvis, mandibles and are mostly calcaneus [1]. Multiple intraosseous lipomatoses have also been reported [2].

Macroscopic Pathology

Lipomas are well circumscribed and sometimes lobulated. The lesion is best described as a glistening yellow, soft mass of adipose tissue. The gross findings are determined by the stage of the lesion. In 1988 Milgram et al. [3] reported the largest series of bone lipomas and defined three progressive stages. The principal findings are: stage I lesions, the adipose tissue predominates with a few bony trabeculae; stage II lesions have more calcifications or ossifications; and stage III lesions consists of adiponecrosis, well-formed cysts, sometimes extensive calcification and an sclerotic rim of reactive bone.

Microscopic Pathology

Intraosseous lipomas are made of mature adipocytes with scattered intertwining bone trabeculae. They may be missed because median age normal bone marrow has prominent adipose tissue. Moreover, the lesion is curetted in the majority of cases, and without information regarding the radiological aspect of the lesion it is very difficult to identify a lipoma. As it occurs with the gross finding the microscopic features vary with the stages. Stage I lesions are predominantly adipose; stage II lesions show partially calcified focal adiponecrosis or isquemic bone formation; and stage III lesions demonstrate extensive adiponecrosis, massive isquemic bone formation and dark purple calcification, and cysts.

Microscopic Differential Diagnosis

Intraosseous lipoma differential diagnosis includes fatty bone marrow and bone infarct. The roentgenographic information is most useful in making the right diagnosis. The calcification is similar to that seen in infarcts, but in infarcts it is peripheral. Most of them are found incidentally or with local pain.

Imaging

An X-ray shows a well-defined lytic bone lesion with a surrounding osteosclerotic border around. MRI shows a typical high signal in T1; also in T2 if there is central

A. Solar (✉)
Pontificia Universidad Católica de Chile, Santiago, Chile
e-mail: asolar@med.puc.cl

necrosis and no signal in STIR [4], characteristic MRI signals for fat.

Treatment

This consists of observation if the tumor is asymptomatic and located in a region without risk of fracture. Curettage and filling the cavity with bone graft is the definitive treatment.

References

1. Narang S, Gangopadhyay M. Calcaneal intraosseous lipoma: a case report and review of the literature. J Foot Ankle Surg. 2011;50 (2):216–20.
2. Rehani B, Wissman R. Multiple intraosseous lipomatosis, a case report. Cases J. 2009;2:7399.
3. Milgram JW. Intraosseous lipomas: radiologic and pathologic manifestations. Radiology. 1988;167:155–60.
4. Blacksin MF, Ende N, Benevenia J. Magnetic resonance imaging of intraosseous lipomas. Skeletal Radiol. 1995;24(37):41.

Liposarcoma

19

Antonieta Solar

Abstract

Liposarcoma is a malign bone tumor, with growth like a mass intraosseous destroying the cortical and giving rise to metastasis. Variant types have different behaviors. Wide resection treatment and chemotherapy can be necessary.

Keywords

Malign bone tumor • Liposarcoma

Liposarcoma is a rare malignant introsseous bone tumor, histologically similar to soft tissue liposarcomas. It is formed by cells forming fat cells with diferent grades of atypias. Variants of liposarcoma are well-differentiated, myxoid and pleomorphic. Well-differentiated and myxoid variants have a better prognosis [1–3] than pleomorphic types.

Inmunohistochemically, liposarcomas are MDM2/CDK4 positive.

They are usually located in the femur and tibia metaphysis or diaphysis.

Imaging shows a X-ray with ill-defined radioluscent lesion, and can have cortical destruction and invasion of soft tissue. The study with MRI shows a isosensitive or high T1and T2 signal and STIR positive (Short-T1Inversion Recovery, null the signal from fat).

The diagnosis needs a biosy to classify the variant type and differential diagnosis with other pleoformicsarcomas.

Macroscopic Pathology

Usually the tumors are large with a lobular appearance, soft, fleshy, sometimes rubbery. The cut surface can show bright yellow to white or gray.

Microscopic Pathology

Most cases of liposarcomas are of the pleomorphic type. Other variants seldom reported are myxoid liposarcoma and well-differentiated lipoma-like liposarcoma. Pleomorphic liposarcoma type [4] as its soft tissue counterpart is very cellular, composed of sheets of large pleomorphic cells, which have eosinophilic cytoplasm or a clear citoplasmic vacuole. Mitotic activity is typically very high. Lipoma-like liposarcoma consists of sheets of mature adipocytes with scattered lipoblasts, which show clear cytoplasmic vacuoles, and an scallop nucleus. Myxoid liposarcoma consists of stellate and spindle cells immersed in a myxoid matrix with subtle arborizing blood vessels; also scattered lipoblasts can be seen.

Special Techniques: the intracitoplasmic droplets of fat can be demonstrated with oil red O staining.

Microscopic Differential Diagnosis

The differential diagnosis includes other pleomorphic sarcomas: malignant fibrous histiocitoma, leiomyosarcoma, sarcomatoid carcinoma, among others. In order to make the right diagnosis lipoblasts should be found. Immunohistochemical markers might prove useful to rule out other pleomorphic sarcomas.

Treatment

Surgery with wide block must be done, if not amputation. Pleomorphic types need pre-op chemotherapy plus surgery [5].

A. Solar (✉)
Pontificia Universidad Católica de Chile, Santiago, Chile
e-mail: asolar@med.puc.cl

© Springer-Verlag London Ltd., part of Springer Nature 2021
J. Paulos and D. G. Poitout (eds.), *Bone Tumors*,
https://doi.org/10.1007/978-1-4471-7501-8_19

References

1. RetzL D. Primary liposarcoma of bone: report of a case and review of literature. J Bone Surg Am. 1961; 43: 123–129. https://doi.org/10.2106/00004623-1961143010-00010.

2. Larsson SE, Lorentzon R, Boquist L. Primary liposacoma of bone. Acta Orthop Scand. 1975;46:869–76. https://doi.org/10.3109/17453677508989275.

3. Cremer H, Koischwitz D, Tismer R. Primary osteoliposarcoma of bone. J Cancer Res Clin Oncol. 1981;101:203–11. https://doi.org/10.1007/BF00413314.

4. Coindire J, Pedeutour F. Pleomorphic liposarcoma. In Fletcher CDM, Bridge JA,Hogendoorn PCW, Mertens F editors. WHO classification of bone tumors and soft tissues. Lyons: IARC; 2013, p. 42–43.

5. Sanfilippo R, Bertulli R. High dose continous infusion ifosfamide in advanced well differentiated/dedifferentiated liposarcoma. Clin Sarcoma Res. 2014;4(1):16. https://doi.org/10.1186/2045-3329-4-16.

Fibrous Dysplasia

20

Jaime Paulos

Abstract

Fibrous dysplasia is a benign deforming lesion involving one or several bones in which the structure of bone is replaced with altered osteofibrous tissue. It appears in a mono or polyostotic form. Treatment is based on biphosphonates and also by surgery when deformed bones occur.

Keywords

Fibrous dysplasia • Tumor-like bone lesions • Fibrous bone lesions • McCune–Albright syndrome

Fibrous dysplasia produced bone lesions with altered structure of the bone as a tissue and organ in which the bone is replaced with fibrocystic zones. The bone is transformed becoming wider and with thin corticals. The bone becomes deformed and fragile [1–3]. Fractures in the proximal femur and the Shepherd's crook deformity are characteristics (Fig. 20.1).

The etiology is unknown, but associated chromosomal abnormalities have been found, probably a mutation in the gen GS alpha in the human chromosome 20q13. It is not a inherited disease. The high production of FGF-23 can lead to hypophosphatemia.

It can compromise one bone, as in the monostotic form, or many bones, as in the poliostotic form. The skull, jaw, ribs, pelvis, femur and tibia are mainly involved. In the poliostotic form there is a trend of the lesions to be placed towards one half of the body. The monostotic form makes up about 80% of the cases.

Early puberty (mostly in women), skin spots, coffee and milk markings as in the coast of Maine pattern, and poliostotic fibrous dysplasia constitutes the Albright syndrome or McCune–Albright syndrome (20% of cases of fibrous dysplasia).

J. Paulos (✉)
Pontificia Universidad Católica de Chile, Santiago, Chile
e-mail: paulos.jaime@gmail.com

The combination of poliostotic fibrous dysplasia and soft-tissue intramuscular myxomas is named the Mazabraud syndrome.

The age of diagnosis is between the first and third decades of life. Although the genetic lesion is present at birth, most times it remains asymptomatic until adolescence.

Clinical Symptoms

For many years patients can be asymtomatic or have a casual finding. The progression of the lesions can frequently produce swelling and deformation of the segment, without any pain or few pain except when a pathological fracture is produced.

Deformations of the lower extremities are very notorious with bowing of the thigh and or leg produced by the plastic deformity of the femur and tibia which curve the bones induced for the body weight.

Craniofacial bone affections produce deformation of the skull cap or facial asymetry and neurological symptoms of the cranial nerves produced by obstruction of the cranial hollows in the base of the skull.

The progression of the lesions sometimes halts with the end of skeletal growth. That is an important consideration for the treatment.

Malignant transformation can occasionally occurs [4].

Rx Imaging

The radiological aspect is characteristic, with zones of cysts with different sizes rounded with areas of fibrous dense bone. Sometimes the image resembles "frosted glass". The bones frequently compromised are femur, tibia, ribs, maxilla and craniofacial bones (Figs. 20.2 and 20.3).

The cranial bones show very calcified zones, which explains the closing of the hollows of the cranial nerves in the skull base.

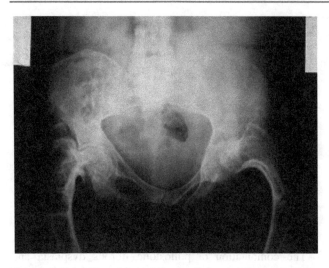

Fig. 20.1 Pelvis X-ray bilateral Shepherd's crook deformity in fibrous dysplasia

Fig. 20.2 Rx of a patient 23 years old, previous surgery at 15 years old; cystic images, frosted glass aspect, varus deformity

Scintigraphy (with Tc99)

It is very useful to detect the distribution of the affected bones showing an hypercaptation of the radioisotope. Also it can be useful to measure the diminution of the activity of the lesion.

Magnetic Resonance

The signal is low in T1 but high in T2 in the affected bones.

Histology

The normal bone is changed into new bone with deformed bone trabeculaes, fibrous tissue with fibroblastos, osteoid tissue and giant cells replacing the normal bone marrow.

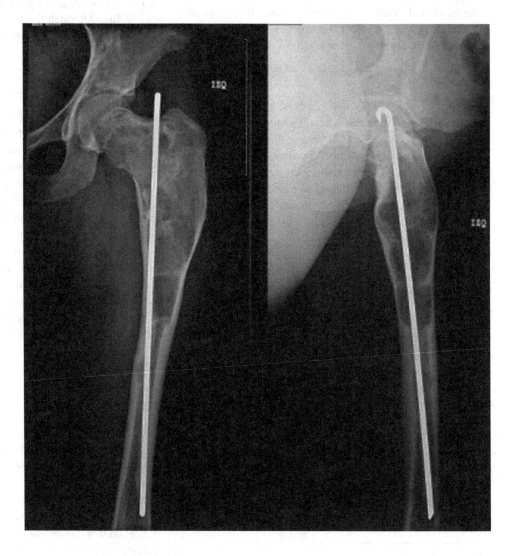

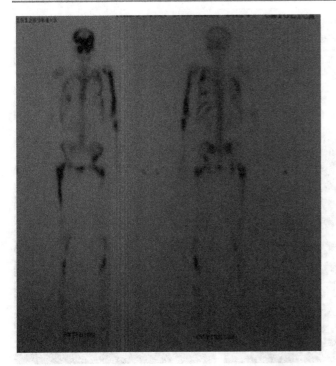

Fig. 20.3 Bone scan of patient with polyostotic fibrous dysplasia

There is fibroblast proliferation surrounding islands of woven bone. The truncated dysplastic trabeculaes are named as the "soup of Chinese alphabet." Another typical finding is the lack of osteoblasts around the bone trabeculaes.

Diferential Diagnosis

When there is an image of cartilage enchondroma can be proposed and if it is poliostotic, Ollier disease can be proposed. Poliostotic lesions can be proposed with neurofibromatosis but in these cases the typical intramedular bone findings of fibrous dysplasia are not present. A solitary cyst can be also be proposed.

If there is a lonely tibia lesion the diferential diagnosis will be with osteofibrous dysplasia or adamantinoma [12].

Treatment

A biopsy is useful to define the diagnosis.

Observation is indicated in asymptomatic pre-adolescent patients. In painful, big monostotic lesions intramedular fixation is indicated [8] Curretage alone has a high incidence of relapse, so must be combined with a structural cortical bone graft (fibula) or cancellous allograft and endomedular synthes according to the case. Autogenous bone graft is not useful because it quickly turns into fibrous dysplastic bone.

Coxa vara deformity is an indication for intertrocanteric osteotomy [6].

In adults with deformity and extensive proximal femur lesions a hip endoprosthesis can be indicated (Figs. 20.4 and 20.5).

The medical treatment with pamidronate disodium [5, 7, 9–11] can be useful in painful cases. Doses: 0,5 to 1,5 by

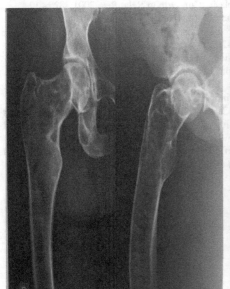
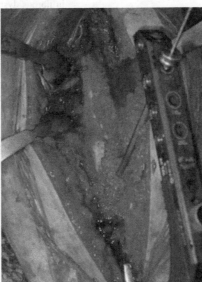
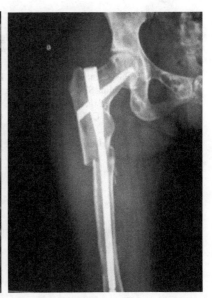

Fig. 20.4 Left: Rx showing fibrous dysplasia in the right femur; Center: intraoperative cancellous allograft; Right: OTS with endomedulary system (TFN)

Fig. 20.5 Rx proximal femur:
reconstruction with a
non-cemented endoprosthesis
stem and cup full-porous coated,
trocanter osteotomy and proximal
lateral osteotomy

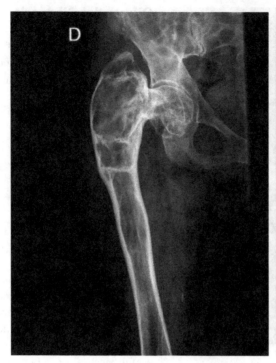 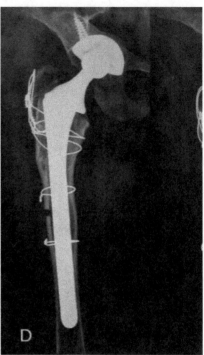

each kg of weight of the patient Iiv in three days repeated
every three or four months.

There is no indication for radiotherapy. There is a risk of
long term secondary malignant lesions.

References

1. Pitcher JD, Weber KL. Benign fibrous and histiocytic lesions. In: Schwartz HS, editor. Orthopedic knowledge update musculoskeletal tumors. 2nd ed. Rosemont, IL: American Academy of Orthopedic Surgeons; 2007. p. 121–32.
2. Fibrous dysplasia. In: Campanacci M, Bertoni F, Bacchini P, Enneking W, Notini S, editors. Bone and soft tissue tumors. New York: Springer-Verlag;1990. p. 391–418.
3. Hillock R, Zuppan C. Fibrous dysplasia. Orthop Knowl. 2007; 5 (4).
4. Ruggieri P, Sim FH, Bond JR, Unni KK. Malignancies in fibrous dysplasia. Cancer. 1994;73(5):1411–24.
5. Chapurlat RD, Hugueny P, Delmas PD, Meunier PJ. Treatment of fibrous dysplasia of bone with intravenous pamidronate: Long-term effectiveness and evaluation of predictors of response to treatment. Bone. 2004;35(1):235–42.
6. Guille JT, Kumar SJ, MacEwen GD. Fibrous dysplasia of the proximal part of the femur: Long-term results of curettage and bone-grafting and mechanical realignment. J Bone Joint Surg Am. 1998;80(5):648–58.
7. Lane JM, Khan SN, O'Connor WJ, et al. Bisphosphonate therapy in fibrous dysplasia. Clin Orthop Relat Res. 2001;382:6–12.
8. Ozaki T, Hamada M, Sugihara S, Kunisada T, Mitani S, Inoue H. Treatment outcome of osteofibrous dysplasia. J Pediatr Orthop B. 1998;7(3):199–202.
9. Boyce AM, Chong WH, Yao J, et al. Denosumab treatment for fibrous dysplasia. J Bone Miner Res. 2012;27(7):1462–70.
10. DiMeglio LA. Bisphosphonate therapy for fibrous dysplasia. Pediatr Endocrinol Rev. 2007;4(Suppl 4):440–5.
11. Mansoori LS, Catel CP, Rothman MS. Bisphosphonate treatment in polyostotic fibrous dysplasia of the cranium: Case report and literature review. Endocr Pract. 2010;16(5):851–4.
12. Most MJ, Sim FH, Inwards CY. Osteofibrous dysplasia and adamantinoma. J Am Acad Orthop Surg. 2010; 18(6):358–366.

Osteofibrous Dysplasia

21

Jaime Paulos

Abstract

Osteofibrous dysplasia is a rare bone fibrous dysplasia occurring in children, infancy and childhood. The tibia is the most common site involved. Differential diagnosis is made with adamantinoma.

Keywords

Osteofibrous lesions • Tumor-like bone lesions

Osteofibrous dysplasia is an uncommon form of bone fibrous dysplasia confined to the cortices affecting the tibia [8]. It is also known as ossifying fibroma [1] or as the Kempson–Campnacci lesion. The difference with fibrous dysplasia is that there is no Gs alpha activated mutation and trisomies 7, 8, 12 have been reported.

It is found in children, most of them younger than 10 to 15 years old. The lesions can regress in adulthood. Family cases have been reported [2].

Clinical Symptoms

The most common symptoms are a painless swelling and the bowing of the tibia.

Imaging

It usually shows an anterior eccentric lytic diaphyseal tibia lesion with a tibia bowing without periosteal reaction. It can be found in the fibula.

Histology shows a fibroblast proliferation surrounding islands of woven bone with osteoblastic rimming (a difference with fibrous dysplasia).

Pathologic Differential Diagnosis is needed because adamantinoma and fibrous dysplasia are also common locations in the tibia [3–5].

Adamantinoma

An epithelial component predominates in a classical adamantinoma. The so-called well-differentiated adamantinoma contains clusters of keratin-positive epithelial cells. In a small specymen biopsy, the differential may be extremely difficult.

Fibrous Dysplasia

This is an intramedullary lesion. The immature bony trabeculae lack the osteoblastic prominent rimming.

J. Paulos (✉)
Pontificia Universidad Católica de Chile, Santiago, Chile
e-mail: paulos.jaime@gmail.com

© Springer-Verlag London Ltd., part of Springer Nature 2021
J. Paulos and D. G. Poitout (eds.), *Bone Tumors*,
https://doi.org/10.1007/978-1-4471-7501-8_21

Treatment

Observation is indicated for most patients. If deformity is present, bracing is indicated [6, 7]. Corrective osteotomy can be indicated after skeletal maturity.

References

1. Mirra JM, Picci P, Gold RH, editors. Osseous tumors of intramedullary origin, bone tumors: clinical, radio-logic and pathologic correlations. Philadelphia/London: Lea and Febiger; 1989, p. 143–438.
2. Karol LA, Brown DS, Wise CA, Waldron M. Familial osteofibrous dysplasia: A case series. J Bone Joint Surg Am. 2005;87(10): 2297–307.
3. Most MJ, Sim FH, Inwards CY. Osteofibrous dysplasia and adamantinoma. J Am Acad Orthop Surg. 2010;18(6):358–66.
4. Ramanoudjame M, Guinebretière JM, Mascard E, Seringe R, Dimeglio A, Wicart P. Is there a link between osteofibrous dysplasia and adamantinoma? Orthop Traumatol Surg Res. 2011;97(8):877–80.
5. Adamantinoma and osteofibrous dysplasia. In: Mirra JM, Picci P, Gold RH, editors. Bone tumors: clinical, radiologic and pathologic correlations. Philadelphia/London: Lea and Febiger; 1989. p. 1203–32.
6. Moretti VM, Slotcavage RL, Crawford EA, Lackman RD, Ogilvie CM. Curettage and graft alleviates athletic-limiting pain in benign lytic bone lesions. Clin Orthop Relat Res. 2011;469(1): 283–8.
7. Ozaki T, Hamada M, Sugihara S, Kunisada T, Mitani S, Inoue H. Treatment outcome of osteofibrous dysplasia. J Pediatr Orthop B. 1998;7(3):199–202.
8. Campanacci M, Bertoni F, Bacchini P, Enneking W, Notini S, editors Osteofibrous Dysplasia of Long Bones Bone and Soft Tissue Tumors. New York: Springer-Verlag; 1990, p. 419–432.

Non Ossifying Fibroma

Jaime Paulos

Abstract

Non ossifying fibroma is a well defined benign lesion with a metaphyseal subcortical location, small in size, frequent in children. It can disappear spontaneously after puberty.

Keywords

Benign bone tumor • Non ossifying fibroma • Metaphyseal lacoon • Metaphyseal fibrous defect

Non ossifying fibroma is also known as "metaphyseal fibrous defect." It is a painless benign fibrous lesion common in childhood, most of the time found incidentally. The X-ray shows a well-defined subcortical lytic lesion about 1 or 2 cms in the metaphysis of long bones: the distal femur, proximal tibia or fibula. Most lesions disappear spontaneously, so only observation is the first line treatment. Some cases can present bigger lesions up to 7cms that can produce a pathological fracture (Fig. 22.1). Surgery for the bigger cases is indicated: curettage and bone grafting [1].

Reference

1. Gouin F, Noailles T, Waast D, Crenn V. Fibrome non ossifiante. EM Consulte Bone Tumor 13/11/18 [14-172-A]. https://doi.org/10.1016/s1286-935x(18)41471-2.

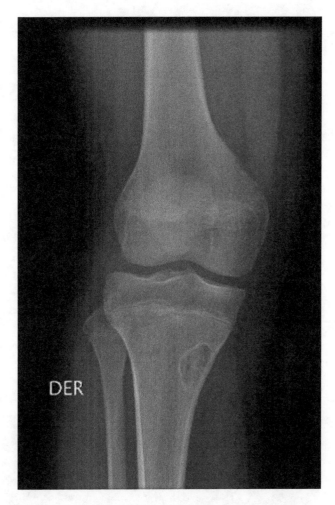

Fig. 22.1 A 13 years old child, X-ray taken after a simple fall

J. Paulos (✉)
Pontificia Universidad Católica de Chile, Santiago, Chile
e-mail: paulos.jaime@gmail.com

© Springer-Verlag London Ltd., part of Springer Nature 2021
J. Paulos and D. G. Poitout (eds.), *Bone Tumors*,
https://doi.org/10.1007/978-1-4471-7501-8_22

Aneurysmal Bone Cyst

Pierre-Louis Docquier and Christian Delloye

Abstract

Aneurysmal bone cyst is a benign lesion occurring most often in excentric position in the long bone metaphysis, pelvis and spine. It may cause pain and swelling which becomes obvious in cases of blowing tumors. In the long bones, pathological fracture is mostly produced in central blowing aneurysmal bone cyst, and in the spine, vertebral fracture. A standard radiograph may be sufficient for diagnosis, and magnetic resonance imaging is also performed for differential diagnosis. A biopsy is mandatory as aneurysmal bone cyst may be secondary to a malignant lesion as telangiectasic osteosarcoma. The most accepted etiopathogenic theory is the one of a reactional process following a venous malformation. The neoplastic theory is now evoked since the translocation t (16;17) (q22;p13) has been discovered that is recurrent in primary aneurysmal bone cysts. Most often a surgical treatment is needed. As aneurysmal bone cyst is a benign condition, radiotherapy has to be avoided. A lot of minimal invasive surgical techniques are nowadays available and have shown their efficiency.

Keywords

Aneurysmal bone cyst • Pseudotumor • Bone cyst • Benign bone lesion

Introduction

Aneurysmal bone cysts are lesions which look like a bone tumor but they are not. Bone cysts are a common example of this. However there are a lot of bone lesions that can simulate a bone tumor from the clinical, image or pathological point of view.

Aneurysmal bone cyst (ABC) is not really a tumor but rather a pseudotumor. It is a lytic bone lesion located most often in metaphyseal position in the long bones, in the pelvis or the spine. ABC may have different aspects.

Classical ABC: This is a primitive bone lesion, lytic, in metaphyseal position, with multiple cavities separated by septa. The cavities are filled with blood and aggregates of solid tissues (Fig. 23.1).

Other possible precursors are osteoblastoma, non ossifying fibroma, chondromyxoid fibroma, fibrous histiocytoma, or eosinophilic granuloma. It may also be secondary to a malignant lesion such telangiectasic osteosarcoma (Fig. 23.2), angiosarcoma, chondrosarcoma or fibrosarcoma.

Multiple cavities and septa are present. The biopsy should demonstrate malignancy.

Secondary ABC: This may be secondary to a traumatism or another pre-existing lesion such a simple bone cyst, fibrous dysplasia, or brown tumor of primitive hyperparathyroidism. It may be secondary to another benign tumor, most often a giant cell tumor.

Solid variant ABC or giant cell resorption granuloma: These ABC are more compact and do not contain cavities.

Soft tissue ABC may develop in the muscles, perivascular areas, the susclavicular or inguinal spaces without bone involvement. The radiographic aspect may evoke myositis ossificans.

Epidemiology

Incidence: ABC is a rare lesion. Incidence is about 1.4 per million people each year. ABC represents 1% of bone tumors.

Age: ABC may occur at every age but mainly during the two first decades of life and becomes rare after 30 years of age (Fig. 23.3).

P.-L. Docquier (✉) · C. Delloye
Cliniques Universitaires Saint-Luc, Brussels, Belgium
e-mail: pldocquier@gmail.com

© Springer-Verlag London Ltd., part of Springer Nature 2021
J. Paulos and D. G. Poitout (eds.), *Bone Tumors*,
https://doi.org/10.1007/978-1-4471-7501-8_23

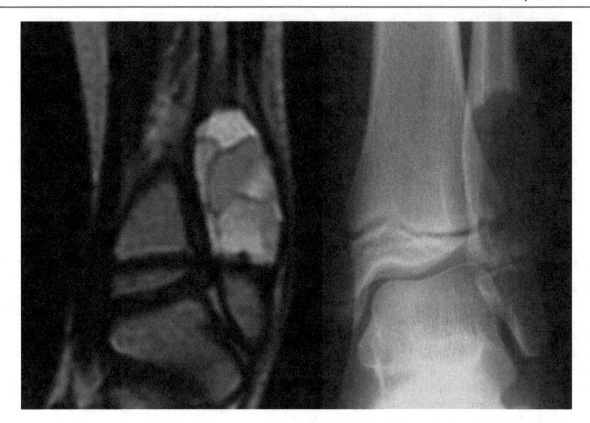

Fig. 23.1 Classical ABC involving a long bone metaphysis, with multiple cavities separated by septa

Location

ABC is generally a single lesion, but rare multiple lesions have been described. ABC may involve adjacent bone, which is often the case at the spine level with progression of the tumor to a rib or another vertebra by the articular apophysis. The most frequent location is the long bones of the lower limbs, next the upper limbs, and finally the axial skeleton and flat bones (Fig. 23.4). Location at hands and feet are quite rare and limited to the tubular bones.

Long Bones

ABC is usually excentric in metaphysis (Fig. 23.1) or in the metaphyso-diaphysis and ABC may rarely be located in the diaphysis. ABC is never primarily epiphyseal but may involve secondarily the epiphysis by extension from the metaphysis.

Spine

Vertebral ABC usually first involves the posterior arch of the vertebra (Fig. 23.5). Most often, it progresses to the vertebral body (71% of cases) Fig. 23.6. Transmission to a rib or an adjacent vertebra is possible. Articular cartilage does not really constitute a barrier at the difference of the intervertebral disc. Weakening of the vertebra may lead to a flattening (vertebra plana).

For most authors, the lumbar location is the most frequent whereas for others, it is the thoracic and cervical location.

Pelvis

The pelvic location is very frequent (11.6%) (Fig. 23.7). ABC is usually initially located in the obturator ring and secondarily may involve the acetabulum or iliac wing.

Sacrum

The sacral involvement is often anterior and posterior (Fig. 23.5). Several sacral vertebrae may be involved. Extension may occur by the sacral to the iliac wing and to the whole pelvis.

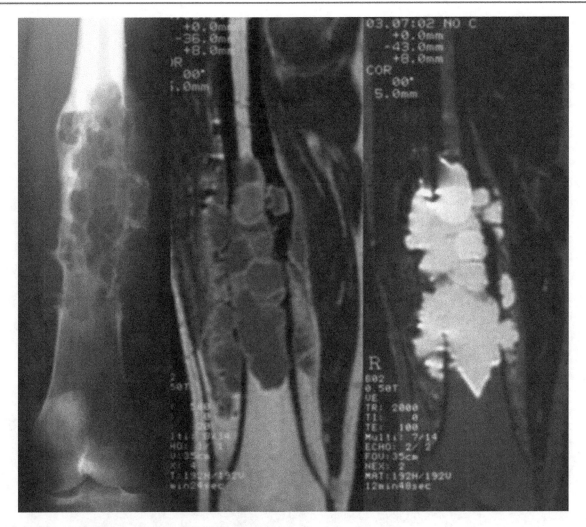

Fig. 23.2 Telangiectasic osteosarcoma may mimic ABC appearance

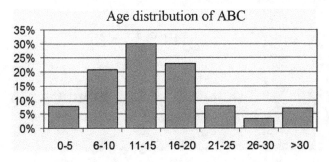

Fig. 23.3 Age distribution of ABC

Etiopathogeny

Several theories have been proposed for the pathogenesis of ABC [1]. The most widespread theory considers ABC as a reactional process secondary to an intraosseous subperiosteal hemorrhage. This hemorrhage should be secondary to a local circulatory abnormality with increased venous pressure and dilatation of the local vascular network. This venous malformation may be primitive or secondary. Szendroï et al. found venous abnormalities but no arteriovenous fistulae based on an angiographic study of 20 ABC cases. ABC should be a reactional tissue to this hemorrhage with osteoclast activation. This theory may also explain the secondary ABC as some tumors may lead to a circulatory perturbation and may contain some area histologically comparable with ABC. Recent studies propose a purely neoplastic etiology to ABC. Panoutsakopoulos et al. demonstrated a chromosomal translocation t(16;17)(q22;p13) recurrently found in primary ABC. Other authors have confirmed that translocation 17p13 is a frequent chromosomal aberration in primary ABC. Oliveira showed that translocation 17p13 locates USP6 oncogen under the regulatory influence of the very active CDH11 promotor. Pathogenesis of most primary ABC should be a up-regulation of the transcription of USP6. On the contrary secondary ABCs do not have this chromosomal aberration.

Fig. 23.4 Bone distribution of ABC

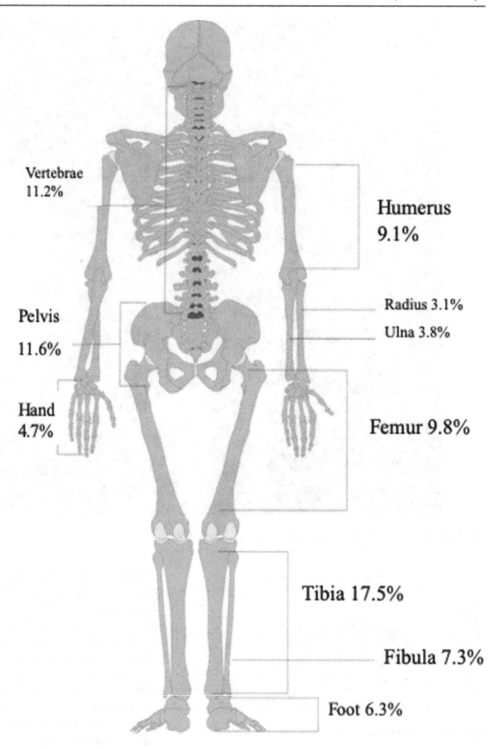

A hereditary factor has been evoked by some authors. DiCaprio et al. reported a case of ABC involving T12 vertebra in a father and another involving L1 in his daughter. Power et al. reported a case of ABC in two monozygotic twins but at different locations.

Clinical Features

The main symptoms associated with ABC are pain and swelling. Pain comes from microfissures due to cortical weakening by the ABC. Swelling may be important and due

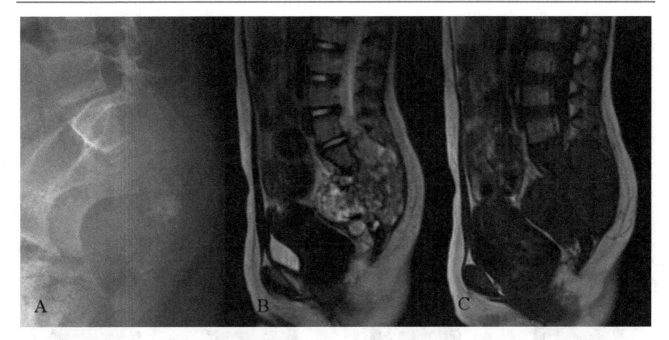

Fig. 23.5 Sacral ABC in a 7-year-old girl; the sacral involvement is often anterior and posterior; several sacral vertebrae are involved

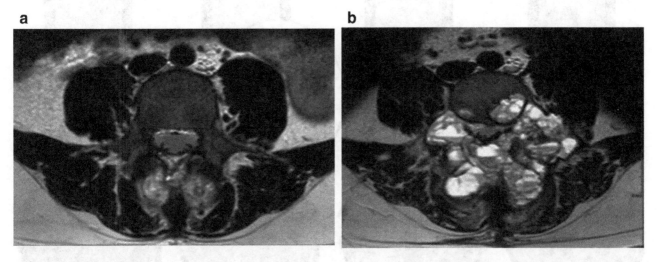

Fig. 23.6 ABC of the fourth lumbar vertebra in a 13-year-old child: **A** Initial lesion is limited to the posterior arch (spinous process); **B** six months later, the lytic process has expanded to the vertebral body

to the blowing aspect of the lesion. Sometimes symptoms appear or worsen during pregnancy. Pathological fractures are quite rare at long bones and more frequent for central ABC than for excentric ABC. Pathological fractures are more frequent at the spinal column. At that location, pain may cause segmental stiffness with scoliosis or torticolis and neurological impairment can appear (45% of cases).

Imaging

Standard radiograph. Maturation stages of ABC. The ABC evolution shows several maturation stages with radiographic typical aspects [2] (Fig. 23.8).

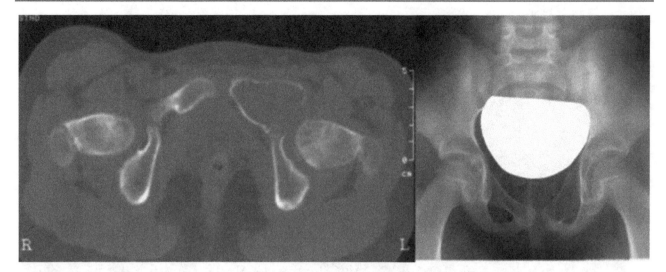

Fig. 23.7 Pelvis ABC

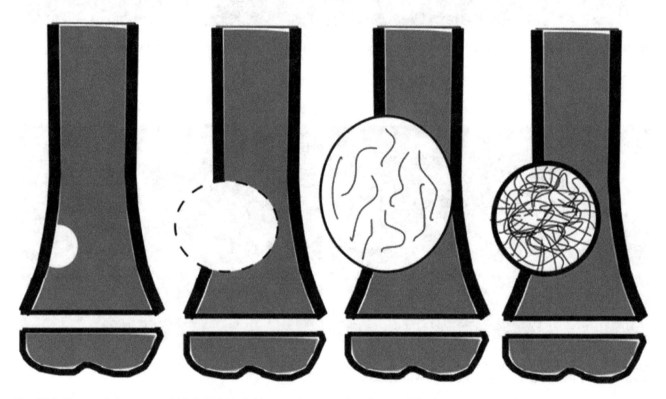

Fig. 23.8 Four evolutive stages of ABC: initial lytic phase, active expansion phase, stabilization phase and healing phase

Early lytic phase: a lytic well-defined area appears often excentric or subperiosteal.

Active expansion phase: it is the typical blowing aspect of ABC that is entered in an aggressive stage (stage 3 of Enneking) (Fig. 23.9). At this stage ABC is difficult to distinguish from a malignant lesion. The periosteum may be lifted with Codman's triangle but no peripheral shell is obvious. The limit between ABC and soft tissue is not clear.

Stabilization phase: a peripheral bony shell appears as well as internal septa giving a "soap bubble" aspect. The periosteum has produced bone that delimits ABC with a thin border. Codman's triangle is often visible at the diaphyseal side of the periosteal lifting.

Late healing phase: progressive ossification of ABC results in a bony dense irregular lesion. The peripheral shell and the septa are enlarged. The border is more clearly

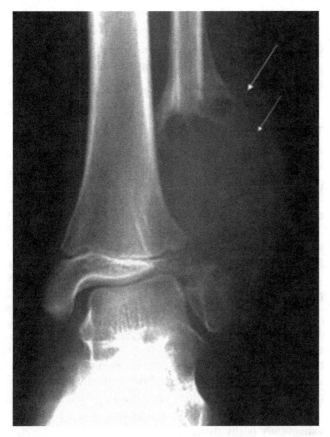

Fig. 23.9 ABC in an active expansion phase; the periosteum is lifted to soft tissue but is not yet ossified; Codman triangles are present at diaphyseal side; at this stage, ABC looks like a malignant tumor

defined. ABC enters into a latent phase (stage 1 of Enneking). At this stage recurrence is not possible.

ABC is usually discovered at expansion or stabilization phases (stage 2 or 3). Healing is usually obtained after treatment but spontaneous healings have been reported (45).

Radiographic Classification of ABC

In 1985, Capanna et al. proposed an interesting classification for the juxtaepiphyseal ABC of long bones (Fig. 8.1.11):

Type I: central ABC, not blowing, metaphyseal or metaphyso-diaphyseal.

Type II: central ABC extending to the whole breadth of the bone, with the blowing aspect. It is usually observed at metaphysis or metaphyso-diaphysis of small diameter long bones (fibula, radius, ulna) or at the flat bones.

Type III: excentric ABC, intraosseous, often metaphyseal.

Type IV: subperiosteal ABC, extraosseous, often diaphyseal (rare).

Type V: subperiosteal ABC intra- and extra-osseous, often metaphysodiaphyseal.

The "fallen fragment sign" is never present in the ABC following a fracture, at the difference of simple bone cyst.

Angiography

This radiographic study shows usually venous malformation with persistence of the contrast inside ABC. No arterial malformation or arteriovenous fistula is observed. This is usually performed for therapeutic or pre-operative embolization but not for diagnosis.

Tomodensitometry

Fluid-fluid levels may be visible at CT-scanner and are due to blood sedimentation (serum is separated from blood cells). CT-scanner may show the limit of the blowing expansion and may show the possible cortical destruction.

Magnetic Resonance Imaging

The liquid component is high signal T2 and low signal T1. T2-weighted MRI mainly shows fluid component and fluid-fluid levels. T1-weighted MRI better shows bony cortex. Fluid-fluid levels are present in 66–84% of the cases but presence of fluid-fluid levels is not specific to ABC. It is only due to the presence of liquids with different densities. In case of blood, the cellular component has a more important density than the plasma, so the plasma constitutes the upper layer. These levels may change their orientation following the patient position.

Other lesions such as fibrous dysplasia, simple bone cyst, malignant fibrous histiocytoma, osteosarcoma may also present fluid-fluid levels.

In ABC fluid-fluid levels are mainly present at the expansion or stabilization stages but absent at the early stages. The presence of multiple cavities separated by septa is much more constant (100% of cases).

Technetium Bone Scan

The bone scan will show hyperfixation at the border of ABC whereas the center will fix moderately or not at all.

Differential Diagnosis

The differential diagnosis has to be made with other metaphyseal lesions:

Simple Bone Cyst

The simple bone cyst is more often central [3]. It involves mainly the proximal humerus or proximal femur. It is filled with serum and no blood, except in cases of fracture or microfracture. Fluid-fluid levels are possible but rarer. Septa are absent, except after fracture. Epiphyseal involvement is not frequent. Evolution is slower. The blowing aspect is rare but possible after multiple fractures and a fibrous dysplasia lesion involvement of the callus by the cyst.

Eosinophilic Granuloma

Isolated eosinophilic granuloma could be confused with ABC. Its borders are often irregular and blurred. In the multiple disease, several osteolytic lesions are present (Langerhans histiocytosis).

Non Ossifying Fibroma

Non ossifying fibroma or cortical defect is the most frequent benign tumor. The cortex is the point of birth of the lesion. It is surrounded by a dense line and is multilocular with multiple septa separating lobules. The diagnosis is usually easy.

Fibrous Dysplasia

This may mimic ABC. The borders are often blurred and radiolucency is typically veiled by a "ground glass" opacity due to the delicate trabeculae of woven bone. The MRI will show hyposignal T1 and T2 and should distinguish the two lesions.

Chondromyxoid Fibroma

This is usually also located in the metaphysis and occurs within the same age range. It is often excentric. Its borders are polycyclic and well demarcated. MRI shows no fluid-fluid levels and no septa.

Giant Cell Tumor

Giant cell tumor is rare in open-physis patients as it is usually a tumor of adults. It is located in the metaphysis and can extend to the epiphysis.

Telangiectasic Osteosarcoma

Radiographic and MRI features may be very similar compared with ABC [4]. Fluid-fluid levels are frequent as well as the septa. It is due to this difficult distinction that a biopsy is mandatory to give the diagnosis of ABC.

Pathology

Gross Anatomy

The tumor is surrounded by an intact periosteum and soft tissues are not invaded. In case of opening of an ABC, hemorrhage may occur with venous blood that can persist as long as the time of the surgery. ABC is filled with a spongy tissue constituted by cavities surrounded by thick septa. The cavities are filled with blood sometimes clotted. In the solid variant only fleshy tissue is present.

Histological Aspect

Three main components are present in ABC (Fig. 23.10) [2].

Cellular Component

The cellular component includes stromal cells and giant cells. Giant cells are easily detected as they contain several nuclei. Stromal cells are mononuclear, with a round or oval nucleus and a scarce or absent intercellular matrix.

Fibrillar Component

The fibrillar component is comprised of fibroblasts and collagen. Fibroblasts are elongated cells characterized by an oval nucleus and a spindle cytoplasm, embedded into a collagenous extracellular matrix. Dense collagen is occasionally present, with abundance of enlarged thick collagenous fibers.

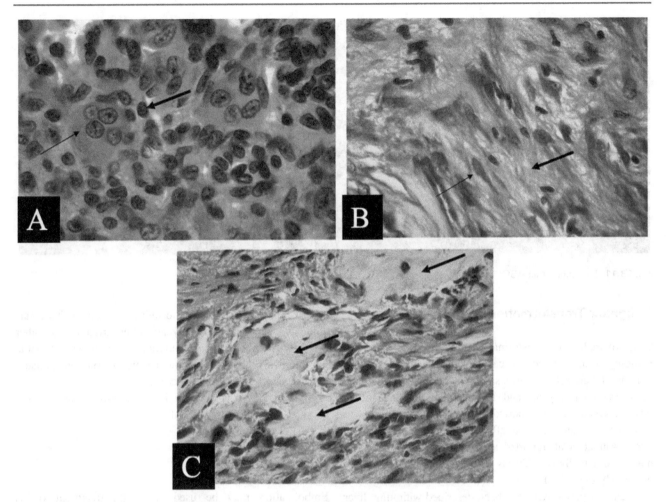

Fig. 23.10 Three histological components of ABC: **A** cellular component: stromal cell (small large arrow) and giant cells (large small arrow); **B** fibrillar component: fibroblasts (small arrow) and collagene (large arrow); **C** osteoid component: osteoid tissue (arrow) and osteoblasts

Osteoid Component

The osteoid component is made of organic bone matrix deposited by osteoblasts.

- **Immunostaining:** A cluster of differentiation 68 (CD68) is a glycoprotein that binds to low-density lipoprotein and is expressed only on macrophages. Commercially available antibodies (anti-CD68) are available to detect macrophage (giant cells and stromal cells). Proliferating cell nuclear antigen (PCNA) is an antigen that is expressed in the nucleus during the DNA synthesis phase of the cell cycle. Commercially available antibodies (anti-PCNA) are able to detect proliferating cells.

Natural History

Spontaneous Healing

Cases of spontaneous healing have been reported. These cases occur most often in adults and in the pelvic location. Healing after biopsy has also been described (Fig. 23.11).

Fracture Risk

The fracture risk is minimal for ABC of long bones by comparison with simple bone cysts. It is the central blowing ABC that may lead to a fracture. In the spine, vertebral fracture is more frequent.

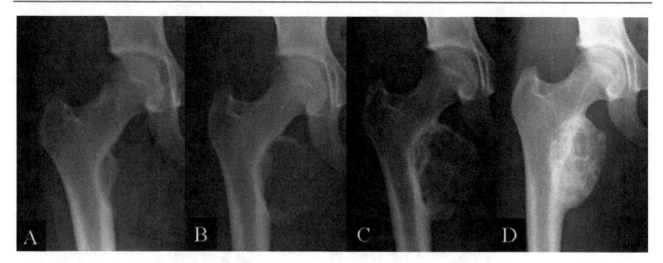

Fig. 23.11 Evolution of an ABC

Malignant Transformation

Cases of malignant transformation have been reported [5]. Brindley et al. reported two cases of malignant transformation to telangiectasic osteosarcoma and to fibroblastic osteosarcoma five years and 12 year after curettage of an ABC. Kyriakos et al. reported a case of transformation to Pleomorphic osteosarcoma after multiple curettage of an ABC. Anract et al. reported a case of malignant transformation to a malignant fibrous histiocytoma at the site of a previously treated ABC.

A case of pelvic ABC has been described with lung, liver and kidney metastasis.

Growth Perturbation

In the growing child, ABC may alter the bone growth. When the ABC is close to the growth plate (juxtaepiphyseal ABC) it may invade it (23% of the cases). In 60% of the cases of invasion, a premature epiphysiodesis occurs with leg length discrepancy or axial deviation.

Treatment

First of all, it must be kept in mind that ABC is a benign lesion. To avoid confusion with a malignant tumor, a biopsy is mandatory.

Radiotherapy

Radiotherapy has been shown to be efficient in the treatment of ABC but numerous complications may occur, the most severe being the risk of radio-induced sarcoma. This sarcoma appears two to 28 years after irradiation. Other reported complications are vertebral fractures with possible neurological impairment, growth plate destruction, gonadal lesions, and femoral head necrosis.

This treatment is only used in exceptional cases where surgical access is very difficult.

Selective Embolization

Embolization may be used as single treatment or as pre-operative treatment to decrease post-operative bleeding.

Cases of healing after embolization used as a unique treatment have been reported for ABC involving cervical vertebra, thoracic vertebrae or the sacrum [11]. De Cristofaro et al. obtained a healing in 17 cases out of 19 (89%). Ossification occurred very slowly and after more than one year. Embolization has to be repeated (two to four times). The main danger is embolization of vital arteries with ischemia of visceral or nervous structures (spinal cord). Somesthetic evoked potential are mandatory during the procedure. Sometimes embolization may not be performed as no afferent artery is evident.

Ethibloc® Injection

Ethibloc is an emulsion of zein (a corn protein), alcohol, oleum papaveris, propylene glycol, and a contrast medium. It induces fibrosis and secondary ossification of ABC. It is introduced into the cyst under fluoroscopy or CT-scanner. George et al. obtained a complete healing in 58% and a partial healing in 35.5% of cases in a series of 33 patients [6]. Following injection an inflammatory response occurs with pain and sometimes fever. The major risk of Ethibloc is the risk of multiple pulmonary embolisms if the fibrosing agent goes intramedullary. Topouchian et al. reported a high complication rate in his series: severe pulmonary embolism (7%), early aseptic fistulization needing surgical debridement and curettage (27%), transient inflammatory reaction with temperature (33%). A case of fatal embolism in the vertebrobasilar system has been described after Ethibloc injection into a cervical vertebra. For Mascard and Adamsbaum, Ethibloc injection is a safe, efficient and non invasive treatment for ABC if precautions are respected. ABC opacification has to be performed and in case of venous drainage the use of Ethibloc is contra-indicated. The filling of ABC has to be slow and not complete. A preventive antipyretic treatment has to be given. In view of the possible complications numerous centers have forsaken this technique.

Alcohol

An alternative to Ethibloc is absolute alcohol which has good fibrosing properties. It is very cheap and easily available. It is used at 95% or 100% strength. It acts by injuring the vascular endothelium and by denaturing the blood proteins leading to thrombosis. Injections are performed by transcortical puncture under general anesthesia and fluoroscopy with two or three 18 or 19 gauges needles depending on the size of the cyst. Sclerotherapy is performed with 5 or 10 ml of alcohol in each needles without increase of the pressure. The results seems to be comparable to Ethibloc without local inflammatory reaction.

Cryotherapy

Cryotherapy may be used alone or as adjuvant treatment to decrease the recurrence rate. The surgical technique consists of curettage of the cyst followed by one or more cycles of freeze-thaw by introducing liquid nitrogen into the cyst. It is also possible to produce a liquid nitrogen spray with a machine. A temperature less than $-50°C$ in the cavity is considered as lethal for tumoral residual cells. Post-operative complications such as pathological fracture or soft tissue healing problems are possible.

Surgical Curettage

In the literature review, Schreuder et al. reported the following recurrence rate after surgical treatment (all recurrences occurring in the two post-operative years): 14.2% for curettage and radiotherapy

- 30.8% for curettage and bone grafting
- 12.8% for curettage and cryotherapy
- 7.4% for marginal resection
- 0% after wide resection
- 11.4% for radiotherapy alone.

Only a wide resection may guarantee the healing without recurrence but at what price? To avoid surgical aggressiveness, numerous minimal invasive techniques are now available [6–9].

Percutaneous Injections

This is demineralized bone matrix mixed with bone marrow (Fig. 23.12).This treatment is interesting because is it not invasive. The bone matrix has to be demineralized to acquire induction power. Bone marrow aspirated at the iliac crest may bring osteoblast progenitor cells. Muschler et al. recommends aspirating no more than 2 ml of bone marrow at the same puncture site to maximize the number of osteoblast progenitor cells and avoid contamination by peripheral blood. The osteogenic power of bone marrow is increased by mixing it with the demineralized bone matrix (synergetic effect). The particle size of demineralized matrix has been decreased to be able to inject it with a normal syringe without any surgical approach.

Calcitonin and Methylprednisolone

Numerous cases of healing after percutaneous injections of calcitonin and methylprednisolone have been reported. Calcitonin acts as osteoclastic inhibitor whereas corticoid acts as angiostatic. Szendroi et al. recommend injections of calcitonin alone in case of hypovascularized ABC. They obtained healing in six out of seven cases. The recurring cases were hypervascularized ABCs.

Calcium Sulfate

An injectable type of calcium sulfate cement has been used by Clayer. The cement is fully resorbed in eight weeks. The first response is a bony peripheral shell followed by a progressive ossification of the cavity. Two patients out of 15 had a recurrence.

Sclerotherapy by Polidocanol Injection

Intralesional 3% polidocanol administration may be used percutaneously under fluoroscopy. In the Rastogi series, the

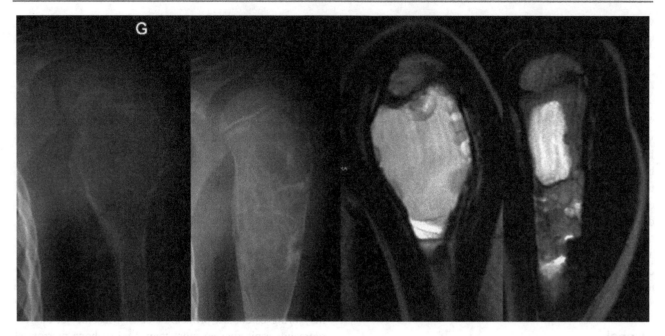

Fig. 23.12 Percutaneous injection of demineralized bone matrix mixed with bone marrow: **A** voluminous ABC of proximal humerus in a 7-year-old boy; a swelling is visible and the child has pain; right: two years after percutaneous injection of demineralized bone matrix mixed with bone marrow, swelling has disappeared and the child is asymptomatic; ABC has become latent, only small cavities are persisting

mean number of injections was three. This technique may be used for surgically inaccessible sites [10].

Factors for Recurrence After Treatment

Different factors may be associated with a higher recurrence rate after treatment.

Young Patients

Patient less than 15 years of age with open growth plate have more recurrence risk. Cottalorda et al. in a retrospective review found that the recurrence rate was not increased in children of less than five years of age.

Male Sex

The male sex could be associated with greater recurrence.

Location

Central locations are prone to recurrence (Capanna types I and II)

Stage

Aggressive (Enneking stage 3) or active ABC (stage 2) may recur after treatment whereas latent ABC (stage 1) do not recur.

Histology

Mitotic index of 7 or more is associated with a important recurrence rate (Fig. 23.13). Freiberg et al. did not observe this correlation.

The cellular component is a factor of bad prognosis if important, whereas osteoid and fibrillar components are factors of good prognosis. A healing index may be calculated by histomorphometry. It corresponds to addition of osteoid (O) and fibrillar (F) components divided by the cellular component (C). If the ratio (O + F)/C is equal or more than 1:2 ABC is prone to heal [2].

Abundant immunostaining with CD68 (macrophage marker) is a factor of bad prognosis.

Conclusion

Aneurysmal bone cyst is a benign lesion that develops commonly in children and young adults. The usual symptoms are pain and swelling in cases of blowing tumors.

Fig. 23.13 Prognostic factors: typical picture of a ABC prone to recur after treatment; it is mainly compound of cellular component (giant cells and stromal cells (white arrows); osteoid tissue and fibrous tissue are scarce

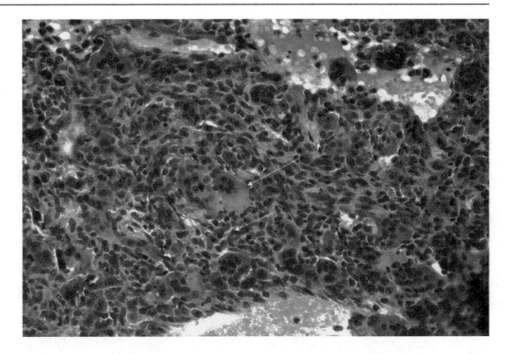

Diagnosis may be probable with a standard radiograph but magnetic resonance imaging is more useful in the differential diagnosis. A biopsy is mandatory as aneurysmal bone cyst may be secondary to a malignant lesion such as the telangiectasic osteosarcoma. Cases of spontaneous healing after biopsy have been reported but remain rare. Most of the cases require surgical treatment. As it is a benign lesion, invasive treatment and radiotherapy has to be avoided. Numerous minimal invasive treatments are now available.

References

1. Cottalorda J, Bourelle S. Modern concepts of primary aneurysmal bone cyst. Arch Orthop Trauma Surg. 2007;127(2):105–14.
2. Docquier PL, Delloye C, Galant C. Histology can be predictive of the clinical course of a primary aneurysmal bone cyst. Arch Orthop Trauma Surg. 2010;130(4):481–7.
3. Capanna R, Campanacci DA, Manfrini M. Unicameral and aneurysmal bone cysts. Orthop Clin North Am. 1996;27(3):605–14.
4. Murphey MD, wan Jaovisidha S, Temple HT, Gannon FH, Jelinek JS, Malawer MM. Telangiectasic osteosarcoma: radiologic-pathologic comparison. Radiology. 2003; 229(2):545–553.
5. Van de Luijtgaarden AC, Veth RP, Slootweg PJ, et al. Metastatic potential of an aneurysmal bone cyst. Virchows Arch. 2009;455 (5):455–9.
6. George HL, Unnikrishnan PN, Garg NK, Sampath JS, Bass A, Bruce CE. Long-term follow-up of Ethibloc injection in aneurysmal bone cysts. J Pediatr Orthop B. 2009;18(6):375–80.
7. Gibbs CP Jr, Hefele MC, Peabody TD, Montag AG, Aithal V, Simon MA. Aneurysmal bone cyst of the extremities: Factors related to local recurrence after curettage with a high-speed burr. J Bone Joint Surg Am. 1999;81(12):1671–8.
8. Basarir K, Piskin A, Gulu B, Yildiz Y, Saglik Y. Aneurysmal bone cyst recurrence in children: a review of 56 patients. J Pediatr Orthop 2007; 27(8):938–943.
9. Steffner RJ, Liao C, Stacy G, et al. Factors associated with recurrence of primary aneurysmal bone cysts: Is argon beam coagulation an effective adjuvant treatment? J Bone Joint Surg Am. 2011;93(21):e1221–9.
10. Varshney MK, Rastogi S, Khan SA, Trikha V. Is sclerotherapy better than intralesional excision for treating aneurysmal bone cysts? Clin Orthop Relat Res. 2010;468(6):1649–59.
11. Rossi G, Rimondi E, Bartalena T, et al. Selective arterial embolization of 36 aneurysmal bone cysts of the skeleton with N-2 butyl cyanoacrylate. Skeletal Radiol. 2010;39(2):161–7.

Unicameral Bone Cyst

24

Dominique G. Poitout

Abstract

Unicameral bone cysts are benign bone lesions, also called simple bone cysts, located on the metaphysis of long bones. Presentation usually occurs within the first two decades of life, and are usually asymptomatic until they become a pathological fracture.

Keywords

Bone cyst • Benign lesion • Pseudotumor • Pathological fracture

The unicameral bone cyst is an intraosseous cyst, also called a "simple bone cyst." A cyst is a cavity surrounded by a membrane. Considered a growing dystrophy, most of them are found within the first two decades of life (two to 20 years of age) [1, 2]. There is a slight predominance in males. Its pathogeny is unknown; some authors think they can be secondary to trauma while others support an enzymatic mechanism [3–5]. Most of them are asymptomatic or present with abrupt pain associated to a pathological fracture (80% of the cases). The most frequent localizations are the proximal metaphysis of the femur and humerus (80% of the cases). Very rarely they can be found in the diaphysis of the long bones. They can be found incidentally in x-rays. Occasionally, on physical examination, a painful mass can be found. The hematologic study is normal.

X-ray images: these look like a lonely oval shaped lagoon, central with well-limited contours, under the growing plate; sometimes they present trabeculation.The adjacent cortical bone can be thinned but not affected. A pathological fracture is often found, usually a non displaced fracture (Fig. 24.1).

There is no periosteal reaction. The proximal pole can be in contact with the growing plate bur never cross it. Multi-loculars aspects can be observed in recurrences. Sometimes, the inferior or distal pole is cup shaped.

Evolution

It is a local benign lesion, with a high potential for recurrence.

These cysts grow longitudinally in the bone and they migrate to the diaphysis during growth (Fig. 24.2).

Cysts of the great trochanter, called "active cysts", can grow through the femoral neck. When they grow to the diaphysis they are termed "inactive" cysts. They can also be found in the diaphysis [6]. In the femoral neck they can be distal to the growing plate of the great trochanter, the femoral epiphysis or the lesser trochanter. Other locations are less frequent like in the calcaneus or fingers [7] (Fig. 24.3).

Differential diagnosis must be made with the aneurysmal bone cyst, fibrous dysplasia, giant cell tumor (most of these are in an higher age range), and chondromyxoid fibroma (Fig. 24.4).

Biopsy: not usually required as images are characteristic. Biopsies are suggested if surgery is indicated for other reasons.

Pathology

Macroscopic findings: the cavity has thinned walls and contains a citrine colored serohematic liquid. A conjunctive membrane lines the cavity, which contains giants cells. The distal pole ends in a hard layer of bone.

D. G. Poitout (✉)
Aix Marseille University, Marseille, France
e-mail: dominique.poitout@live.fr

© Springer-Verlag London Ltd., part of Springer Nature 2021
J. Paulos and D. G. Poitout (eds.), *Bone Tumors*,
https://doi.org/10.1007/978-1-4471-7501-8_24

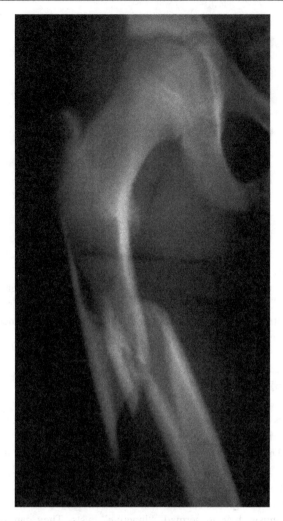

Fig. 24.1 Unicameral displace bone cyst fracture

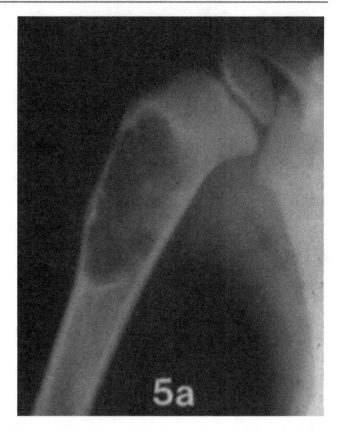

Fig. 24.2 Unicameral bone cyst in a 5 yera-old male

3. Treatment or prevention of a fracture (very important in the femoral neck). In these cases curettage with spongious bone graft and osteosynthesis, special consideration for the epiphyseal growth plate [10] (Fig. 24.7).

Treatment

The fracture of a simple bone cyst can heal. In the past, Professor Imhausser did an osteotomy and fixed it with crossed kirschner wired with good results (Fig. 24.5).

Treatment alternatives are:

1. Local injections of corticoids. Works well in the humerus. The suggested technique requires draining the cyst and injecting 40 to 80 mg of acetate of methylprednisolone
2. Curettage and padding with spongy bone [6, 8, 9] (Fig. 24.6).

Evolution

It is difficult to get a complete restitution and disappearance of the cyst; sometimes a residual cicatrized image persists with some smaller lacunar images (residual cyst). The cyst can undergo a continuous slow growth, that produces bone embrittlement and risk of a pathological bone fracture. The fracture of a cyst always consolidates [11]. But it can evolve with deformations (coxa vara), dysmetria or vicious callus.

The radiological surveillance must be continuous till the end of the young patient's growth. A recurrence is always possible.

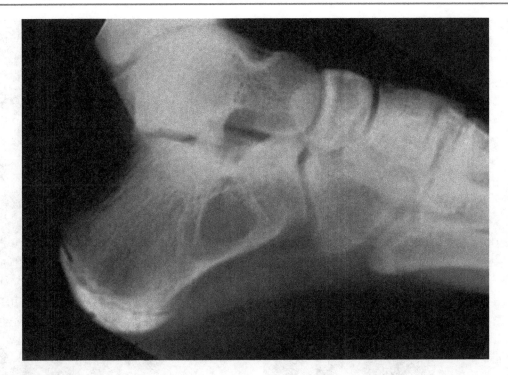

Fig. 24.3 Calcaneus bone cyst

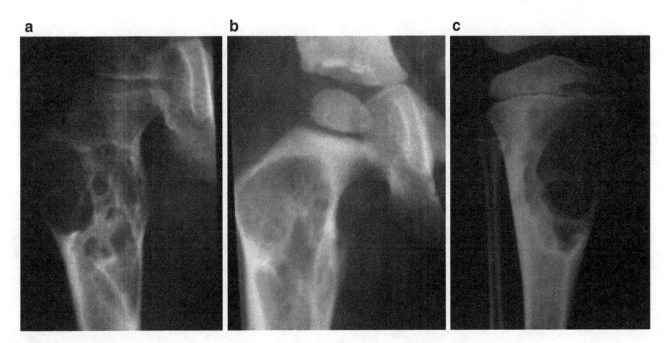

Fig. 24.4 Differential diagnosis of: **a** unicameral bone cyst; **b** aneurysmal cyst; **c** chondromyxoid fibroma

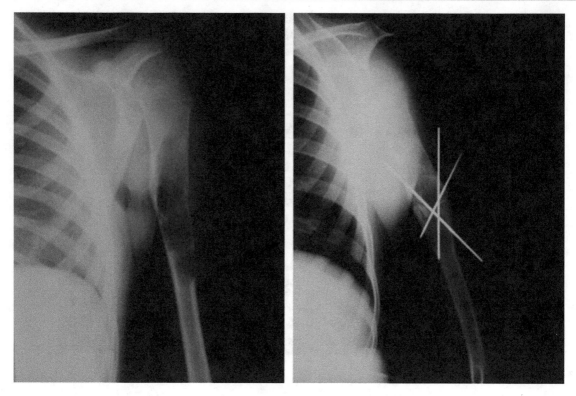

Fig. 24.5 Imhausser technique of treatment

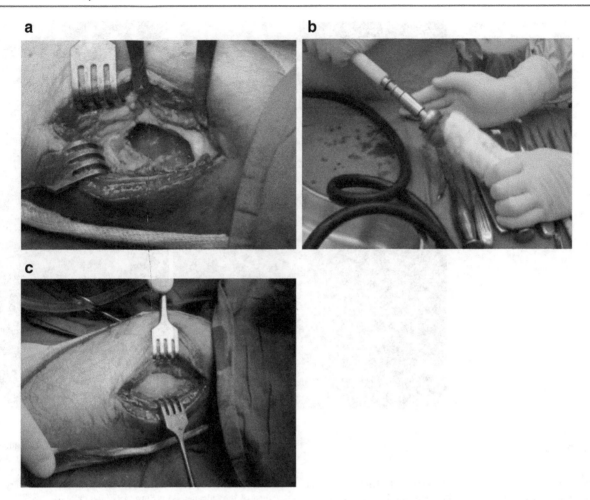

Fig. 24.6 Surgical treatment of UBC, curettage plus allograft of femoral head: **a** curettage; **b** femoral allograft; **c** bone defect covered with allograft

Fig. 24.7 Unicameral bone cyst treatment with curettage, bone filling and osteosynthesis (DHS)

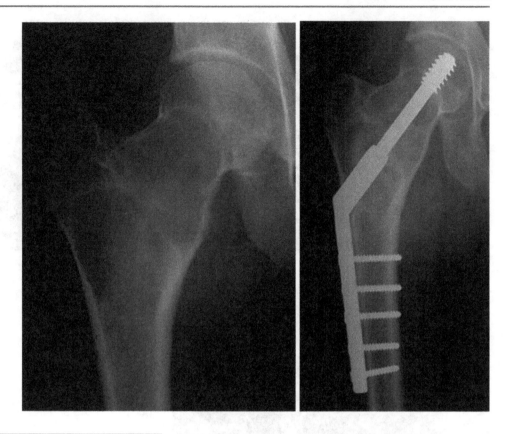

References

1. Capanna R, Campanacci DA, Manfrini M. Unicameral and aneurysmal bone cysts. Orthop Clin North Am. 1996;27(3):605–14.
2. Kaelin AJ, MacEwen GD. Unicameral bone cysts. Int Orthop. 1989;13(4):275–82.
3. Harnet JC, Lombardi T, Klewansky P, Rieger J, Tempe MH, Clavert JM. Solitary bone cyst of the jaws: a review of the etiopathogenic hypotheses. J Oral Maxill ofac Surg. 2008;66 (11):2345–8.
4. Komiya S, Kawabata R, Zenmyo M, Hashimoto S, Inoue A. Increased concentrations of nitrate and nitrite in the cyst fluid suggesting increased nitric oxide synthesis in solitary bone cysts. J Orthop Res. 2000;18(2):281–8.
5. Pretell-Mazzini J, Murphy RF, Kushare I, Dormans JP. Unicameral bone cysts: general characteristics and management controversies. J Am Acad Orthop Surg. 2014;22(5):295–303.
6. Pedzisz P, Zgoda M, Kocon H, Benke G, Górecki A. Treatment of solitary bone cysts with allogenic bone graft and platelet-rich plasma: a preliminary report. Acta Orthop Belg. 2010;76(3):374–9.
7. Symeonides PP, Economou CJ, Papadimitriou J. Solitary bone cyst of the calcaneus. Int Surg. 1977;62(1):24–6.
8. Hou HY, Wu K, Wang CT, Chang SM, Lin WH, Yang R Sen. Treatment of unicameral bone cyst: Surgical technique. J Bone Jt Surg Ser A. 2011; 93 (Suppl. 1): 92–99.
9. Pogoda P, Priemel M, Linhart W, et al. Clinical relevance of calcaneal bone cysts: a study of 50 cysts in 47 patients. Clin Orthop Relat Res. 2004;424:202–10.
10. Sung AD, Anderson ME, Zurakowski D, Hornicek FJ, Gebhardt MC. Unicameral bone cyst: A retrospective study of three surgical treatments. Clin Orthop Relat Res. 2008;466(10):2519–26.
11. Urakawa H, Tsukushi S, Hosono K, Sugiura H, Yamada K, Yamada Y, et al. Clinical factors affecting pathological fracture and healing of unicameral bone cysts. BMC Musculoskelet Disord. 2014;15(1):1–9.

Langerhans Cell Histiocytosis

25

Pedro Valdivia and Cristián Carrasco

Abstract

Langerhans cell histiocytosis is considered as a neoplastic disease and has a wide range of lesions, mainly bone and cutaneous lesions. It occurs at any age, from newborns to the eighth decade of life. It is currently considered as myeloid neoplasm. Treatment strategies are based on the extent and location of the disease. The cancer treatment model is essential to improve outcomes for both adult and child patients with Langerhans cell histiocytosis.

Keywords

Langerhans cell • Myeloid neoplasm • Cancer treatment

Definition

Langerhans cell histiocytosis is a probable neoplasic clonal proliferation of pathological Langerhans cells [1–7]. It is a myeloproliferative disorder characterized by lesions composed of pathological dendritic cells CD207+, with inflammatory infiltrate. It is a poorly understood hematologic disorder, with a wide range of clinical presentations, characterized by granulomatous lesions, composed of clonal pathological histiocytes CD207+ [8].

The terms eosinophilic granuloma and histiocytosis, have been used as synonymous however, the name currently accepted by the WHO is Langerhans cell histiocytosis [6, 7, 9].

It has three clinical variant forms:

(1) Eosinophilic, monostotic or polyostotic granuloma. Usually a single and curable lesion (81%).

(2) Hand–Schüller–Christian disease. Characterized by osteolytic lesions of the skull, exophthalmos and diabetes insipidus.

(3) Letterer–Siwe disease. This shows disseminated lesions with multisystem compromise, and is rapidly fatal in younger infants.

The disease can be located in any bone, but it is mostly found in the skull, femur and pelvis.

It occurs at any age, from newborns to the eighth decade of life, but it is more common before the age of 30 years (up to 80% of cases). It is more common in men, with a male: female ratio of 2:1.

The coincidence of Langerhans cell histiocytosis and myelodysplastic syndrome, with other malignant pathologies, plus the evidence that the Langerhans histiocytosis cells are clonal, support the theory that this disease has a neoplastic origin. BRAF-V600E remains the only recurrent mutation reported in Langerhans cell histiocytosis [3–5]. A very important finding has been the identification of aberrant activation pathways of activated mitogenic protein kinase (MAPK), due to the acquisition of somatic mutations in the myeloid lineage precursors, as the basic mechanism of Langerhans cell histiocytosis [2, 10]. This has not only established the pathogenesis matter in favor of a neoplastic process of Langerhans cell histiocytosis, but it has also opened the door for the incorporation of selective agents for the treatment of the disease.

The range of potential symptoms of this pathology and the overlapping with common pathologies in children and adults, bring about important differential diagnosis challenges. Symptoms can range from self-limited lesions in a single organ to disseminated multi-organ disease, with mortality between 10 and 20%.

Bone (75%) and cutaneous lesions (34%), are the most common lesions. Bone lesions are preferentially located in

P. Valdivia (✉) · C. Carrasco
Universidad Austral de Chile, Valdivia, Chile
e-mail: pavaldiviac@gmail.com

C. Carrasco
e-mail: Cristian.carrascohv@redsalud.gob.cl

© Springer-Verlag London Ltd., part of Springer Nature 2021
J. Paulos and D. G. Poitout (eds.), *Bone Tumors*,
https://doi.org/10.1007/978-1-4471-7501-8_25

the skull, but any bone can be affected either alone or in multiple forms. They appear as irregular osteolytic lesions with or without periosteal reaction and may show soft tissue mass. They can be confused with traumatic lesions, with or without local pain. Skin lesions are very variable in appearance and similar to common lesions; dry scaly appearance on the scalp may be similar to seborrheic dermatitis. Other times, it simulates Candida albicans dermatitis in the axillary or inguinal intertrigo, with erythematous eruptions. Diffuse lesions are also seen with red or purple papules on the chest, back and extremities. The compromise of the external auditory canal skin can be confused with otorrhea.

The disease can compromise the mucous membranes; gingival lesions in the mouth can reach the mandibular bone, appearing as "floating teeth." The intestinal tract involvement can show chronic diarrhea, hypoalbuminemia, weight loss and/or alteration of the normal pondo-estatural growth.

Risk Organs

A severe and characteristic outbreak appears as diffuse or focal infiltration of the spleen, liver or bone marrow, being more frequent in patients younger than two years old. These patients are considered at high risk because they have a more severe clinical presentation and higher death risk. Hepatic involvement is shown by hepatomegaly, elevated transaminases, hyperbilirubinemia or hypoalbuminemia. A bone marrow biopsy shows cytopenia and lack of differentiated CD207+histiocytes.

Pulmonary involvement may also occur with pleurodynia, shortness of breath and spontaneous pneumothorax. In the high-resolution computed tomography (CT) examination of the thorax and lungs show a nodular cystic pattern.

Lymph nodes are often involved in high-risk patients, but lymphatic infiltration per se does not increase clinical risk.

Central nervous system involvement can be manifested by the presence of a mass, diabetes insipidus (10–50%), or by the development of progressive neurodegenerative symptoms. Magnetic resonance imaging may show a mass or thickening of the hypophysial stem. Langerhans histiocytic cell masses elsewhere in the brain may produce long-term symptoms, such as tremors, ataxia, dysmetria, dysphagia, behavioral changes, and learning disabilities. The permanent consequences can be severe, even in patients with low risk disease. Patients with diabetes insipidus are at risk of developing permanent dysfunction of the anterior pituitary gland, with growth hormone deficiency.

Among the orthopedic problems associated with Langerhans cell histiocytosis is the vertebral collapse or "flat vertebra" (Fig. 25.5), scoliosis, facial asymmetry, and limb asymmetry.

Other problems associated with this disease are ophthalmological alterations such as persistent exophthalmos, dental problems such as floating teeth, liver disease such as sclerosing cholangitis or liver failure, and pulmonary fibrosis [11].

Radiology

Cranial lesions predominate in patients younger than 20 years, while solitary lesions in the ribs and mandible are seen in patients over 20 years old. Long bone injuries are more frequent in the femur, pelvis and humerus (Fig. 25.1).

In addition you can see injuries to the pelvis and vertebrae. In multiple lesions, the most affected bones are the skull and the femur, therefore it is necessary to request an X-ray of both bones when lesions are found in one of them. It is necessary to remember that any bone in the body can be affected. The most frequent radiographic findings are relatively well-defined osteolytic lesions with irregular borders, without sclerosis. The lesions of the skull are variable in size, multiple and confluent, with jagged edges, and in the case of Letterer–Siwe disease, they are small and with extensive involvement of the entire skull. They may also have the appearance of a hole in a hole due to the different destruction of the two boards of the bone. Mandibular lesions are located in the alveolar ridge producing lack of support to the teeth, which appear to as floating teeth (Fig. 25.2).

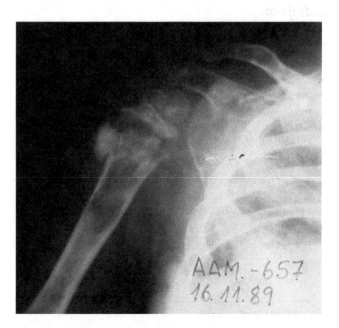

Fig. 25.1 AP radiograph of right humerus: extensive osteolytic, diaphyseal and metaphyseal lesions, with thinning of the cortical bone, with aspect of reparative process in the proximal third; male patient 29 months old

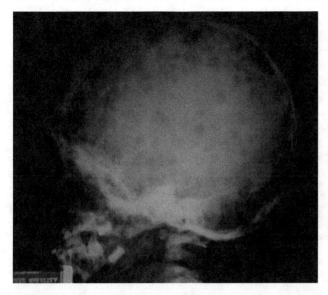

Fig. 25.2 Lateral X-ray of the skull: multiple rounded osteolytic lesions of different sizes and some coalescents; extensive mandibular involvement with dental involvement, and "floating teeth" appearance

The long bones X-rays show rounded, medullar and diaphyseal osteolytic lesions, with erosion of the cortical bone, with slight bulging and an onion cataphylls reaction, simulating Ewing's sarcoma or osteomyelitis. The spine shows the vertebral body partially or totally collapsed, leaving a flat disc, described by Calvè in 1925 as "flat vertebra," and identified as an eosinophilic granuloma by Compere in 1954 (Fig. 25.3).

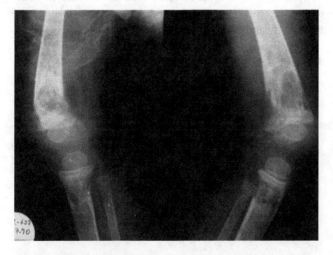

Fig. 25.3 AP and lateral X-rays of both knees: extensive osteolytic lesions of the metaphysis and diaphysis of both femurs and both tibias, with medullar and medial and lateral cortical bone involvement; no periosteal reaction or soft tissue involvement

Pathology

Langerhans cell histiocytosis is currently considered as a myeloid neoplasm, originating in the dendrite cells precursors of the bone marrow, according to the new model "Misguided Myeloid Dendritic cell precursor."

Regardless of the clinical manifestation of the disease, the histopathological findings are similar. The diagnosis is based on the identification of the Langerhans cell, which corresponds to a 15-25 µm major axis cell with irregular cytoplasmic borders, clear or eosinophilic cytoplasm, indented and pleated nucleus, small or non-existent nucleolus and fine chromatin. These cells are arranged in nests and/or accumulations accompanied by an inflammatory component composed of a variable amount of eosinophils ranging from very few to very abundant (Charcot–Leyden crystals may also be observed), in addition, there are small lymphocytes mainly surrounding the Langerhans cells Plasmatic cells are not a characteristic of the disease. Polymorphonuclear neutrophils and macrophages can also be observed, which are more abundant in cases associated with necrosis or fracture (Fig. 25.4).

Confirmation of the presence of Langerhans cells in the lesion may be done on the basis of ultrastructure or immunophenotype. The first one is based on the identification of Birbeck granules corresponding to tennis racket structures present in the cytoplasm of Langerhans cells of normal epithelia, as well as in Langerhans cell disease. These granules are part of the subdomain of the endosomal recycling compartment that is formed when langerine accumulates. Confirmation by immunophenotype is based on the expression of CD1a on the surface of the cells, CD207 (langerin) in the cell's cytoplasm and surface, and S-100 in cytoplasm and nucleus; these cells also express vimentin, HLA class II cytoplasmic and paranuclear CD68, whereas CD45 is negative (Fig. 25.5).

Treatment

Treatment strategies are based on the extent and location of the disease. When the disease is limited to the skin or the bone lesion is unique, systemic therapy is not required. Some patients have received low-dose radiation therapy, with good clinical response [12]. The symptomatic treatment for the skin limited disease, includes topic treatment with corticosteroids, nitrogen mustards, imiquimod and phototherapy. Systemic therapies have also been reported with methotrexate, 6-mercaptopurines, vinca alkaloids, thalidomide, cladribine, and cytarabine.

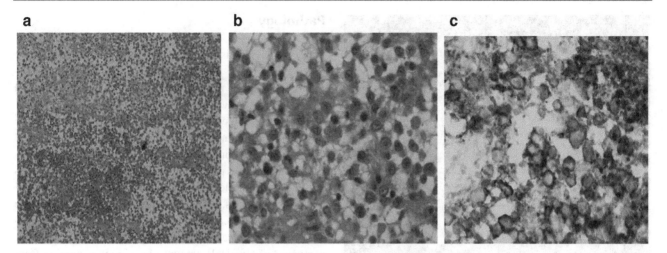

Fig. 25.4 **a** Biopsy: staining Hematoxylin-Eosin (HE) 20x: abundant histiocytic-like cells, broad eosinophil cytoplasm, arranged in mantles next to polymorphonuclear neutrophils and eosinophils; **b** HE 40x: detail of the previous photograph.;histiocytic cells with nuclear clefts and small nucleolus; eosinophils, are also observed; **c** IHC CD1a: positive membrane and cytoplasmic staining in histiocytic cells (Langerhans)

Limited skin lesions, skin may be surgically resected and simple bone lesions can be treated with local curettage and corticoids.

A study from 2013 showed that prolongation of the 12-month treatment with vinblastine/prednisone resulted in a decrease in early relapses. The response to treatment is an important prognostic factor. According to the literature, the survival of patients with high-risk disease, according to the response to therapy at six weeks is 95% when there is a good response, 83% when there is an intermediate response, and 57% when the disease progresses despite the treatment. However, mass-type lesions in the central nervous system cannot be reversed either clinically or by imaging, so the symptoms of neurodegenerative disease appear to be irreversible.

With the current concept of the Langerhans cell histiocytosis, as a myeloid stem cell disease, the use of agents with activity against acute myeloid leukemia may be a reasonable strategy. Many patients who did not improve with vinblastine/prednisone have been cured with salvage therapies used in the treatment of acute myeloid leukemia, such as cytarabine, cladribine, and clofarabine. Vemurafenib, a BRAF inhibitor, has been used with good clinical response in patients with BRAF-V600E mutations.

Langerhans cell histiocytosis has been reclassified according with the progress of our understanding of its pathophysiology, being represented as a common cell of unknown origin, which connects the different phenotypes of the disease. There may be multiple levels of differentiation, leading to manifold clinical manifestations. The current understanding of Langerhans cell histiocytosis allows reclassifying it as a myeloid neoplasm. The cancer treatment management model, with prospective clinical collaborative trials and related biological studies, is essential if we are to continue to improve outcomes for our adult and children patients with Langerhans cell histiocytosis. A record of all patients in a database (such as the Histyiocyte Society since the late 1980s) is highly recommended in order to better define the natural history of the disease and the optimal therapy for these patients.

- Female patient, 19 months old, who presented extensive cutaneous involvement in the anterior and posterior face of the thorax and abdomen, in addition to scalp lesions, similar to seborrheic dermatitis.

Abdominal distension is observed due to liver and spleen involvement in the patient's anterior view.

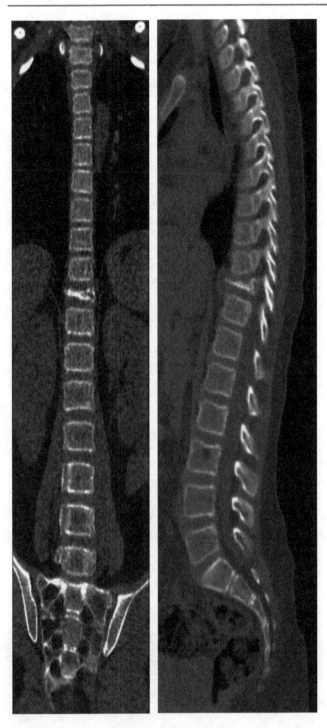

Fig. 25.5 Computed tomography of the dorsal and lumbar vertebral column that shows a significant decrease in the height of the T10 vertebral body, corresponding to the so-called "flat vertebra" of Calvé; decrease of the bone trabeculation of the L3 lumbar vertebra; osteolysis of the right half of the sacral vertebra S1 and S2

References

1. Nezelof, C., Basset, F., Rousseau, M. Histiocytosis X histogenetic arguments for a Langerhans cell origin. *Biomedicine* (publiée pour I'AACIG) 1973; 18: 365.
2. Mc Dermontt R, Ziylan U, Spehner D et al. Birbeck granules are subdomains of endosomal recycling compartment in human epidermal Langerhans cells, which form where Langerin accumulates. Mol Biol Cell. 2002; 13:317–335.
3. Badalian-Very G, Vergilio JA, Degar BA, et al. Recurrent BRAF mutations in Langerhans cell histiocytosis. Blood. 2010;116 (11):1919–23.
4. Sahm F, Capper D, Preusser M, et al. BRAFV600E mutant protein is expressed in cells of variable maturation in Langerhans cell histiocytosis. Blood. 2012;120(12):e28–34.
5. Chakraborty R, Hampton OA, Shen X, et al. Mutually exclusive recurrent somatic mutations in MAP2K1 and BRAF support a central role for ERK activation in LCH pathogenesis. Blood. 2014;124:3007–15.
6. Krishnan UK, Inwards CY. Dahlin's bone tumors, vol. 26, 6th edn. Philadelphia, PA: Lippincott Williams & Wilkins; 2011. p 358–361.
7. De Young B, Egeler RM, Rollins BJ. Langerhans cell histiocytosis. In: Bridge J, Fletcher C, Hogendoorn PCW, Mertens F, editors. World health organization classification of tumors, pathology & genetics: tumors of soft tissue and bone, 4th edn. 2013; 25: 356–357.
8. Schajowicz F, Sundaram M, Gitelis S, McDonald J. Tumors and tumorlike lesions of bone, 2nd edn. Springer-Verlag; 552–566.
9. Berres ML, Merad M, Allen CE. Progress in understanding the pathogenesis of Langerhans cell histiocytosis: back to Histiocytosis X? Br J Haematol. 2015; 169(1): 3–13.
10. Allen CE, Li L, Peters TL et al. Cell-specific gene expression in Langerhans cell histiocytosis lesions reveals a distinct profile compared with epidermal Langerhans cells. J Immunol. 2010; 184:4557–4567.
11. Zinn DJ, Chakraborty R, Allen C. Langerhans cell histiocytosis: emerging insights and clinical implications. J Clin Oncol. 2016; 30 (2):122–132, 139.
12. Abla O, Egeler RM, Weitzman S. Langerhans cell histiocytosis: Current concepts and treatments. Cancer Treat Rev. 2010;36 (4):354–9.

Bone Hydatidosis

26

Jaime Paulos

Abstract

Bone hydatidosis is a bone infection due to equinococosis granulosus. It is a rare condition, similar to a multilocular osteolytic lesion. It occurs in endemic regions with that infection.

Keywords

Bone hydatidosis · Equinococosis infection

Bone hydatidosis is a rare condition and also not very frequent among all the cases of hydatidosis (estimated at 0,5–3% of the cases). It is a zoonosis whose aethiology is the equinococosis granulosus in the larval stage. In Chile [1], the cases come from the cattle in the southern region. The spine, long bones and pelvis are the most frequent bone locations. The conventional Rx shows an osteolytic multilocular lesion. Inmuno diagnosis is useful. Its treatment combines surgery [2] together with antiparasitic drugs (albendazol, mebendazol).

References

1. Oscar T, Vidal A, Bellolio E, Roa JC. Bone hydatidosis, report of five cases. Rev Med Chile 2010;138: 1414–1421. https://doi.org/10.4067/SOO34-98872010001200011
2. Gorun N. Necessary hip disarticulation in extended echinococosis of the femur. Rev Chir Orthop Reparatrice Appar Mot. 1992;78:255–7. www.higiene.edu.uy/parasite/teo09/hidatid.pdf

J. Paulos (✉)
Pontificia Universidad Católica de Chile, Santiago, Chile
e-mail: paulos.jaime@gmail.com

© Springer-Verlag London Ltd., part of Springer Nature 2021
J. Paulos and D. G. Poitout (eds.), *Bone Tumors*,
https://doi.org/10.1007/978-1-4471-7501-8_26

Osteomyelitis

27

Jaime Paulos

Abstract

The clinical features and images of osteomyelitis can look like a bone tumor. A differential diagnosis must sometimes be made from local osteolytic lesions and malign bone tumors.

Keywords

Osteomyelitis • Tumor-like bone lesions • Brodie's abscess

Although the diagnosis of osteomyelitis can be well defined, some cases can propose a differential diagnosis from a bone tumor [2].

Brodie's abscess: this is a subacute osteomyelitis with most cases located in the metaphysis of long bones (tibia, femur) [1, 3]. It is a monostotic lytic lesion surrounded with sclerosis, with few inflammatory signs and frequently the germen is not found (bacteriological and histological studies must be made).

Some other cases can show a periosteal reaction wich looks like an onion bulb, confusing it with a bone tumor such as Ewing's sarcoma or osteosarcoma mostly seen in children or adolescents [4] (Fig. 27.1).

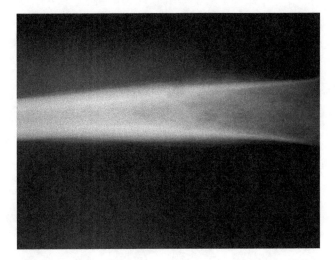

Fig. 27.1 Periosteal reaction

References

1. Pranshu Agrawal, Anshul Sobti. Brodie's abscess of femoral neck mimicking osteoid osteoma: diagnostic approach and management strategy. Ethiop J Health Sci. 2016;26(1):81–4.
2. Lindenbaum S, Alexander H. Infections simulating bone tumors: a review of subacute osteomyelitis. Clin Orthop. 1984; 184:193–203.
3. Cabanela AE, Franklin H, Beabout JW. Osteomyelitis appearing as neoplasms. Arch Surg. 1974; 109:68–72.
4. McGuinness B, Wilson N, Doyle AJ. The penumbra sign on T1 weighted Mri for differentiating musculoskeletal infection from tumor. Skeletal Radiol. 2007;36(417):421.

J. Paulos (✉)
Pontificia Universidad Católica de Chile, Santiago, Chile
e-mail: paulos.jaime@gmail.com

© Springer-Verlag London Ltd., part of Springer Nature 2021
J. Paulos and D. G. Poitout (eds.), *Bone Tumors*,
https://doi.org/10.1007/978-1-4471-7501-8_27

Bone TBC

28

Jaime Paulos

Abstract

Most TBC osteoarthritis cases involve the joints, but in rare occasions they appear as an intraosseous bone lesion.

Keywords

Osteoarthritis TBC • Tumor-like lesions

Isolated bone tuberculosis is very rare. Most cases show osteoarthritis involving the joint, but it can sometimes be seen as an intraosseus lytic lesion (calcaneus) [1, 2].

References

1. Rafiki K, Yousri B, Ahiri M, Bjitro M, Abomaarouf M, Andaloussi M. Localisations inhabituelles de la tuberculose osteoarticulaire chez l'enfant. Revue de Chirurgie Orthopedique et Traumatologie. 2013; 99(3):297–303.
2. Gonzalez H, Farrington DM, Angulo G. Peripheral osteoarticular tuberculosis in children: tumor-like bone lesion. J Pediatr Orthop B. 1997;6:274–82.

J. Paulos (✉)
Pontificia Universidad Católica de Chile, Santiago, Chile
e-mail: paulos.jaime@gmail.com

© Springer-Verlag London Ltd., part of Springer Nature 2021
J. Paulos and D. G. Poitout (eds.), *Bone Tumors*,
https://doi.org/10.1007/978-1-4471-7501-8_28

Osteopoikilosis

29

Jaime Paulos

Abstract

Most cases of osteopoikilosis are incidental findings because they are asymptomatic. An X-ray shows multiple little dense bone foci, which are characteristic.

Keywords

Osteopoikilosis • Osteopathia codensans • Benign bone tumor-like lesions

Osteopoikilosis is a rare disease, also called osteopathia condensans disseminate or spotted bone disease. It can be sporadic or inherited by an autosomal dominant inheritance. Its main characteristics are hyperostotic lesions in the metaphysis and epiphysis of long bones. An X-ray shows multiple round dense foci of small diameter of only 1 or 2 mm [1, 2]. Usually they are asymptomatic and they are diagnosed incidentally. Differential diagnosis can be presented with bone prostate metastasis; Tc-99 m bone scan in osteopoikilosis shows little or no uptake. The treatment is observation.

References

1. Di Primio G. Benign spotted bones: a diagnostic dilemma. CMAJ. 2011;183:456–9.
2. Carpintero P, Abad JA, Serrano P, Serrano JA, Rodríguez P, Castro L. Clinical features of ten cases of osteopoikilosis. Clin Rheumatol. 2004;23:505–8.

J. Paulos (✉)
Pontificia Universidad Católica de Chile, Santiago, Chile
e-mail: paulos.jaime@gmail.com

© Springer-Verlag London Ltd., part of Springer Nature 2021
J. Paulos and D. G. Poitout (eds.), *Bone Tumors*,
https://doi.org/10.1007/978-1-4471-7501-8_29

Paget's Disease of Bone

30

Jaime Paulos

Abstract

Paget's disease of bone is very common in older people, secondary to an altered remodeling, deforming bone structure. X-rays are characteristic. Most cases are asymptomatic, but can attain pathological fractures and long term infrequent cases of secondary sarcomas.

Keywords

Paget'S disease • osteitis deformans

Paget's disease (osteitis deformans) is a skeletal disease that results from an altered bone remodeling with accelerated resorption in some areas and abundant new bone formation in others [1–3]. The most common form of presentation is poorly localized bone pain and additionally it can present itself with pathologic bone fractures. The pelvis, spine, skull, and proximal long bones are most frequently affected. The X-ray is characteristic [4, 5]. Serum alkaline phosphatase is elevated because of the high bone turnover rate. It is a common finding in older people. It can be mono or poliostotic. The mixed (middle) phase of Paget's disease combine characteristics of both the lytic (initial) and the blastic (late) phases. Most patients present in the mixed phase when decreased osteoclastic activity and increased osteoblastic activity are encountered. Symptomatic cases can be treated with bisphosphonates. The most advanced form is the malignant transformation to a secondary sarcoma (osteosarcoma) [2] that has a poor prognosis.

References

1. Kaplan FS, Singer FR. Paget's disease of bone: pathophysiology, diagnosis, and management. J Am Acad Orthop Surg. 1995;3(6):336–44.
2. Wick MR, Siegel GP, McLeod RA. Sarcomas of bone complicating osteitis deformans (Paget's disease): fifty years experience. Am Pathol J Surg. 1981; 5:47–59.
3. Resnick D. Paget's disease, diagnosis of bone and joint disorders. 4th ed. Philadelphia, PA: Saunders; 2002. p. 1947–2000.
4. Whitehouse RW. Paget's disease of bone. Semin Musculoskelet Radiol. 2002;6:313–22.
5. Mirra JM, Brien EW, Tehranzadeh J. Paget's disease of bone: review with emphasis on radiologic features—part I. Skeletal Radiol. 1995;24:173–84.

J. Paulos (✉)
Pontificia Universidad Católica de Chile, Santiago, Chile
e-mail: paulos.jaime@gmail.com

© Springer-Verlag London Ltd., part of Springer Nature 2021
J. Paulos and D. G. Poitout (eds.), *Bone Tumors*,
https://doi.org/10.1007/978-1-4471-7501-8_30

Hyperparathyroidism

Jaime Paulos

Abstract

Hyperparathyroidism is a disease produced by excessive parathyroid hormone. Affects the bones metabolism developing lytic lesions known as brown tumors.

Keywords

Hyperparathyroidism • Brown tumor • Hypercalcemia

Bone disease in hyperparathyroidism is characterized by bone resorption, osteopenia and brown tumors [1, 2]. Classically called osteitis fibrosa cystica, it can present itself as bone pain, deformities and fractures. Laboratory tests show elevated levels of serum parathyroid hormone and hypercalcemia. In severe forms of the disease renal compromise can be a great danger with high elevations of serum calcium and medical complications. In the long bone imaging shows lucent bone tumors (brown tumors) and in the pelvis the images could resembled an aneurysmal bone cyst, giant cell tumor, myeloma or metastatic carcinoma [3]. Other findings are subperiostic reabsorption of medial and distal phalanges. Primary and secondary hyperparathyroidism results in elevated levels of serum parathyroid hormone, a finding that helps differentiate this disease process from malignant hypercalcemia.

References

1. Parisien M, Silverberg SJ, Shane E, Dempster DW, Bilezikian JP. Bone disease in primary hyperparathyroidism. Ethiop J Health Sci. 2016; 26(1): 81–84. PMCID: PMC4762963.
2. Silverberg SJ, Shane L, De La Cruz D et al. Skeletal disease in primary hyperparathyroidism. J Bone Miner Res. 4, 1989: 283–291.
3. Ullah E, Ahmad M, et al. Primary hyperparathyroidism having multiple brown tumors mimicking malignancy. Ind J Endocrinol Metab.

J. Paulos (✉)
Pontificia Universidad Católica de Chile, Santiago, Chile
e-mail: paulos.jaime@gmail.com

© Springer-Verlag London Ltd., part of Springer Nature 2021
J. Paulos and D. G. Poitout (eds.), *Bone Tumors*,
https://doi.org/10.1007/978-1-4471-7501-8_31

Chordoma

Franklin H. Sim

Abstract

Chordomas are slow-growing, locally destructive, rare primary malignant bone tumors located in the neural axis [1, 2]. Once the diagnosis is made (with a combination of clinical, imagenological and histological aspects), the tumor has to be staged in order to provide the best treatment option. These tumors are challenging to treat, with many questions left open about their optimum treatment. Wide surgical resection with a 1 cm tumor-free margin remains the standard of care for achieving curative resection. Other complementary therapies described and in development are adjuvant radiotherapy, proton beam therapy and newer chemotheraspy agents such as imatinib.The most important prognostic factor in these patients is to perform a resection with adequate margins, thus achieving oncological survival of up to 20 years. Recurrences have a worse prognosis and continue to be a greater challenge in the treatment of this type of bone tumor.

Keywords

Chordoma • Malignant bone thumor

Introduction

Chordoma is a rare primary malignant tumor of bone found along the neural axis. The notocord is an embryonic structure which induces segmentation of vertebral bodies. The remnants are generally obliterated as embryonic maturation occurs; however, notochordal rests may remain and are felt to be the source cells for the development of malignant chordomas.

F. H. Sim (✉)
Mayo Clinic, Rochester, MN 55905, USA
e-mail: sim.franklin@mayo.edu

As outlined below, chordoma is a slow but relentless cancer. The mainstay of treatment for it is wide oncologic resection. In cases when this cannot be achieved, there is a potential role for adjuvant radiotherapy and an investigational role for some chemotherapy regimens.

Presentation

The Sundfoordistribution of chordoma roughly parallels that of notochordal rests. Approximately 25–30% occur in the spheno-occipital region, 10–15% occur in the mobile spine, and the remainder occur in the sacrococcygeal area. The most common presentation of chordoma is a deep-seated pain which begins insidiously with gradual progression. Although the pain may initially appear to be intermittent, it ultimately progresses to a constant pain which is often sensed by the patient to be worse in the evening. True night pain, that is pain which awakens the patient from a sound sleep, is a common finding.

Other symptoms vary with the location of chordoma along the spinal axis. As the majority occur in the sacrococcygeal region, patients may experience bowel, bladder, or sexual disfunction as the associated nervous structures are impinged upon.

Constipation is a common presenting symptom. This may be due to impingement on the lower cauda equina or from mechanical obstruction of the rectum rather than true destruction of the nerves whichh innervate it.

When presenting in the mobile spine or in the spheno-occipital region, neurologic symptoms are more frequent. Additionally, patients who present with chordomas at the craniocervical junction may have airway compromise, dysphasia, or Horner's syndrome as a part of their presentation.

Because of a non-specific manner in which these tumors present and the fact that the majority occur deep in the pelvis, they may reach a large size prior to diagnosis. Fuchs

© Springer-Verlag London Ltd., part of Springer Nature 2021
J. Paulos and D. G. Poitout (eds.), *Bone Tumors*,
https://doi.org/10.1007/978-1-4471-7501-8_32

et al. reported a mean two-year delay from symptom onset to diagnosis [3]. However, it is relatively rare for patients with chordoma to present with overt metastatic disease at the time of diagnosis. As tumors generally arise in the mid-line, radicular involvement tends to occur relatively late in the presentation of this tumor.

Epidemiology

The incidence of chordoma is estimated at 0.8 per million persons in the population [4]. It appears to be more common in male patients and in Caucasians compared to other minorities. The median age at presentation in a recent series was 58.5 years; less than 5% of tumors present in the pediatric age group. There may be a slight predilection to skull-based tumors in pediatric patients.

Overall, chordoma is probably the most common primary bone tumor along the spinal axis. In tumors presenting in the mobile spine, the lumbar spine appears to be the most commonly affected site.

Imaging

Chordomas present as expansile, lytic lesions which are centered in the mid-line of the vertebral bodies. They exhibit a lobular growth pattern on imaging studies and gross examination. Amorphous calcification is detected in between 30 and 90% of tumors, usually best viewed on CT imaging.

Because of the common location of chordomas in complex anatomical areas, they are poorly viewed upon plain film radiographs. Axial imaging with CT and MRI scans are the mainstay of diagnosis in imaging for these tumors. On MRI scans, chordomas are iso- or hypointense compared to muscle on T1 weighted sequences. They are hyperintense on T2 weighted sequences and demonstrate contrast enhancement on gadolinium-enhanced images (Fig. 32.2).

When large, chordomas may have internal cystic changes or hemorrhagic regions. Chordomas characteristically arise at or near the mid-line with an expansile growth pattern from this region.

On CT images, chordomas appear to be purely lytic with occasionally small foci of amorphous calcification noted. Soft tissue masses are frequently encountered. The presacral fascia and posterior longitudinal ligament in the mobile spine are usually strong natural barriers to tumor extension. However, in advanced cases, chordomas can frequently break through normal fascial barriers.

Chordomas are readily detected upon bone scans. The use of positron emission tomography (PET) scans remains investigational at this time. Because of the relatively low metabolic rate of these tumors, PET scans are probably an unreliable mechanism for detection and monitoring of chordomas with current technologies.

Differential Diagnosis

As the median age of presentation with chordoma is nearly 60 years of age, it is important to remember that metastatic disease, multiple myeloma, and lymphoma are far more common tumors which will present in the spine in this age group. Often times the nature of these tumors may be suspected based on a multifocal nature as imaged through the spine. Additionally, standard staging studies will usually identify metastatic and hematopoietic tumors and differentiate them from chordomas. In the case of a solitary plasmacytoma arising in the sacrum, the diagnosis may be difficult to exclude on imaging studies alone.

Chondrosarcoma is a primary bone tumor commonly encountered in the sacrum which on imaging studies can mimic chordoma. Chondrosarcomas are not necessary located in the mid-line as are chordomas. As well, their imaging studies will often implicate a greater degree of myxoid change within the lesion than a chordoma will. Additionally, the pattern of stippled calcification present in chondrosarcomas will frequently suggest this diagnosis over that of chordoma.

Myxopapillary ependymoma is a rare tumor which can arise from the filum terminale within the sacral region. A biopsy readily distinguishes chordoma from myxopapillary ependymoma. Other tumors which may arise characteristically in the sacrum include teratoma; however, these generally have a significantly more complex appearance on axial imaging studies than do chordomas. Benign notochordal rest may be imaged within the sacrum or elsewhere along the spinal axis. These generally have no associated bony destruction in contrast to chordomas. Additionally, there is no soft tissue mass and no cortical violation in a patient with a benign notochordal rest. These lesions are generally felt to be asymptomatic.

Other tumors which may arise in the sacrum (such as aneurysmal bone cyst, or other sarcomas) can often be excluded from chordomas based upon imaging studies.

Biopsy

Biopsy confirmation of chordoma is obtained prior to definitive surgical treatment. Core needle biopsy is the mainstay of diagnosis for these tumors. Chordoma is an extremely implantable tumor; open biopsies or poorly planned biopsies can significantly change the outcome for patients with this disease. As such, a near mid-line posterior biopsy which samples the tumor well but avoids contamination of the epidural compartment is a key aspect of diagnosis. Such a biopsy is readily excisable at the time of definitive surgical treatment and will not adversely impact the ability for the patient to undergo curative surgery. It should be very strongly cautioned that a transrectal biopsy is always contraindicated in the evaluation of a mass which is expected to be chordoma. As well, the use of open biopsies should be approached with great caution given the very high propensity for chordoma to seed along a biopsy tract and any subsequent hematoma.

Histology/Pathology

Chordoma demonstrates a lobular growth pattern both grossly and on low power microscopy. On higher power images, syncytial strands of cells are seen within a mucus background. Physaliferous cells ("soap bubble") are the hallmark finding of chordomas [5]. These are cells which contain intracellular vacuoles and bubbly cytoplasm giving them a characteristic appearance (Fig. 32.1). Giant noto-chordal rests [6–8] can at first glance appear similar to chordomas; however, these benign lesions generally lack the surrounding myxoid stroma, have no mitotic figures, and do not exhibit any areas of necrosis when compared with chordomas. This, in conjunction with imaging findings, will generally allow differentiation of the two lesions.

Two subtypes of chordoma which bear mention are chondroid chordoma and dedifferentiated chordoma. In chondroid chordoma, hyaline cartilage is seen within the lesion. Dedifferentiated chordomas have a high grade sarcomatous component in conjunction with the malignant chordoma [9]. The high grade sarcoma may have evidence of osteogenic differentiation or more closely resemble an undifferentiated pleomorphic sarcoma.

Chordomas stain S-100 positive on immuno-histo chemistry studies, and this can help distinguish them from metastatic adenocarcinomas [5]. A positive cytokeratin CAM 5.2 immunohistochemistry study is sensitive but not specific for the detection of chordoma. As well, chordomas may demonstrate epithelial membrane anagen positivity which can help differentiate them from chondrosarcoma.

Staging

Staging of chordomas falls into two categories: systemic staging and local surgical staging. Systemic staging seeks to define the extent of the disease within the body to detect any metastatic foci. This is most commonly performed with a computed tomography scan of the chest, abdomen, and pelvis as well as a bone scan. As mentioned earlier, the sensitivity of PET scans to adequately stage chordoma is not

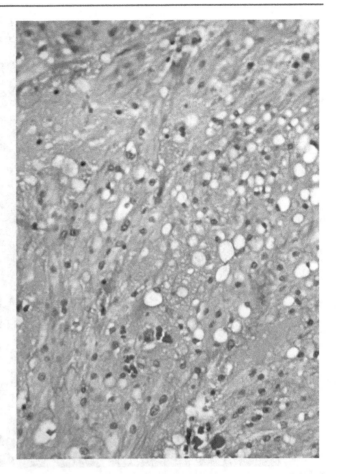

Fig. 32.1 Histology of chordoma demonstrating syncytial strands of cells within a mucinous background and physaliferous cells with intracellular vacuoles and bubbly cytoplasm

known at this time. Based upon the low metabolic activity of this tumor, it may not be a reliable staging mechanism.

Local surgical staging is provided by three plane imaging studies of the tumor. Magnetic resonance imaging in three planes is very helpful to define the extent of the tumor. Axial, sagittal, and coronal images are used for surgical planning. When dealing with tumors in the sacrum, coronal oblique images (coronal images obtained within the plane of the sacrum) are quite helpful in defining the local extent of tumor with respect to the neural foramina in this complex anatomic area. MRI imaging is the most useful modality to define the location of tumors and the integrity of standard fascial planes in the resection. In addition, it provides ready imaging of the neural elements to detect areas where surgical resection may safely take place. Particularly when dealing with tumors in the sacrum, plain film radiographs are obtained to help plan intraoperative localization. Since as many as 11% of patients do not display the standard 12 thoracic/5 lumbar vertebral configuration, it is critical to define a priori the counting scheme to allow proper intraoperative localization.

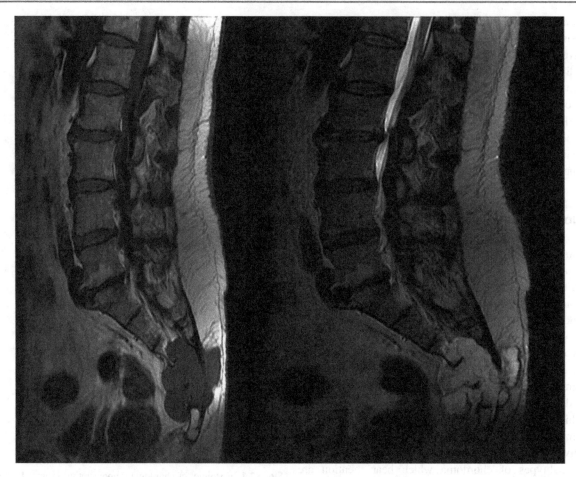

Fig. 32.2 Imaging features of chordoma on MRI; demonstrates the lobulated nature of the tumor and penetration through dorsal fascia; gross specimen following resection

Additionally,, in the case of resections which require spinal instrumentation, these radiographs allow detection of any abnormalities which might influence the reconstructive process.

Treatment

Wide surgical resection is the mainstay of treatment for chordomas [10–12]. It is critical in the treatment of these tumors that surgeons respect a proper margin around the lesion. A well-meaning attempt to "save" nerve roots which are close to the tumor is almost always doomed to ultimate failure. Marginal resection along nerve roots almost guarantees that some microscopic residual tumor is left behind. This tumor inevitably regrows and recurs in an unpredictable fashion. In doing so, it destroys the nerve root which was attempted to be saved (and thus there is no benefit to trying to do this for the patient).

Also, as the pattern of recurrence is often unpredictable, it may be difficult to achieve curative treatment of the patient following such an exercise. As such, resections for chordoma frequently involve deliberate neurologic sacrifice which will erase bowel, bladder, and sexual functions for patients. Although this is disappointing and difficult to pursue, it is critical in the appropriate treatment of the tumor and undertaken with the recognition that the natural history of the tumor, whether untreated or poorly treated, is to destroy the neurologic function of any local nerve roots. This fact is highlighted by the finding of Dr. Fuchs in that the most important predictor of survival in an analysis of 52 patients with chordoma was the ability to obtain a wide surgical margin. The details of surgical resection in the sacrum are outlined in chapter 41 on sacral surgery [13]. Interestingly, the anterior sacral fascia appears to provide a strong natural barrier for chordomas. As such, recurrences in this region are relatively rare, and concurrent resection of visceral structures is not often needed. We seek to obtain a minimum 1 cm tumor-free margin at the site of bony osteotomies and fascial barriers around the remainder of the tumor. For tumors which extend into the pyriformis muscle, we seek a 4 cm margin of uninvolved muscle given the poor compartmentalization of this region.

The use of adjuvant radiotherapy is developing in the treatment of chordoma. Chordomas are relatively resistant to standard radiotherapy techniques. The use of proton beam therapy for the treatment of these tumors is maturing.

Recent data from the Massachusetts General Hospital demonstrated that high dose photon/proton radiotherapy delivered in doses in excess of 70 cobalt Gray equivalent showed five-year recurrence-free survival of 63% when applied to chordomas and other spinal sarcomas [14]. When tumors arise in areas where a tumor-free margin of resection cannot be obtained (such as at the craniocervical junction), treatment of this nature is used to assist in tumor control. In cases where an en bloc margin of resection can be obtained, the use of adjuvant radiotherapy remains a matter of debate, with different centers employing different treatment protocols.

There are no known standard effective chemotherapy regimens for chordoma. Recent results demonstrate that imatinib may have efficacy in treating patients with chordoma.

Imatinib is an inhibitor of the platelet drive growth factor receptor beta (PDGFR-beta) [15], and PDGFT-beta activation and over-expression have been demonstrated in chordomas [16].

A small series of 18 patients with chordoma demonstrated symptomatic improvement as well as decreased contrast enhancement on MR scans in patients treated with one year follow-up [17]. These results are promising, and further studies with imatinib and other agents are clearly indicated [18].

In the case of dedifferentiated chordoma, chemotherapy is directed at the high grade sarcomatous component of the tumor [9].

Outcomes

Assessing prognosis in chordoma is difficult, given the long natural history of the disease. A minimum five year follow-up has been suggested by Dr. Boriani in the evaluation of these patients.

It appears that adequacy of surgical resection is critical in the treatment of patients with chordoma. In reporting on the Mayo Clinic series, Fuchs et al. showed that survival was 100% in patients in whom a wide surgical margin could be obtained; but with patients for whom less than a wide surgical margin was obtained, salvage and survival were much more challenging [3]. Similar reports come from other large centers; Dr. Bergh reporting the series from Gottenberg has shown a 21-fold increased risk of death in patients who experience local recurrence [19]. These findings again highlight the critical nature of appropriate and aggressive surgical treatment from the onset in patients presenting with chordoma. Similar results have been seen in large studies

from other centers [20, 21] with a ten-year survival rates of 50–60%.

Examining chordoma of the mobile spine, Boriani and colleagues found similar results. All patients treated with radiation and/or intralesional resection alone developed recurrence within two years. The only treatment in this series associated with continuous disease-free survival beyond five years was uncontaminated en bloc resesction [22, 23].

Given the long natural history of chordoma, it is difficult to know for certain how recent advances in radiotherapy and potential chemotherapy regimens may affect the ultimate survival of patients. The results appear promising for these mechanisms to be used for patients in whom an adequate surgical margin cannot readily be obtained.

Metastatic disease is generally a relatively late finding in patients with chordoma. Metastatic sites are most commonly seen in the lungs, soft tissue, and bone of chordoma patients. They are present in up to two-thirds of patients at autopsy.

Post-operative Management and Surveillance

Patients undergoing treatment for chordoma require long-term oncologic surveillance [24]. One recommended protocol includes a CT of the chest, abdomen, and pelvis, as well as an MR scan of the operative site every four months for one to two years based upon the surgeons assessment of risk of local and distant recurrence. For up to five years surveillance studies are obtained every six months and after that annually. At ten years, surveillance studies may be changed to every two years up to a minimum 20-year follow-up. Technetium bone scans are obtained annually through to year five and then every two years through approximately ten years of follow-up and then every three to five years thereafter.

In patients who do demonstrate recurrence of chordoma, treatment is carefully individualized. If an isolated recurrence is noted and is amenable to surgical resection, aggressive treatment is performed to resect all detectable disease. In patients who have multifocal areas of recurrence, consideration is given to radiotherapy to the region to slow or halt the disease process. Additionally, the use of imatinib or other chemotherapy adjuvants is heavily considered.

If patients have solitary or oligo metastatic disease in areas which are difficult to resect, cryo or radiofrequency oblation may be used to ablate these local areas of tumor.

Conclusions

Chordoma is a rare malignant tumor which occurs along the spinal access, arising from notochordal rests. Aggressive surgical treatment remains the mainstay for curative resection of these patients. The role of advanced radiotherapy, techniques and newer chemotherapy agents is promising in the treatment of these patients. However, aggressive en bloc surgical resection is generally considered necessary for curative treatment of these patients. As tumors may present late, this often requires surgeries of large magnitude.

Post-operatively, the prognosis for patients is guardedly optimistic provided adequate surgical margins were obtained. Because of the slow growing nature of chordoma, oncologic surveillance is extended out to a minimum of 20 years. In patients that demonstrate recurrence of disease, treatment is individualized but often aggressive to provide long-term survival for patients.

References

1. Walcott BP, Nahed BV, Mohyeldin A, Coumans JV, Kahle KT, Ferreira MJ. Chordoma: current concepts, management, and future directions. Lancet Oncol. 2012;13(2):e69–76.
2. Chugh R, Tawbi H, Lucas DR, Biermann JS, Schuetze SM, Baker LH. Chordoma: the nonsarcoma primary bone tumor. Oncologist. 2007;12(11):1344–50.
3. Fourney DR, Gokaslan ZL. Current management of sacral chordoma. Neurosurg Focus. 2003;15:E9.
4. Maclean FM, Soo MY, Ng T. Chordoma: radiological-pathological correlation. Australas Radiol. 2005;49:261–8.
5. Llauger J, Palmer J, Amores S, et al. Primary tumors of the sacrum: diagnostic imaging. AJR Am J Roentgenol. 2000;174:417–24.
6. Yamaguchi T, Suzuki S, Ishiiwa H, et al. Benign notochordal cell tumors: a comparative histological study of benign notochordal cell tumors, classic chordomas, and notochordal vestigious of fetal intervertebral disks. Am J Surg Pathol. 2004;28:756–61.
7. Kyriakos M. Benign notochordal lesions of the axial skeleton: A review and current appraisal. Skeletal Radiol. 2011;40(9):1141–52.
8. Amer HZ, Hameed M. Intraosseous benign notochordal cell tumor. Arch Pathol Lab Med. 2010;134(2):283–8.
9. Fuchs B, Dickey I, Yaszemski M, Inwards C, Sim F. Operative management of sacral chordoma. J Bone Joint Surg Am. 2005;87:2211–6.
10. Fleming GF, Heimann PS, Stephens JK, et al. Dedifferentiated chordoma: response to aggressive chemotherapy in two cases. Cancer. 1993;72:714–8.
11. Sciubba D, Cheng J, Petteys R, et al. Chordoma of the sacrum and vertebral bodies. J Am Acad Orthop Surg. 2009;17:708–17.
12. Osaka S, Kodoh O, Sugita H, et al. Clinical significance of a wide excision policy for sacrococcygeal chordoma. J Cancer Res Clin Oncol. 2006;132:213–8.
13. Hulen CA, Temple HT, et al. Oncologic and functional outcome following sacrectomy for sacral chordoma. J Bone Joint Surg Am: 1532–1539.
14. DeLaney T, Liebsch N, Pedlow F, et al. Phase II study of high dose proton/photon radiotherapy in the management of spine sarcomas. Int J Radiation Oncology Viol Phys. 2009;74:732–9.
15. Tamborini E, Miselli F, Negri T, et al. Molecular and biochemical analyses of platelet derived growth factor receptor (PDGFR) beta, PDGFRA, in KIT receptors in chordomas. Clin Cancer Res. 2006;12:6920–8.
16. Sciubba DM, Chi JH, Rhines LD, Gokaslan ZL. Chordoma of the spinal column. Neurosurg Clin N Am. 2008;19:5–15.
17. Casali PG, Stacchiotti S, Messina A, et al. Imatinib mesylate in 18 advanced chordoma patients. J Clin Oncol. 2005;23:9012.
18. Schwab JH, Boland PJ, Agaram NP, et al. Chordoma and chondrosarcoma gene profile: Implications for immunotherapy. Cancer Immunol Immunother. 2009;58(3):339–49.
19. Bergh P, Kindblom L, Gunterberg B, et al. Prognostic factors in chordoma of the sacrum and mobile spine: a study of 39 patients. Cancer. 2000;88:2122–34.
20. Hanna SA, Tirabosco R, Amin A, et al. Dedifferentiated chordoma: a report of four cases arising "de novo". J Bone Joint Surg Am. 2008;90:652–6.
21. McMaster ML, Goldstein AM, Bromley CM, et al. Chordoma: Incidence and survival patterns in the United States, 1973–1995. Cancer Causes Control. 2001;12:1–11.
22. Boriani S, Schevalley F, Weinstein JN, et al. Chordoma of the spine above the sacrum: treatment and outcome in 21 cases. Spine. 1996;21:1569–77.
23. Boriani S, Bandiera S, Biagini R, et al. Chordoma of the mobile spine: 50 years of experience. Spine. 2006;31:493–503.
24. Chambers PW, Schwinn CP. Chordoma: a clinicopathologic study of metastasis. Am J Clin Pathol. 1979;72(5):765–76.

Adamantinoma

33

Jaime Paulos

Abstract

Adamantinoma is a malignant, slow-growing bone tumor. It has an epithelial origin and is commonly located in the diaphysis and metaphysis of long bones, mainly the tibia. It affects typically adolescents and young adults. The term adamantinoma has been given to this tumor due to its histological resemblance to ameloblastoma of the jaws. It is commonly confused with osteofibrous dysplasia, and the definitive diagnosis is established mainly by histopathological examination, which shows small epithelial islands in a fibrous stroma, without cytological atypia. The mainstay of treatment is block resection and reconstruction, but due to the high recurrence rate, some authors recommend amputation.

Keywords

Adamantinoma • Malignant bone tumor

Adamantinoma is an infrequent malignant bone tumor of the long bones of epithelial origin. It is located in 90% of cases in the tibia (Fig. 33.1), sometimes in the fibula and very rarely in other long bones. Its epithelial origin has been confirmed in studies through immunohistochemical and electron microscopy studies [1].

Most cases appear between the second and fifth decades of life, in adolescents and young adults, although there are cases in the first decade of life and also older people over 70 years of age [2–6].

Adamantinoma is so-named because of its resemblance to the ameloblastoma of the jaw bones.

The clinical course indicates a slow speed of growth. Pain is the principal symptom and also a painful mass. Most cases have a long evolution.

Pathological fracture is uncommon. Only about 20% of cases develop metastasis in the long term.

Imaging

The most typical X-ray appeareances are multiple lucent defects of different sizes in the anterior cortical tibia. A bigger lytic lesion can be found with a zone of sclerotic margin or many lytic defects configuring a bubble or lobulated aspect. It can invade the cortical and penetrate the soft tissues.

Histopathology

It is a gray or white tumor delimited peripherally, often lobulated, and varies in consistency from a firm tissue to a brain-like tissue. The typical histologic appearance is a small epithelial islands in a fibrous stroma and islands with peripherical palisading containing stellate-shaped cells that are also seen in ameloblastomas. Some cases show islands of squamous cells with central keratin formation. One important feature in adamantinoma is the lack of cytological atypia. The most frequent differential diagnosis is osteofibrous dysplasia [4, 5, 7–12].

Treatment

Local excision has a high range of recurrence and many of these recurrences evolved in metastasis and death. Block resection and reconstruction is the logical surgical option. Some authors conclude that amputation is the treatment of choice based in the high percentage of recurrence after local excision. Chemotherapy is not indicated.

Metastasis occurrs through hematogenous or lymphatic routes.

J. Paulos (✉)
Pontificia Universidad Católica de Chile, Santiago, Chile
e-mail: paulos.jaime@gmail.com

© Springer-Verlag London Ltd., part of Springer Nature 2021
J. Paulos and D. G. Poitout (eds.), *Bone Tumors*,
https://doi.org/10.1007/978-1-4471-7501-8_33

Fig. 33.1 X-ray of tibia adamantinoma

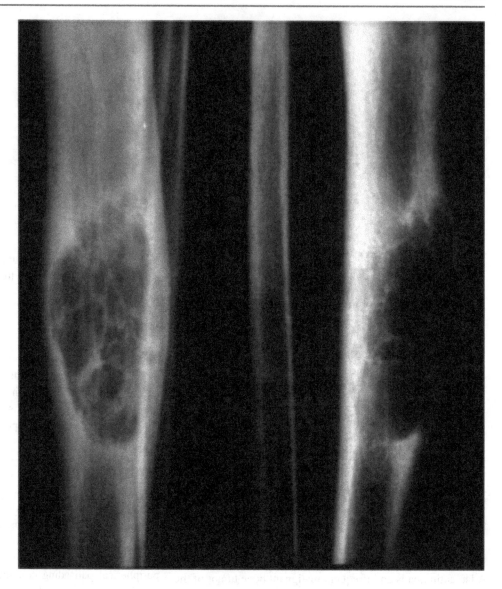

References

1. Jain D, Jain VK, Vasishta RK, Ranjan P, Kumar Y. Adamantinoma: A clinicopathological review and update. Diagn Pathol. 2008;3:8.
2. Papagelopoulos PJ, Mavtogenis AF, Galanis EC, Savvidou OD, Inwards CY, Sim FH. Clinicopathological features, diagnosis, and treatment of adamantinoma of the long bones. Orthopedics. 2007; 30(3): 211–215, quiz 216–217.
3. Bethapudi S, Ritchie DA, Macduff E, Straiton J. Imaging in osteofibrous dysplasia, osteofibrous dysplasia-like adamantinoma, and classic adamantinoma. Clin Radiol. 2014;69(2):200–8 Epub 2013 November 5.
4. Kitsoulis P, Charchanti A, Paraskevas G, Marini A, Karatzias G. Adamantinoma. Acta Orthop Belg. 2007;73(4):425–31.
5. Gleason BC, Liegl-Atzwanger B, Kozakewich HP, et al. Osteofibrous dysplasia and adamantinoma in children and adolescents: A clinicopathologic reappraisal. Am J Surg Pathol. 2008;32(3): 363–76.
6. Maki M, Athanasou N. Osteofibrous dysplasia and adamantinoma: Correlation of proto-oncogene product and matrix protein expression. Hum Pathol. 2004;35(1):69–74.
7. Most MJ, Sim FH, Inwards CY. Osteofibrous dysplasia and adamantinoma. J Am Acad Orthop Surg. 2010;18(6):358–66.
8. Czerniak B, Rojas-Corona RR, Dorfman HD. Morphologic diversity of long bone adamantinoma: The concept of differentiated (regressing) adamantinoma and its relationship to osteofibrous dysplasia. Cancer. 1989;64(11):2319–34.
9. Kahn LB. Adamantinoma, osteofibrous dysplasia and differentiated adamantinoma. Skeletal Radiol. 2003;32(5):245–58.

10. Ishida T, Iijima T, Kikuchi F, et al. A clinicopathological and immunohisto-chemical study of osteofibrous dysplasia, differentiated adamantinoma, and adamantinoma of long bones. Skeletal Radiol. 1992;21(8):493–502.

11. Markel SF. Ossifying fibroma of long bone: Its distinction from fibrous dysplasia and its association with adamantinoma of long bone. Am J Clin Pathol. 1978;69(1):91–7.

12. Springfield DS, Rosenberg AE, Mankin HJ, Mindell ER. Relationship between osteofibrous dysplasia and adamantinoma. Clin Orthop Relat Res. 1994; 309:234–44.

High Degree Undifferentiated Pleomorphic Sarcoma

34

Pedro Valdivia and Cristián Carrasco

Abstract

High degree undifferentiated pleomorphic sarcoma primary of the bones is a malignant neoplasm with low incidence that compromises mainly adults but can also affect children. It is located mainly in long bones like the femur, tibia and humerus. The most common symptoms are increased volume and pain. On images, it appears as osteolytic lesions with badly defined borders of metaphyseal location, destroying the cortical bone. Histopathologic diagnosis of undifferentiated pleomorphic sarcoma is a diagnosis of exclusion and requires a large panel of immunohistochemistry. Treatment is as used in osteosarcoma with chemotherapy and extensive surgical resection.

Keywords

High degree sarcoma • Undifferentiated sarcoma • Pleomorphic sarcoma • Bone sarcoma

Definition

High degree undifferentiated pleomorphic sarcoma is a high degree malignant neoplasm characterized by tumor cells with diffuse pleomorphism, in the absence of a specific line of differentiation. The name fibrous malignant histiocytoma of the bones is accepted as a synonym in the past.

In the past, many undifferentiated pleomorphic sarcomas were classified as liposarcomas, pleomorphic fibrosarcomas, osteolytic osteosarcomas, anaplastic reticulosarcomas or giant cell malignant tumors.

P. Valdivia (✉) · C. Carrasco
Universidad Austral de Chile, Valdivia, Chile
e-mail: pavaldiviac@gmail.com

C. Carrasco
e-mail: Cristian.carrascohv@redsalud.gob.cl

Clinical Findings

This is a rare tumor that represents less than 2% of the malignant primary bone tumors.

According to the different series, the authors report either slight female or male predominance. The age of appearance varies from between six to 88 years, with an average age of around 50 years. It is rare to find patients under ten years of age, and less than 15% of them are under 20 years old.

This tumor can be located in any bone but predominates in long bones especially the femur, tibia and humerus. In the axial skeleton a preferred location is the pelvis, but it can also be found in the spine and scapulae (personal series). It can be a primary lesion of the bone or, exceptionally, appear as as multiple injuries, (personal series). It may be a primary lesion of the bone or appear as a secondary one, associated with Paget's disease, bone infarction or irradiated bone in up to 28% of the cases. It may also occur on bones treated with total knee or hip prosthesis.

The most common symptoms are increased volume and pain that can exist from a few weeks to three years at the time of diagnosis, with an average of seven to nine months from the onset of symptoms.

This is a neoplasia that, like osteosarcoma, shows frequent metastases to the lungs (45–50%).

Imaging

The tumors appear as osteolytic lesions with badly defined borders of metaphyseal location, destroying the cortical bone and invading the soft tissues. They can also appear as a cystoid lesion and in other cases as a moth-eaten bone. The fracture in pathological bone is not uncommon. It is rare to find periosteal reaction. Computer-based axial tomography is useful to assess the spinal cord involvement and the destruction of cortical bone, as well as the extension to soft tissues.

© Springer-Verlag London Ltd., part of Springer Nature 2021
J. Paulos and D. G. Poitout (eds.), *Bone Tumors*,
https://doi.org/10.1007/978-1-4471-7501-8_34

Differential diagnosis should be made with osteosarcoma, fibrosarcoma, lymphoma, myeloma, and metastasis.

Histopathology

Undifferentiated pleomorphic sarcoma is a diagnosis of exclusion. The neoplasia is heterogeneous and consists mainly of cells that are fused with variable amounts of large epithelial or polygonal cells with eosinophilic cytoplasm; nuclear atypias that are accentuated with abundant mitosis, and aberrant mitotic figures are not unusual. Atypical multinucleated giant cells and variable degree of accompanying inflammatory infiltrate of the lymphocytic and histiocytic type, together with the presence of neutrophils, are frequently identified in areas of necrosis or fracture.

Since it is a diagnosis by exclusion, it is necessary to correlate it with the clinical and image evidence, to guide the different diagnostic possibilities, to make a broad mapping of the sample, in the cases of biopsies by puncture, the multiple levels study and to carry out immunohistochemical study. The genetics study is not the front line. The large/multiple levels mapping is basically aimed at the identification of osteoid, to rule out osteosarcoma. It should be considered that in cases of fracture there may be bone neoformation that should not be misinterpreted as osteoid.

The immunohistochemical study is the rule, and it should include a panel to rule out sarcomatoid carcinomas, melanoma and some hematological malignancies [1]. It should be considered that many undifferentiated sarcomas express epithelial markers but they generally do that as isolated cells; a diffuse staining and of more than one marker, would lead to think of a metastatic carcinoma [1]. Positivity for p63 leads to carcinoma metastasis and it would be useful to rule out those sarcomas that normally express epithelial markers such as synovial sarcoma, where p63 is expressed only in the epithelioid component and in the epithelioid sarcoma, where the staining is weak [2].

Undifferentiated pleomorphic sarcomas express myogenic markers, mainly SMA but they may also express desmin or h-caldesmon. When there is an expression of only one marker, the diagnosis is undifferentiated pleomorphic sarcoma, mentioning that it presents incomplete myogenic differentiation. In the case of showing two or more markers, the diagnosis of undifferentiated pleomorphic sarcoma is excluded, because it corresponds to a leiomyosarcoma [3].

Treatment

There is sufficient information that supports clinicians to carry out the same treatment as used in osteosarcoma with chemotherapy and extensive surgical resection. Occasionally, amputation is necessary in very advanced lesions or to perform radiotherapy on unresectable lesions of the pelvis and spinal cord.

The survival prognosis is similar to that of the osteosarcoma, as long as the requirements for a favorable chemotherapy response and a wide margin of resection are met. Another favorable prognostic factor is the presentation of the disease in patients under 40 years of age.

References

1. Goldblum John R. An approach to pleomorphic sarcomas: can we subclassify, and does it matter? Mod Pathol. 2014;27:S39–46.
2. Jo MD VJ, Fletcher MD CD. Immunohistochemical staining is limited in soft tissue tumors. Am J Clin Pathol 2011;136: 762–766. (FRCPath. p. 63).
3. Romeo Salvatore, et al. Malignant fibrous histiocytoma and fibrosarcoma of bone: a re-assessment in the light of currently employed morphological, immunohistochemical and molecular approaches. Virchows Arch. 2012;461:561–70.

Glomus Tumor

35

Sergio Morales

Abstract

Glomus tumor is an infrequent benign tumor usually located on subungueal tissue on the distal phalanx of hands. Pain with temperature changes and pressure on the fingertips make the diagnoses.

Keywords

Glomus tumor • Fingertip tumor

Glomus tumor is an infrequent benign tumor affecting the glomus body, an neuromyoarterial apparatus involved in thermo-regulation of the cutaneus microvasculature [1]. This is a soft tissue tumor, most frequently located in glomus bodies rich areas such the distal phalange of the hands in the subungueal soft tissue. Recently many others presentation areas has been described like toes, forearm, wrist, thigh and even out of musculoskeletal system [2–5].

Characteristic clinical symptoms, such as paroxysmal and intense pain with temperature changes or contact pressure on the distal finger (or involved area) are described. Subcutaneous nodules may be observed or palpated according to the depth of the injury [3].

Usually imaging test are not required and diagnosis is made clinically. Some imagenological features can help diagnostic process in unusual presentations. On plain radiographs a well-limited notch (resorbed bone) in cortical bone of the phalange could be seen (Fig. 35.1).

On MRI, this tumor presents a low signal tumor on T1-weighted images and high signal on T2-weighted images [6] (Fig. 35.2).

Pathology

Glomus tumor is considered an hamartoma, frequently around 1 cm in size. Histology images shows small round cells with dark nuclei and no cellular atypia or mitotic activity. Small vessels are associated in a hyaline stroma [4].

Treatment

Surgical treatment consist on marginal excision; the approach must be selected based on location. For most frequent location (hands), onisectomy is necessary to reach the tumor located under the nail matrix (Fig. 35.3). With a fine curette the tumor it is gently dissected in totality.

Complications

Recurrence is rare [7] and post-surgical deformity of the nail can appear. Malignancy is very rare, but there are some reports of it in the literature [8].

S. Morales (✉)
Pontificia Universidad Católica de Chile, Santiago, Chile
e-mail: slmorales@uc.cl

© Springer-Verlag London Ltd., part of Springer Nature 2021
J. Paulos and D. G. Poitout (eds.), *Bone Tumors*,
https://doi.org/10.1007/978-1-4471-7501-8_35

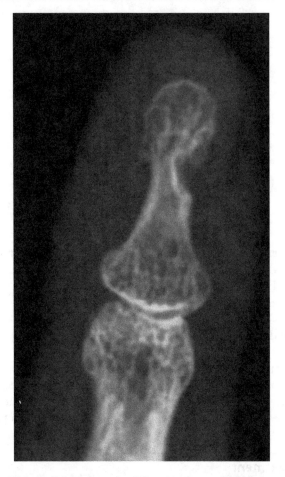

Fig. 35.1 Radiological aspect of glomus tumor on distal phalanx

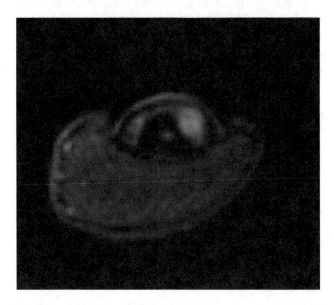

Fig. 35.2 Axial view on MRI of distal phalanx showing high signal on T2 of the on dorsal aspect of phalanx

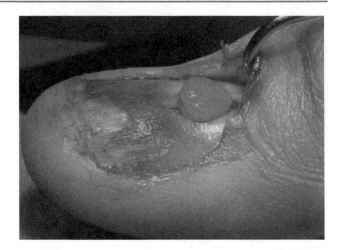

Fig. 35.3 Macroscopic aspect of glomus tumor of distal phalanx after onisectomy

References

1. Lee W, Kwon SB, Cho SH, Eo SR, Kwon C. Glomus tumor of the hand. Arch Plastic Surg. 2015;42(3):295–301. https://doi.org/10.5999/aps.2015.42.3.295.
2. Kurohara K, Michi Y, Yukimori A, Yamaguchi S (2018) The glomus tumor resorbed bone and teeth in the mandible: a case report. Head and Face Med 14(1). https://doi.org/10.1186/s13005-018-0175-3
3. Lui TH, Mak SM (2014) Glomus tumor of the great toe. J Foot Ankle Surg 53(3):360–363. https://doi.org/10.1053/j.jfas.2013.05.011
4. Gombos Z, Zhang PJ (2008, September) Glomus tumor. Archives of pathology and laboratory medicine. https://doi.org/10.5858/2008-132-1448-gt
5. Beksaç K, Dogan L, Bozdogan N, Dilek G, Akgul GG, Ozaslan C (2015) Extradigital glomus tumor of thigh. Case Rep Surg 2015:1–3. https://doi.org/10.1155/2015/638283
6. Glazebrook KN, Laundre BJ, Schiefer TK, Inwards CY. Imaging features of glomus tumors. Skeletal Radiol. 2011;40(7):855–62. https://doi.org/10.1007/s00256-010-1067-1.
7. Sanna M, De Donato G, Piazza P, Falcioni M. Revision glomus tumor surgery. Otolaryngol Clin North Am. 2006 https://doi.org/10.1016/j.otc.2006.04.004.
8. Folpe AL, Fanburg-Smith JC, Miettinen M, Weiss SW. Atypical and malignant glomus tumors: Analysis of 52 cases, with a proposal for the reclassification of glomus tumors. Am J Surg Pathol. 2001;25(1):1–12. https://doi.org/10.1097/00000478-200101000-00001.

Bone Metastasis

36

Jaime Paulos and Dominique G. Poitout

Abstract

Bone metastasis is a frequent secondary bone tumor. Primary malignant tumors from the breast, kidney, lung, thyroid and prostate are the most frequent ones giving metastasis to bone, although any malign tumor can eventually spread to bone, mostly through a vascular route. Local osteoarticular pain, pathological fracture and general constitutional symptoms are frequent forms of presentation. Imaging study and biopsy are necessary. Treatment will depend of the origin of the tumor, location, and condition of the patient. Stabilization and reconstructive surgery will be necessary to achieve a better quality of life.

Keywords

Bone metastasis · Osteolysis · Pathological fracture · Bone pain · Reconstructive surgery · Bifosfonato

Definition

Bone metastasis is the spread of an extraosseus malign primary tumor to bone. It is the most frequent malignant bone tumor, and it is 4 times more frequent than a primary bone tumor [1].

The spread of a primary tumor is usually through a vascular route; although in rare cases it can be via the lymphatic system [2, 3].

Most of the primary tumors giving bone metastasis are breast cancer, kidney, lung, thyroid, and prostate malignant primary tumors [4]. Less frequent are bone metastases from digestive primary tumors and gynecological malignant tumors.

However, any primary malignant tumor can give rise to bone metastasis. Although bone metastasis from malignant tumors in children are extremely rare, their presence can seen in retinoblastoma or a malignant tumor of the rhino-pharynx.

Malignant cells of the primary tumor enter into the venous system arriving at the cava vein and then to the right heart, and then giving lung metastasis [5]. From there they spread to the left heart and to the arterial vascular system to the bones. The metastatic cells must be implanted and grow in the new environment of the lung or later in the bone.

The lung represents a special environment that works like a filter and is a very vascular tissue: for that reason most patients with bone metastasis have also lung metastasis [6]. Most metastases are groups of cells that stop on their way in this pulmonary filter being first like micro metastasis and then growing in situ giving a macro metastasis which it is possible to see in a chest X-ray study. The Computerized Tomography is more sensitive in finding out lung metastasis.

Hypernephroma (or kidney sarcoma) give monocells to the bloodstream and they do not stop in the lung but they are implanted in the bone. For that reason we can find bone metastasis without the presence of lung metastasis. These are the cases where the first manifestation of a metastasis is in the bone with sometimes a pathological fracture being the first sign of the disease.

Digestive carcinomas give a first metastasis to the liver and then secondarily through the cava vein to the heart, lung, left heart and then to the arterial systemic system. So most patients have symptoms derived from the invasion of the liver and much later bone metastasis can appear.

Bone metastasis can occur in any bone but more commonly occurs in the spine, pelvis and proximal long bones. That is because these bone regions are very vascularized. Metastases in the hands or feet are rare. A hand metastasis must made us think of a lung primary malignant tumor.

J. Paulos
Pontificia Universidad Católica de Chile, Santiago, Chile
e-mail: paulos.jaime@gmail.com

D. G. Poitout (✉)
Aix Marseille University, Marseille, France
e-mail: dominique.poitout@live.fr

© Springer-Verlag London Ltd., part of Springer Nature 2021
J. Paulos and D. G. Poitout (eds.), *Bone Tumors*,
https://doi.org/10.1007/978-1-4471-7501-8_36

Clinical Symptoms and Signs

The most important symptom is pain. Each time a patient has a localized pain in a bone the bone must be studied to find the cause. It can be the first manifestation of the disease. However, it is frequently an asymptomatic finding in a study for another reason. Bone metastases are usually presented in patients over 50 years old.

General symptoms also can be a frequent manifestation, such as weight loss.

The appearance of a mass can be an alert symptom.

A pathological fracture can be an ominous clinical sign and in some cases it can be the first manifestation of the disease. Patients with bone metastasis are frightened to have a pathological fracture [7].

For that the prediction of a fracture is important and when that occurs it is worse than the preventative treatment. Two guidelines are frequently cited: 1. A defect >2,5 cms. in dimension must be considered at risk for fracture 2. >50% cortical destruction is an indication for prophylactic fracture.

Efforts have be done to predict a pathological fracture and the work of Hilton Mirels (1989) is one of the more accepted in spite of critical evaluations of his rating system [8].

Scoring system for diagnosing impending pathological fractures [11]: (Table 36.1)

Each risk factor gives one to three points, providing a maximum of 12 points. As the score increases above seven, the risk of fracture also increases.

Another method to measure the risk of fracture is the Harrington's criteria, which follows:

- 50% or more destruction of diaphyseal cortices;
- 50–75% destruction of methaphysis;
- permeative destruction of the subtrocantheric region;
- persistent pain following irradiation.

Hypercalcemia

The symptoms of hypercalcemia can be confusion, muscle weakness, polyuria, polydipsia, nausea, vomiting, dehydration. It is the consequence of bone destruction.

Neurologic deficits: spine metastases are the most frequent site of bone metastasis and can be the expression of compression of the spinal cord.

An evaluation and search for bone metastasis: imaging, labs exs., and biopsy are required.

Imaging

Plain radiographs (anteroposterior and lateral) from the suspected site of a bone metastasis are needed. Also a chest X-ray in two planes are needed, however, the chest computed tomography (CT) is much more sensitive for this purpose. Bone metastasis in plain x-rays can be lytic in most cases but they also can be osteoblastic like in prostate carcinoma and some breast carcinomas with a fibrous component.

Scintigraphy with technetium Tc99 is very useful when looking for asymptomatic bone metastasis and the screening of the whole skeletal body. In some cases, scintigraphy can result in a false negative test, especially in multiple myeloma and some cases of thyroid carcinoma (Fig. 36.1).

MRI is very useful to define the extension of a bone metastasis. This is relevant in cases where a bone resection or stabilization of a destructive lesion is planned.

PET-CT is also a useful imaging tool for looking for metastasis.

Laboratory

A hematologic study should be made: blood cell count, eritrosedimentation rate, calcium, phosphorus, alkaline phosphatase. Estrogen, progesterone, HER2/neu receptor are

Table 36.1 Mirels' score

	1	2	3
Site	Upper limb	Lower limb	Peritrocanteric
Pain	Mild	Moderate	Functional
Lesion	Blastic	Mixed	Lytic
Size	<1/3	1/3–2/3	2/3

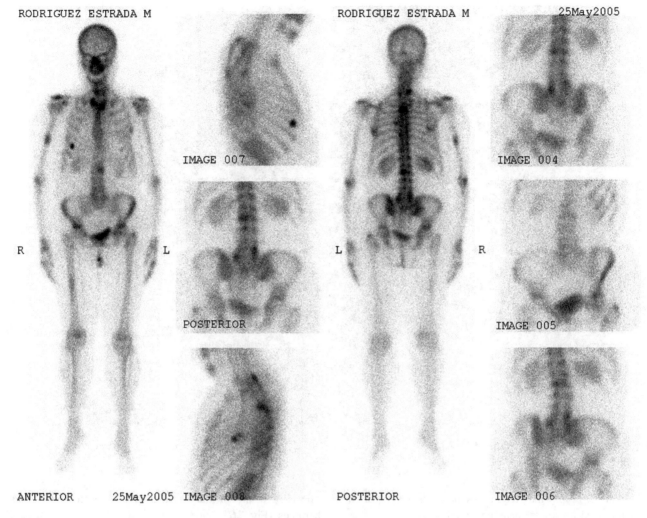

Fig. 36.1 Scintigraphy showing multiple bone metastasis

essential in cases of breast cancer. Also prostatic antigen is needed in prostate cancer study.

Treatment

General measures: treatment is of multidisciplinary management [14].

Bisphosphonate therapy: this is useful in preventing osteoclastic bone destruction. IV pamidronate is commonly used.

Chemotherapy, radiotherapy and hormone therapy is indicated in relation to the type of the origen of the tumor.

Breast cancer is radiosensitive, chemosensitive and hormonesensitive; a oncologic team must define the best indication.

Kidney carcinomas are radio and chemosensitive. In case of surgery pre-op embolization is recommended.

Lung carcinomas, although of bad prognosis, are radio and chemosensitive.

Prostate carcinomas are chemo and radiosensitive.

In thyroid carcinoma radioiodine is useful and also chemotherapy.

Multiple myeloma is radio and chemosensitive.

Surgery: a biopsy is necessary to rule out a primary bone lesion. We should not treat a bone lesion without a tissue

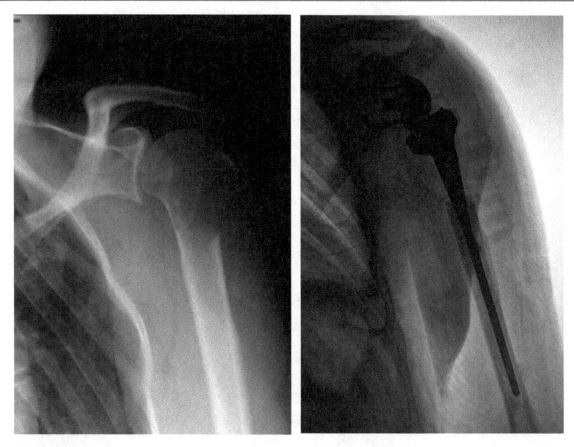

Fig. 36.2 Shoulder X-ray: **a** proximal humerus metástasis of próstata carcinoma, resection proximal humerus and reconstruction with a **b** reverse shoulder endoprosthesis

diagnosis. A biopsy may require a separate incision from the incision used for a intramedullary nailing.

Lesions with risk of fracture or already fractured must have a surgical treatment. Ideally the patient must be in conditions to survive the surgery, immediate weight bearing, and the implant survival should be longer than the expected patient's survival [9]. Another condition is if surgery will relieve the pain.

Two strategies can be used, depending on the site of the lesion that we are treating, the primary cancer and the patient: stabilization and post-operative radiation [10, 13] or reconstructive surgery with osteoarticular implants [14].

Proximal humerus: endoprosthesis (although the shoulder function can be limited). Today a better option is the use of a reverse shoulder endoprosthesis (Fig. 36.2).

Humeral diaphysis: resection with an intercalary spacer is possible. Plates and screws are not ideal,

especially if the primary cancer is not sensitive to other therapies (Fig. 36.3).

Distal humerus: elbow replacement or flexible nails.

Proximal femur: femoral neck and head: hip replacement (hemi, bipolar or total arthroplasty depending on the prognosis) (Fig. 36.4).

Peritrochanteric lesions: intertrochanteric plate, intramedullary nailing or massive endoprosthesis.

Spine metastasis. [10] palliative treatment is indicated in cases of a life expectancy less than six months. Local radiation is indicated for patients who are not surgical candidates [11, 12] (Fig. 36.5).

Patients with neurological deficits have indication for neurological decompression, spinal stabilization and post-operative radiation.

Post-operative radiation will decrease pain, will slow eventual progression and will treat any remaining tumor not removed at surgery.

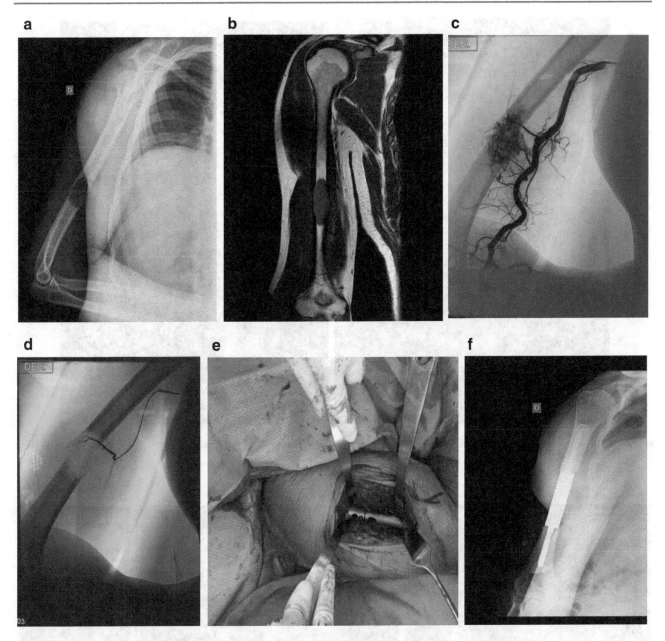

Fig. 36.3 Hypernephroma metastasis: **a** X-ray; **b** MRI; **c** and **d** embolization; **e** surgical treatmet with spacer; and **f** post-operative X-ray

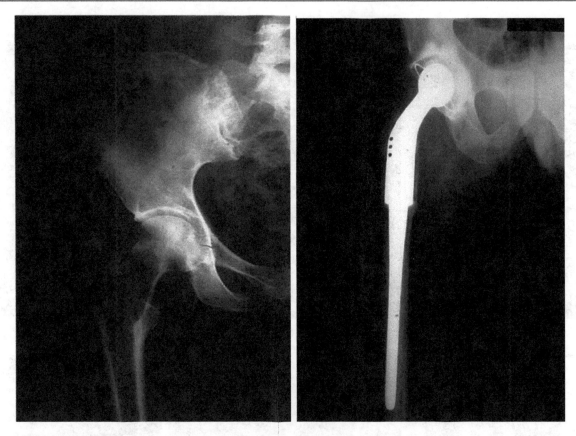

Fig. 36.4 Breast cancer metastasis, resection proximal femur and hip total megaprosthesis replacement

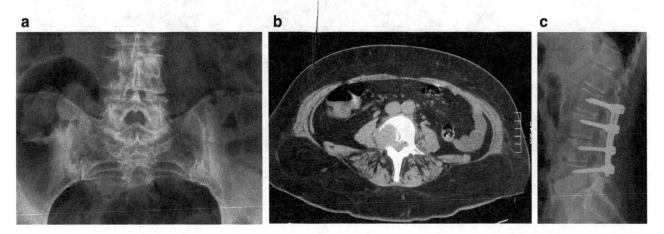

Fig. 36.5 Metastasis lesion of L4; **a** pre-operative X-ray showing a litic metastasis on L4; **b** CT of L4 metastasis; and **c** spine fixation of the lesion

References

1. Hage WD, Aboulafia AJ, Aboulafia DM. Incidence, location, and diagnostic evaluation of metastatic bone disease. Orthop Clin North Am. 2000; 31(4): 515–528, vii.
2. Talmadge JE, Fidler IJ. AACR centennial series: the biology of cancer metastasis: historical perspective. Cancer Res. 2010;70 (14):5649–69.
3. Buijs JT, Van der Pluijm G. Osteotropic cancers: from primary tumor to bone. Cancer Lett. 2009;273(2):177–93.
4. Böhm P, Huber J. The surgical treatment of bony metastases of the spine and limbs. J Bone Joint Surg Am. 2002;84(4):521–9.
5. Coghlin C, Murray GI. Current and emerging concepts in tumor metastasis. J Pathol. 2010;222(1):1–15.
6. Li S, Peng Y, Weinhandl ED et al. Estimated number of prevalent cases of metastatic bone disease in the US adult population. Clin

Epidemiol. 2012; 4: 87–93. This study examines the prevalence of metastatic bone disease in the US population.

7. Coleman RE. Clinical features of metastatic bone disease and risk of skeletal morbidity. Clin Cancer Res. 2006;12(20 Pt 2): 6243s–9s.

8. Talbot M, Turcotte RE, Isler M, Normandin D, Iannuzzi D, Downer P. Function and health status in surgically treated bone metastasis. Clin Orthop Relat Res. 2005; 15(438): 215–220.

9. Nathan SS, Healey JH, Mellano D, et al. Survival in patients operated on for pathologic fracture: Implications for end-of-life orthopedic care. J Clin Oncol. 2005;23(25):6072–82.

10. Coleman RE. Metastatic bone disease: clinical features, pathophysiology and treatment strategies. Cancer Treat Rev. 2001;27(3):165–76.

11. Damron TA, Morgan H, Prakash D, Grant W, Aronowitz J, Heiner J. Critical evaluation of Mirels' rating system for impending pathologic fractures. Clin Orthop Relat Res. 2003; (Suppl 415): S201–S207.

12. Tokuhashi Y, Matsuzaki H, Toriyama S, Kawano H, Ohsaka S. Scoring system for the pre-operative evaluation of metastatic spine tumor prognosis. Spine (Phila Pa 1976) 1990;15(11):1110–1113.

13. Sim FH, Daugherty TW, Ivins JC. The adjunctive use of methylmethacrylate in fixation of pathological fractures. J Bone Joint Surg Am. 1974;56(1):40–8.

14. Poitout D. Bone metastasis: medical surgical and radiological treatment. London: Springer-Verlag; 2002. Chapter 9: Specific surgeries for bone tumors.

Application of Biomechanic Principles to Oncology

Dominique G. Poitout

Abstract

Biomechanical considerations are crucial when treating bone tumors or metastatic conditions. The spine, pelvis and proximal femur are frequent locations where mechanical needs and stability require for surgical interventions in the oncologic patient. Similarly, treatment of impending fractures in the lower extremity are arising as a common scenario given the prolonged survival and better treatments for patients with cancer. This chapter will review specific considerations when treating bone tumors in the appendicular skeleton, with emphasis in some specific body segments.

Keywords

Biomechanic • Impending fracture • Bone tumors • Surgical fixation

Introduction

Malignant metastatic tumors are the most common bone neoplasms. The skeleton is often affected by metastasic cancer, and the discovery of a long bone metastasis may be the first symptom of the primary disease. Nearly every malignant neoplasm has been described as having the capability to metastasize to bone; tumors of breast, prostate, thyroid, lung and kidney are the most common bone-seeking malignant lesions, and between 50 and 85% of affected patients will have bone metastasis at one point of their disease [1–3]. Breast and prostate cancer alone account for more than 80% of metastasic bone disease. The capacity of the neoplastic cells to invade bone is related to the histology and to the aggressiveness of the primary tumor. The axial

skeleton is where the red marrow is situated in adults, and this pattern of distribution suggests that physical properties of the circulation within the bone marrow could assist in the development of bone metastasis. The outcome of metastasis depends on multiple interactions of metastatic cells with homeostatic mechanisms which the tumor cells usurp. The dissemination of cancer cells to vital organs results in eventual multisystem failure and death.

Pathologic fractures are a relatively late complication of bone involvement. Prostate metastases are usually sclerotic lesions, and as such pathologic fractures are less common than litic breast metastasis. Pathologic fractures are devastating complications of metastatic disease; these lesions are associated with considerable morbidity, which includes: unbearable pain, impaired mobility, pathologic fractures, and bone marrow infiltration.

With the advent of improved medical therapies for many types of cancer, life expectancy has dramatically improved in the last two decades, and this makes the orthopedic surgeon more often involved with patient care. This increased patient survival rate has also driven us to a more aggressive management of patients with bone metastasis. It is estimated that 40% of patients with pathologic fractures survive for at least six months after their fracture, and 30% survive for more than one year.

Patients median survival after the first recurrence of carcinoma in patients without extraosseous sites at the time of diagnosis is approximately twenty months, and it varies according to primary cancer type: breast 25 months, prostate 40 months, thyroid 48 months, kidney 12 months, and lung 4 months. Bone metastasis refractory to radiation and chemotherapy have a shorter life expectancy.

Metastasic destruction of bone reduces its load-bearing capabilities, resulting initially in trabecular disruption and microfractures, and subsequently in total loss of bone integrity and pathologic fracture. Clinical trials with bisphosphonates [4] have proved to inhibit tumor induced bone resorption, correct hypercalcemia, reduce pain and diminish

D. G. Poitout (✉)
Aix Marseille University, Marseille, France
e-mail: dominique.poitout@live.fr

© Springer-Verlag London Ltd., part of Springer Nature 2021
J. Paulos and D. G. Poitout (eds.), *Bone Tumors*,
https://doi.org/10.1007/978-1-4471-7501-8_37

the development of new osteolytic lesions and fractures; all leading to potential improvements in quality of life. Even though clinical trials with bisphosphonates in patients with multiple myeloma and breast cancer seem promising, no long-term efficacy of these drugs has yet been proved.

The probability of developing a pathological fracture increases with the duration of the disease, and as such they tend to occur more often in tumors with relatively good prognosis. Pathologic fractures have been reported to occur in 9 to 29% of patients who have bone metastasis. The indications for prophylactic fixation have not been standardized, and will vary according to the size of the lesion, the anatomic location, the bone involved (weight bearing vs. non weight bearing long bones), radiographic appearance and the primary tumor (lung and kidney have a higher incidence of fracture than prostate and breast). There are no biomechanical studies that relate the size and shape of bone defects to the reduction in structural strength in pathologic bone. The most common indications for fixation on impending pathological fractures are increasing pain and cortical destruction (pain is thought to be due to microfractures or to stretching of the periosteum by the increasing tumor size). Sim [2] recommends prophylactic fixation in well defined lytic lesions that are more than 3 cm in diameter and in which 50% or more of the cortex is destroyed. They also consider pain refractory to radiotherapy an indication for fixation. Mirels [5] developed a scoring system for assessing the risks of pathologic fractures in long bones, which takes into account: lesion type, size, site and associated pain. Even though there is no accurate way to predict the risk of fracture; we have found this scoring system useful. With better and earlier diagnosis and with advances and less aggressive surgical techniques and procedures of internal fixation, we are recommending prophylactic fixation in more cases, with smaller lytic lesions. It is technically easier, and results in less morbidity, to stabilize a pathologic bone before it fractures.

The goal of treatment is to prevent bone fracture, and to provide immediate and definitive pain-free usage of the limb, so as to preserve function and to improve quality of life. We have to aim at bringing back the patient to the pre-fracture state; early mobilization and ambulation will ease nursing care, and will shorten hospital stay (realizing life expectancy is short). Relief of pain is also an important goal. Achieving these goals will cause a positive psychological and emotional effect on the patient and their families. This stimulates a more aggressive approach to the management of these patients.

The management of long bone metastasis varies according to the patients' general conditions, the location of the lesion, the extent of bone compromise, and the primary bone tumor. A complete medical examination in order to evaluate the patient's general condition is very important before deciding the definitive management; surgery in general is safe in this group of seriously ill patients. The location of the metastasis, the extent of bone destruction, and the histologic appearance are also important considerations, and will help decide the type of fixation to be used. Since the estimated length of survival cannot be accurately established in this lesion, we do not believe it should be taken into account in deciding the treatment; most of these patients will benefit from surgical treatment.

Biomechanical Considerations

Recognized biomechanical principles used for fracture reduction and stabilization in normal bone do not apply to pathological fractures. In metastatic fractures due to the slow healing capacity of bone, the implants will have to assume a load-bearing role for an extended period of time; this will lead to implant failure if conventional implant fixation techniques are used, consequently different biomechanical guidelines should be applied in the treatment of pathological fractures.

Invasion of metastatic cells in long bones will alter the mechanical properties of bone tissue, this will reduce the ability of the involved bone to carry ordinary functional loads, which will end in failure and fracture. Bone weakness caused by metastatic lesions is generally more extensive than is evident in X-rays, and will decrease screw or intramedullary nail fixation purchase and strength. 50% of the mineral phase must be resorbed before change is evident in X-rays.

The surgical management should provide enough stability to allow immediate full weight bearing. We have to keep in mind that the treatment of these tumors is palliative and not curative (oncologic). Surgical techniques for stabilizing pathologic or impending fractures must be individualized for the area of involvement, the quality of bone, and the potential for involvement of adjacent soft tissue structures. Even though the biomechanical properties are different, implant devices used for pathological fracture fixation are similar to those used in regular fracture management, and include open reduction and internal fixation with plates and screws or endomedullary nails, arthroplasty, allograft plus internal fixation, tumor resection plus segmental bone spacers, and amputations. Fixation devices must be chosen with the understanding that bone union will be delayed or never achieved; in addition most of these patients are not strong enough to restrain themselves from weight bearing; due to these two factors the implant should be sufficiently strong to give the patient a definitive functional painless limb. The implant chosen will be the one that provides the best fracture stability under the individual circumstance. 96% of patients will achieve a good or excellent pain control after adequate fixation of long bone metastasis [6].

Since allograft replacements have yielded poor results in cases in tumor patients where immediate pain free weight bearing is the goal of treatment, this treatment modality has been abandoned for long bone metastasis.

Numerous authors [2, 7] have proved the advantages of using methyl methacrilate to augment the fixation. The technique recommended for diaphysis plating augmented with cement, consist of:

(1) tumor curettage
(2) cement insertion
(3) wait for hardening of the cement
(4) drill and tap through the cement as if it would be normal bone.

We do not recommend waiting until cement hardening in cases of insertion of a compression screw (DHS or DCS) nor in cases where an endomedullary nail has to be introduced. Care should be taken to avoid interpositioning cement between fragments in order to allow fracture healing.

The use of methylmetacrilate to reconstitute large bone defects permits most patients to bear weight immediately. Methylmetacrilate maintains excellent rigidity, especially when compressive load is applied, and is not adversely affected by radiation, nor by antibiotics.

Since the infection rate in these patients is high due to post-operative radiation or to the not-optimal medical general condition, some authors advocate the use of cement impregnated with antibiotics.

Even though the effectiveness of the insertion of chemotherapeutic agents into methylmetacrilate is still to be defined, the addition of an antiblastic drug to the acrylic cement may provide sterilization of the residual tumor cells by the local slow and prolonged release of the drug. This technique along with current anti-mitotic therapy may provide better local control of the neoplasic lesion.

Wedin et al. [8] in a retrospective study of 228 metastatic lesion of long bones treated by resection and reconstruction, intralesional curettage or stabilization only, found a local failure rate of 11%, and the median time to failure was eight months. Local failure was more common in lesion of the femur diaphysis and distal femur (20%), and in kidney cancer (24%). Osteosintesis had a failure rate of 14% while endoprosthesis only 2% (in proximal femur lesions). The most important risk factor for failure was long survival rate.

We favor post-operative rather than pre-operative radiation therapy whenever it is likely that internal fixation will be needed. Post-operative radiotherapy will decrease the risk of local tumor progression but adversely influences union in the absence of rigid internal fixation [9].

Even though surgical stabilization of these lesions is usually indicated, it is not without risks. Thromboembolic complications as well as wound infections risks are higher in these patients. Local as well as systemic dissemination of tumor cells after internal fixation has been proved by Peltier et al. [10]. The importance of the spread of tumor cells along the tract of an intramedullary rod has not outweighted the advantages of this operation.

Patients who have a highly vascular lesion, such as metastatic renal carcinoma (hypernephroma), may present a unique problem of uncontrollable bleeding, and should be treated with arterial embolization before surgery to decrease intraoperative complications.

Nonunion occurs in a high proportion of patients who undergo conventional doses of radiation, but most pathological fractures fixed with adequate internal fixation will heal despite of the adjuvant radiotherapy.

Amputation has few indications in bone metastasis; tumor fungation and infection (common in neglected primary bone tumors) as well as arterial occlusion are rare findings. Amputation is indicated in patients in whom surgical and radiotherapy treatments have failed to alleviate the pain in a functionless extremity, as well as in tumors with significant soft tissue or neurovascular involvement.

Femur

The femur is the most frequently long bone affected by metastasis. Approximately 50% of these lesions affect the proximal femur [11].

The aim of treatment is to obtain a painless limb, and to return the patient to his premorbid state. The decision whether to operate or not depends on the tumor type, location, size, and the patient's general condition. Nonoperative treatment for pathological or impending pathological femur fractures will be recommended only in patients who are not expected to survive a surgical insult, and treatment will consist of radiation, pain medication and immobilization.

Surgical treatment is indicated in most pathological or impending femur fractures. It should provide stable definitive fixation, and should allow immediate weight bearing. Unlike primary lesions, in metastatic lesions a complete tumor resection is not necessary.

Femoral Head and Neck

Due to the high stresses on the proximal femur as well as the low healing potential, replacement arthroplasty is usually recommended [7, 11–14]. Careful examination of the acetabulum should be done in these patients; the choice of hemiarthroplasty versus THA will be given by the involvement of the acetabulum. Commonly a long stem femoral component will be used to prophylactically reinforce the remaining proximal femur. Arthroplasties are always cemented. Even though prosthetic complications after tumor resections include a higher incidence of infections and dislocations, reconstruction based on endoprosthetic replacements as opposed to osteosynthetic devices are safer, and are associated with pronounced better results than osteosynthetic devices. Endoprostheses are not dependent in fracture healing which often is poor in patients with cancer because of systemic and local factors.

Internal fixation in this location has resulted in high failure rates (14 to 40%), and so are usually avoided; common reasons of failure include: poor initial fixation, improper implant selection, and progression of the disease within the operative field [8, 15].

Intertrochanteric Fractures

The treatment varies according to the involvement of the medial cortical bone (lytic lesions that occur in the region of the lesser trochanter are particularly prone to fracture); if these are nil or minimal we prefer ORIF with a compression screw or 95° blade plate, always augmented with cement. In order to prevent the screw cutting out of the femoral head, a lateral window should be opened in the lateral cortex, metastatic bone is removed from the neck of the femur, liquid cement is introduced in the defect, and the compression screw is placed before the cement hardens. The same technique is done when the screws are placed in the proximal femur diaphysis. From the biomechanical point of view, cefalomedullary (load-sharing) devices have proved to have some advantages over DHS since a more medial placement closer to the compression side of the femur and away from the lateral tension side is achieved, also this implants will prophylactically stabilize the rest of the bone, making it more durable.

If the calcar is involved significantly by bone metastasis, or in cases in which internal fixation has failed, or will not achieved a stable fixation due to tumor extension, a cemented, long stem calcar replacement prosthesis is recommended.

Subtrochanteric Fractures

Cefalomedullary devices (such as a long gamma nail) are the treatment of choice for most of these lesions. Cement augmentation is usually not necessary, since the biomechanical properties of these implants will give us stable internal fixation that will allow immediate weight bearing. These implants will also address the whole bone in case intracompartment spread of the tumor occurs. The largest nail possible should be used to fill the femoral canal. When the proximal femur has been weakened in such a way by metastatic disease, that a reconstruction nail is unable to provide stable fixation, or when previous fixation has failed, a cemented megaprosthesis is indicated.

Diaphyseal Fractures

The use of 4.5 mm dynamic compression plates with cement augmentation of this injuries has practically been abandoned by the good results obtained with conventional closed, and locked intramedullary nailing. The surgical technique is less invasive, and as previously stated these implants will protect the long bone in case bone disease progresses. Cephalomedullary devices are recommended when tumor progression is suspected.

Osteosynthetic implants are load sharing and ultimately will fail if the bone does not heal.

Supracondylar Fractures

This is the less frequent site of femur metastasis, and the most technically demanding to treat. These are the fractures with the highest reported failure rate post-operatively [8, 15]. If there is sufficient bone stock, conventional dynamic compression screw/plate devices (DCS) or a locking plate augmented with cement are usually recommended. Distal femoral replacement arthroplasty is also a viable option in lesions with massive destruction of femoral condyles.

Humerus

The humerus is the second most common long bone affected by tumor metastasis.

Complete fracture is more common in the humerus than in the femur or tibia; since the humerus is a non weight bearing bone, the patient does not experience load-related pain suggestive of fatigue before the bone actually fractures.

The treatment of these lesions should aim to restore the patient's function and to relieve pain. Conservative treatment of pathological or impending pathological fractures of the humerus has a more active role than it does in weight bearing bones. Even though each patient has to be individually planned, radiation therapy plus bracing will relieve pain, and might serve as definitive treatment in some terminally ill patients [2]. Overall analysis has shown few satisfactory results in patients treated nonoperatively for humeral fractures [17].

When bone destruction is so extensive that stability cannot be achieved by other methods, surgical treatment is indicated.

Proximal Humerus

Metastasis can be treated conservatively; radiotherapy usually achieves a good degree of pain control and acceptable degree of function. In cases where conservative treatment has failed shoulder resection arthroplasty is recommended. Although the range of motion is usually diminished, endoprosthetic replacement of the proximal humerus provides stability and a predictable and reliable method of reconstruction of the upper limb.

Humeral Diaphysis

If the patient's general condition allows, most diaphysis pathological fractures should be stabilized, particularly in patients who need their upper extremities for ambulation (crutches, cane). The implant of choice is an antegrade or retrograde locked humeral nail (depending on the fracture site and surgeon's preference). Even though augmentation with cement is usually not necessary, the indication of an open technique with tumor curettage, and cement augmentation is a viable option in some lesions. The nail not only stabilizes the fracture, but also acts as a prophylactic stabilizer in cases of the tumor spreading in the humerus. Even though open reduction and internal fixation with plates and screws augmented with cement is advocated by some centers, the bone quality is usually compromised and the screw purchase is poor; this technique has been replaced by the use of closed endomedullary nails [6, 7, 15].

Tumor resection plus humerus shortening and internal fixation is a viable option when a large segment of bone has been destroyed by the lesion.

Distal Humerus

Distal humerus metastases are rare and difficult to treat, unfortunately these lesions do not respond to radiotherapy as well as the proximal humerus does. Three options are available for surgical stabilization, and include: (a) tumor removal plus fixation with plates and screws augmented with cement, (b) tumor removal plus fixation with elastic endomedullary nails augmented with cement, or (c) elbow arthroplasty. Even though from the biomechanical point of view the dual plating technique with two 3.5 mm. reconstruction plates at 90° to each other is the most stable construct in nonpathological fractures, the poor quality of bone as well as the protection of the rest of the bone in case of tumor progression, has made the use of elastic endomedullary nails and cement through a posterior approach the treatment of choice. In cases with important joint infiltration

that have failed radiation therapy, a cemented elbow arthroplasty is the last option before amputation. Morrey et al. [16] reported good results in 13 prosthetic replacements for elbow tumors, six of which were metastatic lesions in the distal humerus.

Tibia

The tibia is not frequently involved in metastatic disease, and when it does occur, it is during the very end stage of the disease. Lung carcinoma is the most frequent primary tumor.

Unlike the femur the tibia can be adequately treated conservatively by radiotherapy plus bracing (PTB).

Surgical Treatment

Proximal Tibia

This is the most common site of lytic lesions in the tibia.

Tumor curettage plus internal fixation with plates and screws augmented with cement is an excellent option when there is no joint involvement. Tumor resection followed by arthroplasty is recommended in patients with tumor joint involvement as well as in tumor recurrence after previous surgical treatment. Preservation of the extensor mechanism is the most common problem encountered with this technique.

Diaphysis

These lesions have more effect on the mechanical strength of the bone. The use of tumor curettage plus cement, plus fixation with plates and screws is a viable option in isolated lesions with good surrounding bone, in more diffuse lesions the indication of an endomedullary nail is preferred. Unlike midshaft femur we believe that the stabilization should be augmented with cement either injected through the reamed medullary canal, or by curettage and cement packing through an open technique.

Distal Tibia

Very few reports of distal tibia metastasis have been published. The principles of distal tibia metaphysis treatment are the same as for proximal tibia, and include curettage plus cement and internal fixation.

Amputation is an indication that must be remembered in metastatic cases with large joint involvement of either the knee or ankle.

Radius and Ulna

Metastases of the forearm bones are very rare; only 0.4% of all metastatic bone lesions occur in the radius, and 0.2% occur in the ulna [18]. The most common primary origin is lung neoplasm; in general intramedullary nailing is the recommended treatment for most diaphiseal lesions. Tension band techniques may be helpful in repairing proximal ulnar lesions; if sufficient bone is present, plating and augmentation with metylmethacrylate can be used. Partial resection with shortening plus plate fixation could be an alternative if it does not produce an important functional deficit.

Something similar occurs with the clavicle and fibula, and distal ulna; in many cases resection of the metastasis is recommended. Resection surgery is used in patients considered to have a good prognosis for long survival, mostly patients with kidney cancer with limited metastatic disease.

In summary, although the clinical presentation may vary according to the patient, the tumor and location of the metastasis; the following surgical treatment guidelines are recommended: (1) cemented prosthesis in the proximal femur and humeral head fractures; (2) locked intramedullary nails for the femur, humerus, tibia and forearm diaphysis; (3) in other locations (proximal and distal methaphysis of long bones), combined osteosynthetic devices with cement; (4) wide resection in patients with long life expectancy.

Successful operative treatment is a feasible option in most pathological or impending fractures, and it depends on achieving a rigid and durable fixation with either internal fixation or prosthetic devices.

Post-operative adjuvant radiotherapy is indicated in most patients, to minimize disease progression and possible implant failure.

References

1. O'Connor MI. Symposium: metastatic bone disease. In: Program and abstracts of the 67th annual meeting of the American Academy of Orthopedic Surgeons; 15–19 March 2000; Orlando, USA.
2. Sim F. Diagnosis and management of metastatic bone disease: A multidisciplinary approach. New York: Raven Press; 1988.
3. Coleman R. Skeletal complications of malignancy. Cancer. 1997;80(suppl 8):1588–94.
4. Diel I, Solomayer E, Costa S. Reduction in new metastasis in breast cancer with adjuvant clodronate treatment. N Engl J Med. 1998;339:357–63.
5. Mirelis H. Metastasic disease in long bones: A proposed scoring system for diagnosing impending pathologic fractures. Clin Orthop. 1989;249:256–64.
6. Harrington K. Orthopedic surgical management of skeletal complications of malignancy. Cancer. 1997;80:1614–27.
7. Harrington K, Sim F, Enis J, Johnson J, Dick H, Gristina A. Methylmethacrilate as an adjunt in internal fixation of pathological fractures: experience with three hundred and seventy-five cases. J Bone Joint Surg Am. 1976;58:1047–55.
8. Wedin R, Bauer H, Wersäl P. Failures after operation for skeletal metastatic lesions of long bones. Clin Orthop. 1999;358:128–39.
9. Janjan N. Radiation for bone metastasis. Cancer. 1997;80:1628–44.
10. Peltier L. Theoretical hazards in the treatment of pathological fractures by the kuntscher intramedullary nail. Surgery. 1951;29:466–72.
11. Swanson K, Pritchard D, Sim F. Surgical treatment of metastasic disease of the femur. J Am Acad Orthop Surg. 2000;8(1):56–65.
12. Lane J, Sculco T, Zolan S. Treatment of pathological fractures of the hip by endoprosthetic replacement. J Bone Joint Surg Am. 1980;62:954–9.
13. Damron T, Sim F. Surgical treatment for metastatic disease of the pelvis and proximal end of the femur. ICL. 2000;49:461–70.
14. Aaron A. Treatment of metastatic adenocarcinoma of the pelvis and the extremities: current concepts review. J Bone Joint Surg Am. 1997;79:917–32.
15. Yazawa Y, Frassica F, Chao E, Pritchard D, Sim F, Shieves T. Metastasic bone disease: A study of the surgical treatment of 166 pathologic humeral and femoral fractures. Clin Orthop. 1990;251:213–9.
16. Sperling J, Pritchard D, Morrey B. Total elbow arthroplasty following resection of tumors at the elbow. Clin Orthop. 2000; (in press).
17. Lancaster J, Koman L, Gristina A. Pathologic fractures of the humerus. South Med J. 1988;81(1):52–5.
18. Sim F, Pritchard D. Metastatic disease in the upper extremity. Clin Orthop. 1982;169:83–94.

Adjuvant Therapy in Bone Tumors

38

Jaime Paulos

Abstract

Adjuvant therapy is used to fill cavities after curettage and to avoid recurrence in bone lesions. Several techniques have been used.

Keywords

Adjuvant therapy • Bone substitute • Bone graft

We consider adjuvant therapy as an adjunctive treatment which is performed secondary to primary surgical treatment (curettage) in aggressive or destructive benign tumors and tumor-like lesions. It is a therapy following the intralesional curettage of these lesions that does not ensure a complete microscopic residual tumor resection.

It is indicated in the following bone diseases:

- giant tumor cell stages 1 and 2 [1–5]
- aneurysmal bone cyst
- simple bone cyst
- fibrous displasia (focal)
- chondroblastoma
- chondrosarcoma low grade (unresectable due to location).

Usable adjuvant methods:

- high speed milling
- compacted milled graft filling (allo- or bone autograft)
- use of phenol in the cavity
- acrylic cement [5]
- liquid nitrogen (cryotherapy)
- bone substitutes
- radiotherapy.

High speed milling: after a thoroughly and careful curettage of the lesion, resection is complemented with a high speed small milling cutter, trying to eliminate the remaining cells in the walls of the lesion that may cause a recurrence of the lesion. This technique is usually associated with compacted bone graft.

Filling made with compacted crushed bone graft: this method is commonly used with two objectives: reduce the possibility of recurrence and also provide the scaffolding necessary for bone restitution. It is used together with an other adjuvant treatment to reduce the risk of recurrence.The best method is the morselized autograft which is removed from another surgical place of the same patient. Therefore allografts are nowadays taken from femoral heads of bone banks.

Phenol: this has been widely used to kill residual cells of the lesion. Literature shows a high effectiveness in terms of decreasing lesion recurrence. It has been less effective in cases of low-grade chondrosarcomas. The toxic phenol for intracavitary cells should be handled carefully to avoid damaging neighboring structures. Literature shows relapses of about 10%.

Acrylic cement: this method widely recommended by Professor Campanacci, Rizzoli Institute (Italy) [1, 2, 6], to fill the cavity with methyl methacrylate after curetage. Increasing temperature removes residual cells and the strength of the cement would give a firm structure and also it would be easier to detect any recurrence around the cement. The use of acrylic cement reduces the possibility of recurrence between 50 and 85%, versus 15% using only curettage.

Liquid nitrogen [7, 8]: its application has been recommended by some authors, but it must be used very carefully as it can highly produce tissue necrosis reaching temperatures of minus 200 degrees celsius limiting its use, considering the risk of damaging neighboring structures. The recurrence rate using it in giant cell tumors reaches only 2.3%.

J. Paulos (✉)
Pontificia Universidad Católica de Chile, Santiago, Chile
e-mail: paulos.jaime@gmail.com

© Springer-Verlag London Ltd., part of Springer Nature 2021
J. Paulos and D. G. Poitout (eds.), *Bone Tumors*,
https://doi.org/10.1007/978-1-4471-7501-8_38

Bone substitutes [9]: they are generally used instead of bone grafts in cavity filling. Depending on the degree of integration they have been effective filling bone cavities. Different products are made in different laboratories based on calciumphosphate $(Ca_3(PO_4)_2$ or hydroxoapathite $(Ca_{10}(PO_4)_6 (OH)_2$. Some labs use low doses of irradiation to decrease the inmunological effect of the graft.

Radiotherapy [10, 11]: in principle, it should not be used in benign lesions due to the risk of inducing sarcomas in the long term. However it is indicated as a palliative treatment for very aggressive lesions in unresectable anatomical locations.

References

1. Campanacci M, Baldini N, Boriani S. Giant cell tumor of bone. J Bone Joint Surg. 1987;69A:106–14.
2. Campanacci M, Capanna R, Fabbri N, Betelli G. Curettage of giant cell of bone: reconstruction with subchondral grafts and cement. Chir Organi Mov. 1990; LXXV(suppl 1):212–213.
3. Capanna R, Fabbri N, Betelli G. Curettage of giant cell tumor of bone. The effect of surgical technique and adjuvants on premises: recurrence rate. Chir Organi Mov. 1990; LXXV (suppl 1): 206.
4. Tomeno B, Forrest M. Tumeurs à cellules géantes. In: Duparc J, editors. Tumeurs Osseuses. Paris: Expansion Scientifique Française; 1994. p. 143–162.
5. Babinet A. Tumeur á cellules géantes: cahier d'enseignement of Sofcot. Paris: Elsevier SAS; 2005. p. 201–19.
6. Fraquet N, Faizon GP, Rosset BJM, Phillipeau ACD, Waast AF, Gouin AC. Traumatology orthopedics: surgery research long bones giant cells tumors: treatment curretage by cementation and cavity filling. 95(6): 402–406 (October 2009) Bone and Joint Unit, Hôtel Dieu teaching medical center, place A. Ricordeau, 44093 Nantes cedex, France B Department of Orthopedics, Hôpital Trousseau, Tours teaching medical center, Tours, France c EA3822, Inserm U957, Bone resorption physiopathology and primary bone tumors therapy, research laboratory, Faculty of Medicine, Nantes University, Nantes, France.
7. Malawer MM, Bickels J, Meller I, Buch RG, Henshaw RM, Kollender Y. Cryosurgery in the treatment of giant cell tumor: a long-term followup study. Washington Cancer Institute, Washington Hospital Center, Washington, D; 2010, USA. Clin Orthop Relat Res. 1999; February(359):176–88.
8. Marcove RC, Weis RH, Vaghaiwalla MR, Pearson R, Huvos AG. Cryosurgery in the treatment of giant-cell tumors of bones: a report of 52 consecutive cases. Cancer. 1978; 41:957–969.
9. Mainard D. Les substitu de l'os du cartilage et du menisque. Sofcot 1990 edit. Romillat.
10. Murray E, Werner D, Greeff E, Taylor D. Postradiation sarcoma: 20 cases and literature review. Int J Radiat Oncol Biol Phys. 1999;45:951–61.
11. Caudell JJ, Ballo MT, Zagars GK, Lewis VO, Weber KL, Lin PP, et al. Radiotherapy in the management of giant cell tumor of bone. Int J Radiat Oncol Biol Phys. 2003;57:158–65.

Reconstruction with Bone Graft and Porous Titanium

39

Dominique G. Poitout

Abstract

Bone grafts and porous titanium for reconstruction currently constitute the new advances in bone replacement. The history of the tissue bank in Marseille, how to prepare the graft, the differents types of bone and cartilage grafts are analyzed, including the use of porous titanium for massive endoprostheses.

Keywords

Bone bank • Bone graft • Porous titanium • Massive endoprostheses • Porous titanium implants

Introduction

Since the time of the Arab physicians Cosmas and Damien, men have tried to graft tissues or tissue groups to replace substance losses of massive tumors, whether traumatic or related to iterative interventions.

Attempts have been made to graft with animal bone, called xenografts, which had a rejection percentage of around 60%.

The story goes that a surgeon had transplanted a dog skull cap onto the skull of a Polish soldier with adequate consolidation.

Grafted humerus transplants and the human femur were attempted, as allografts, with variable results, and a significant number of sepsis cases were recounted.

Many authors have tried to improve the technical procedures and I would cite, for example, one who corresponds to the recent period, our colleague Professor Sicard, who created a bone bank and published much on this issue. I also include Professor Yves Gerard from Reims, Professor Franz Langlais from Rennes, Professor Philippe Chiron from Toulouse, Professor Bejui from Lyon, Professor Bonneviale from Bordeaux, and many others in France; including international boards like Professor Ottolenghi from Buenos Aires, Professor Gérard Mankin and Professor Gary Friedlander from Boston, Professor Rudiger Von Versen from Berlin, Professort Maurice Hinsenkamp and Professor Christian Delloye from Brussels, Professor Capana from Florence, and also Professor Moritoshi Itoman from Japan, Professor Yongjuth Vajaradul from Bangkok and many others.

Wishing to preserve human bone fragments for subsequent transplant, I visited in 1975 the center of blood transfusion which adjoined the Hospital of the Conception where I worked, and after discussion with the head of cryobiology services, Ms. Dr. Gisèle Novakovitch, we chose a technique already used to store white blood cells: tissue preservation by cryobiology, that is to say in liquid nitrogen at −196 °C.

Having no idea of what would happen to the bone and cartilage cells after thawing we made histological studies on these to determine which fall in temperature curve would give the best percentage of conservation of the vitality of the cells after thawing, and what was the best cryo-protecter avoiding intracellular ice formation microcrystals.

We then discussed the proposed techniques and surgical indications in oncology, trauma and during bone reconstruction after iterative operations.

Grafts used since the beginning of our experience are massive grafts preserved in the cold deep of the **bone bank of Marseille** (Fig. 39.1) and not secondarily sterilized.

This technique has given us excellent results that are substantiated with the survival and long-term integration of the grafts whether cortical bone, cancellous bone or cortical-cancellous bone.

If bone cells theoretically do not need to be preserved, the architectural structures of the bone must be preserved along

D. G. Poitout (✉)
Aix Marseille University, Marseille, France
e-mail: dominique.poitout@live.fr

© Springer-Verlag London Ltd., part of Springer Nature 2021
J. Paulos and D. G. Poitout (eds.), *Bone Tumors*,
https://doi.org/10.1007/978-1-4471-7501-8_39

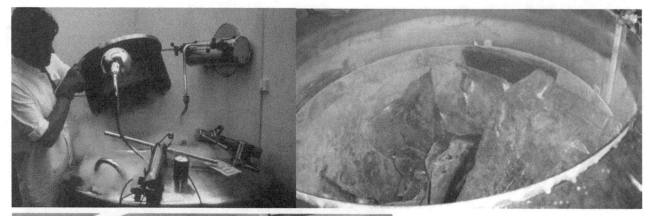

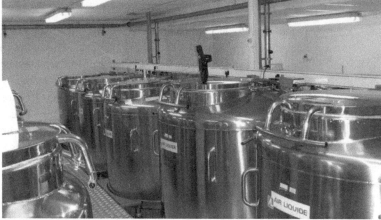

Fig. 39.1 Bone bank, Marseille, France

with the cartilage cells which they, not being replaced by cells of the host and that because of their collagen production which binds hydrophilic proteoglycans, the guarantor of cartilage turgor, must continue to ensure the same function long after the graft has been integrated into the bone.

Conservation Techniques

These techniques are critical to the proper storage of tissues and are critical to the integration thereof. Incomplete use of these techniques invariably results in destruction of graft tissues.

We chose from the beginning of our practice to keep allografts to −196 °C in liquid nitrogen after a four-hour soaking in a cryo-protector which is designed to prevent ice formation at macrocrysts inside cells.

Cryo-Preservatives: several products were tested at the beginning of our experience, but the 10% DMSO (dimethyl sulfoxide) penetrates best into the cells due to its low molecular weight and gives the best results regarding cells survivorship.

The 10% DMSO does not avoid ice microcrystal formations in the cell, but avoids them recombining into macro crystals, which themselves will burst the cell structures as do the other bone macrostructures.

This DMSO is toxic to the tissues at room temperature and must be cooled to less than 8 degrees to be contacted with the tissues themselves and must be refrigerated.

If the tissues are placed directly in a DMSO solution at room temperature there will be a cellular destruction and in the case of articular cartilage destruction of the graft.

DMSO has also an eutectic point that is around −60 °C. This means that this product, which prevents ice macrocrystals forming is especially effective below this temperature. Indeed even if liquid water is in very small quantities at these low temperatures, there still exists a little amount, and that DMSO has its eutectic point to −60 °C indicates that above this temperature it cannot prevent liquid water from turning into macro-ice crystals and thus destroying cells.

Freezers that reach a maximum temperature of −80 °C and should be monitored closely for any temperature rise (door opening, power failure) that can bring this product into its critical phase.

The decrease in temperature is also a determinant of cell conservation. One can not just dip the fabric in liquid nitrogen because it would be burned and destroyed. It must be protected and gradually down their temperature decrease.

A fall in temperature control is necessary so that the temperature falls slowly at first and then more rapidly.

The optimal curve is as follows: 2 °C per minute from +6 °C, then 5 °C per minute to −140 °C.

Then the fragment is placed in vapor nitrogen at −150 °C or directly in the tank of liquid nitrogen at −196 °C.

The effectiveness of this program of the temperature drop is confirmed by the percentage of surviving cells after thawing. Studies were carried out studying the survival of cartilage cells which were subjected to different cryo-preservative and shape descents temperature curves and variable speed.

Cell survival was demonstrated by their ability, after thawing, to fix the methylene blue and produce de novo proteoglycans [19].

The percentage of living cells after thawing was, according to the curves used from 20% to over 82% of living cartilage cells when we use the above methodology.

The Freezing: this is an important step in the conservation of bone and cartilage cells. It must, in contrast to the decrease in temperature, be performed fast so the cells quickly return to normal function and the ice macrocrystals cannot be formed.

Also the cells need to stay in warm saline or Ringer Lactate at 40 °C for about 30 min to allow the graft to get rid of toxic DMSO. The graft may be used on average in the hour following its extraction from the liquid nitrogen container.

In case it needs to be transported it can be thawed in the tissue bank if its use is within hours, or being thawed in the operating room, which seems to me to be preferable for reasons of technical convenience. The transport then takes place in a liquid nitrogen container or in a box containing dry ice. If you plan to use only a portion of the graft, it is possible, having changed your sterile coat and gloves, with new instruments and a specific and isolated operating table, to cut the still frozen graft and return to the container the unnecessary part of the graft, which will be used for another patient. (The bone fragments are so rare and valuable!).

Primary or Secondary Sterilization?

This has long been a subject of controversy [1]. The levies must be sterile, because if there are germs they will be frozen with drawdowns and will reactivate upon thawing.

Multi-organ harvesting is done in the operating room and as it is rare that simple bone samples are taken, there is every reason to take these bone samples in an orthopedic operating room.

To prevent contamination of the harvested bone, it is necessary to transfer the body to another sterile operating room, after other teams have finished.

The subject is again razed and rebuilt, the wall with iodine solution fields replaced as usual for orthopedic operation; new instruments are given to the surgeon.

Samples will be taken from each graft to eliminate the existence or even the mere risk of overt infection.

The Packaging of Grafts: this Is very important and Gambro plastic bags currently appear to be best suited to the preservation of grafts of different sizes in liquid nitrogen.

They are resistant, easy to seal off, do not salt out of toxic chemicals and are resistant to handling and deep cold. Their structure allows us to introduce more cryopreservative and antibiotics.

In order to easily handle the graft in the operating room after thawing or current thereof, two sterile bags placed one on the other allow the sterile handling of the second bag which contains the graft without major difficulties.

The femoral heads, spongy tissue sources, are as they have been collected in sterile plastic boxes and placed in small bags in the Gambro Bone Bank after preparation.

Irradiation of Grafts: never seemed to be a method to remember.

Indeed, for the sterilization to be effective it is necessary to achieve a dose of radiation B or Y of at least 2.6 Mrad, which is the legal dose in France. But this dosage should be higher if one is in the presence of products located in the pasty phase in a frozen aqueous solution as is the case with frozen grafts.

It is easier to perform the irradiation of fresh tissue, but we must wait to have enough and it is difficult to keep bones and especially the cartilage in good condition for several hours or days!

Otherwise, we must accept to freeze the bone, then to thaw and then irradiate and then refreeze. We would not accept that such operations was carried out on our food, neither on those bones used for human transplants!

Also, if one is interested in irradiation sterilization mechanisms of action we note that the rays are effective either when they destroy RNA molecules or viral DNA by direct impact or processing by liquid periviral, so it takes large doses of electrons or ionizing radiation to destroy any viral particles, especially intracellular ones.

Destruction of viruses will never be total and although only a percentage, albeit increasingly important viruses can destroy the cells, increasing the radiation dose helps, but the danger will always remain and radiation does have its prohibitive doses that may be used to sterilize the room.

The protein chains constituting the architecture of the bone and cartilage as well as all the cartilage cells will be destroyed and the graft will become a piece of inert chalk.

With cartilage, the cells will be destroyed, cannot retain their water molecules and due to immunological reactions in connection with the widening of the meshes of the surface layer will disintegrate quickly as osteoarthritis and instability.

It should not then be surprising that the graft so treated does not integrate into the structures on which it is grafted and it disintegrates gradually, unlike grafts simply kept in the deep cold without adding secondary sterilization.

These two types of grafts are very different and can in no way be compared in quality.

Heat Sterilization does not seem to be a recommended method for bone fragments that bear heavy loads.

If the sterility of the grafts by this method is not questionable, the method used results in destruction of all cells and clotting of the whole protein architecture that is thus destroyed.

One cannot therefore use these grafts in areas subject to constraints, and cancellous grafts treated this way will be used only in the case of filling bone cysts or small losses of substances; also for osteosyntheses.

Other methods have been proposed but they have mostly not proven their effectiveness both in the field of mechanical strength (freezing) or their integration (ceramization).

The use of supercritical CO_2 appears to be an interesting method of research, but it is not yet used in clinical practice.

Surgical Indications

The grafts can be used in different circumstances depending on their nature.

The lack of opportunity to perform ostéoformatrice activity for these plugins should be emphasized, since they are made of dead bone.

The material to be grafted, will always graft a devascularized bone fragment that can at best only be a frame and a support to the recolonization of the host cells.

Sponge Grafts are primarily used:

- for attic losses of small-volume substances
- to complete an insufficient volume of autologous grafts (Papineau)
- especially as corners of osteotomies (femoral or tibial)
- and as fillers in acetabular reconstructions with or without total hip replacement.

The Cortical Grafts: it may be necessary to rebuild:

- a vertebral body and it especially will use a portion of the femoral neck

- a shaft fragment to replace a traumatic loss substance
- a more or less substantial portion of the upper or lower end of a long bone
- (femur, tibia, humerus... after traumatic loss of substance).

The Corticocancellous Grafts:

- are extremely useful to rebuild
- the acetabular cup when largely destroyed
- basin, both in the iliac wing as part of the shutter
- epiphyseal and metaphyseal of long bones when you can keep the articular cartilage.

The Osteocartilaginous Transplants: these are used more frequently in place of metal prostheses, either:

- The knee is the favorite place of the use of cartilage allografts to overcome more or less spongy tissues. Reconstructions of cartilaginous fragments condyle, trochlea or tibial plateau has become in a few years of current use and give excellent results remotely.
- At the acetabulum, the use of bone and cartilage fragments more or less voluminous avoids the introduction of metal prostheses and fits quite satisfactorily without clinical or radiological signs of osteoarthritis appearing [2–4].
- The tibial pilon can also be replaced by a massive osteochondral graft often with excellent functional outcome. But the joints of the upper limbs, due to the absence of stresses acting on it, and joint laxity that occurs, do not give the expected results.

The Capsular, Ligament and Tendon Grafts: these grafts pose the problem of revascularization and therefore the end of their mechanical strength due to their elasticity or their necrosis.

Indeed, the grafts having a portion of capsule or ligament attached to the bone and reattached the ligaments or bone of the recipient, seem initially during the months of their introduction, to provide good stability to the joint.

But because of the absence of vascularization, or its necrosis, they progressively distend which is a source of joint laxity and thus alteration of the cartilage due to the progressively unphysiological joint function.

The only exception seems to be the patellar tendon that attaches firmly to the anterior tibial tuberosity and thus enables strong sutures on the extensor apparatus of the recipient.

It is certainly much better to reattach, when possible, ligaments or capsule of the recipient of the allograft than the

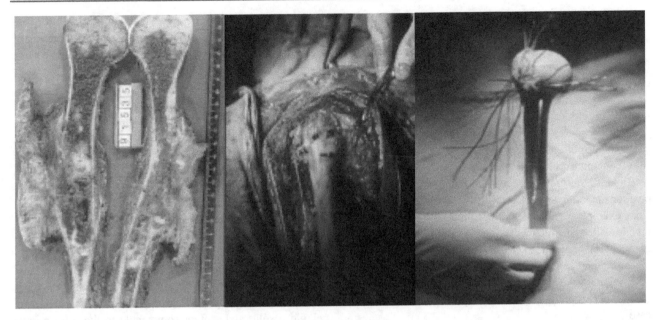

Fig. 39.2 Humeral chondrosarcoma, reconstruction with an osteocartilaginous graft

reverse, that is to say the ligaments or capsule allograft bone on the recipient.

As for the use of preserved tendons they also do not have sufficient mechanical strength to be used alone.

It is therefore necessary when using ligaments, tendons or capsules, to keep doubling the outset with an artificial ligament which will probably break within five years after their introduction, but will have protected their revascularization and their distension.

Terms of Osteosynthesis

It is important when one wants to do a study on the future of grafts to study well the osteosynthesis the arrangements made and analyze the quality of contact between the host bone and allograft and stability mounting, as well as the muscular environment thereof.

Indeed, if the contact between the bone ends is not perfect there will be no creeping substitution but formation of a non-union.

An intramedullary nail, the tail of a prosthesis or a compressing plate will have the best contact if the bone cuts are perfectly congruent.

If an area of the graft is not protected by a nail or plate, we will see the occurrence of fracture of the graft to the bone-plate junction.

If an osteocartilaginous graft will be necessary in addition to grafting a cryo-preserved cartilage (Fig. 39.2), a well vascularized bed is needed in order to achieve union.

The spongy tissue integrates very quickly if the summary is correct; much faster than cortical bone due to its structure, and will add a lot more time to be penetrated by vessels and host cells.

Often when talking about complications (graft fractures, non-union, lysis etc.) they are in fact related to a deficit of osteosynthesis material and poor installation. The graft is often there for nothing!

Outcomes

The transplanted tissue: bone graft; immunology: only the architecture of the bone is grafted. And bone marrow cells have been or will be destroyed. It does not mean that inflammatory reactions and rejection reactions will be nonexistent.

They are found in approximately 9% of cases and especially when you transplant a large amount of tissues as are the synovial or capsule and ligaments (slightly less).

These immunological rejection phenomena, are sometimes confused with an infection of the graft. They translate into effect by a peri-osseous serous effusion sometimes abundant resulting in cutaneous fistula.

This sometimes very productive fistula accompanies the occurrence of a gradual lysis of the graft.

If bacteriological samples are taken from the cutaneous fistula you may find germs that are actually related to the outbreak of cutaneous saprophytic germs. The deep surgical samples are sterile and the liquid contains HLA nonspecific immune groups.

Immunosuppressive therapy such as sandimum like chemotherapy used in the treatment of sarcomas reduce or stop the demonstrations.

Biology: the graft once it is thawed and fixed in correct position in intimate contact with the bone of the recipient (for example cement without interposition) and the junction-allograft recipient bone autografts sleeved, will gradually integrate the skeleton especially if it is surrounded by a muscular sleeve of good quality.

Eventually we will not see the connection between the host bone and graft. This is what we found in 89.8% of our cases.

Indeed the graft vascularization will come from adjacent muscles and the microvessels will enter directly into the superficial portion of the cortex, perpendicularly thereto.

A pseudo-periosteum will surround the graft. It will also surround the ruginer if we want to remove an osteosynthesis material.

This concept is particularly advantageous with regard to the reattachment of certain muscles on the graft (such as the gluteus medius).

This muscular reattachment by removing the peri-prosthetic chamber decreases the lever arm which existed at the junction between a solid metal reconstruction prosthesis and its tail fixed in the bone.

The loosening of the prosthetic stem is exceptional: a mere 1.2% and we have not observed breaking of a reconstruction prosthesis.

Biomechanics [12]: when using frozen bones, even after thawing they are harder but more fragile than normal bone (110 to 125%) so we must be very careful when performing a bore for introducing a intramedullary nail or the drilling a screw hole.

The introduction of the intramedullary nail or stem of the prosthesis must be very low friction if one does not break the bank bones abruptly.

In the case of using a bone bank manchonnant reconstruction prosthesis it seems to be necessary to cement the prosthesis as in the bank of bones in the bone of the recipient.

The use of a prosthesis coated with hydroxyapatite and uncemented is anathema since there is no revascularization of the intra-medullaire part of the bone and therefore no possibility of fixing the prosthesis on the bone death and likely to remain so for some time.

In the 8–18 months after transplantation, the graft goes-through a decline phase of its strength due to penetration of the vessels in the superficial layers of the graft. We must recommend caution to patients who will eventually take over canes.

It takes two years after the graft before it begins to be well integrated into the bone of the recipient. This integration is, however, and for a very long time, very superficial. Only after several years we will be sure of the strength of the limb. The removal of the material cannot be practiced, if it is absolutely necessary, after the fifth year.

Some authors have noticed a gradual lysis of the graft after a few years (particularly in the pelvis). It should be noted that these grafts are generally grafts secondarily sterilized by irradiation or heat.

These grafts whose architecture was destroyed do not possess sufficient mechanical strength to withstand the loads applied to them and do not give the host cells a chance to rebuild a solid architecture comparable to that of a normal bone.

This finding made us persist in the way of conservation of sterile grafts taken in liquid nitrogen without any secondary sterilization method.

Cartilaginous Grafts

Immunology

The cartilage may be grafted if grafted in full, if its cells are not destroyed, and if the hydrophilic proteoglycans are maintained. It is this turgor which decreases the size of the surface pores of the cartilage and prevents immunologically competent macroglobulins to penetrate in this cartilage and destroy chondrocytes.

Since healthy cartilage is avascular, it does not induce any immunological reaction of rejection.

Biology: not requiring vascularization to survive, and chondrocytes included in the cartilage with a turnover of several hundred years, cartilage guard structure and mechanical is quite amazing provided that its cells are maintained during conservation episodes.

The method we use gives about 80% of cell survival, which retrieves a satisfactory cartilage thickness.

The cells contained in the cartilage we find during endoscopic biopsies or when material ablation are the cells initially grafted as no host cell can come to colonize outside (avascular tissue).

Biomechanics: young and healthy cartilage is turgid due to the large amount of water molecules attached to glycoaminoglycans located in the fundamental substance of that particular tissue.

The transplant of a complete cartilage portion with its various structures is therefore a necessity and special cells are responsible to fix these water molecules on glyco-proteins.

It is also vital to ensure that the joint biomechanical condition is perfectly respected as with any abnormality, such as at the onset of joint laxity, the cartilage is destroyed very quickly, much faster than a normal cartilage.

Hence the need to double the graft ligaments by artificial ligaments during the phase of revascularization.

The isolated cartilage transplants and partial osteochondral grafts give excellent results (condyle, trochlea, tibial plateau) in more than 97.4% of cases.

The full-thickness grafts of a part of the joint gives variable results depending on the secondary stability of the joint.

When you can keep ligaments recipient stability is generally excellent in 96% of cases.

When surgeons could not keep the ligaments or the capsule of the recipient, it took a half-graft articulation with its own ligaments that were reattached to the bone of the recipient, the results futures were much worse with only 58% good results.

When we had to practice a rebuild of two parts of a joint with ligaments, the bone healing was set but gained joint instability which forced us to practice a new ligament or a constrained prosthesis in over 87% of cases.

Regarding the transplants in the upper limb (shoulder, elbow). We had only a few good results; often some complication, such as dislocation, prompted us to perform an additional procedure such as an arthroplasty or even an amputation.

Acetabular articular allograft as femoral heads with a frozen articular cartilage have given us excellent results when the dimensions of the articular surfaces were perfectly concordant.

Allografts of the upper femur paired with well-frozen femoral heads gave us great results with pain relief and without loss of cartilage or fracture in the 11 cases we operated.

Complications

When considering the evolution of the grafts outside the complications of the disease treated, it is found that they are integrated quite satisfactorily in over 85% of cases.

Immunological: there is ultimately little own pathology using a graft outside immunological risk (9% of cases). These phenomena often result in serous peri-osseous fluid effusions which can make us believe an infection exists especially in cases of cutaneous fistula, but that is not the case and we simply prescribe immunosuppressive therapy.

Sepsis: these infections are not more frequent in cases of establishment of the immune response.

Fractures and Pseudarthroses of a Graft: in case of establishment of a solid metal prosthesis after extensive tissue resection and protraction (approximately 2.4% of cases).

The graft fractures are related, such as non-union, to and insufficient fixation or the use of inappropriate materials (2% of cases).

Osteoarthritis and Joint Destruction: if the joint is rebuilt and is stable and if the ligaments are good and avoid the occurrence of laxity, articular cartilage will behave quite normally and maintain its thickness and function; if it is not the case it will lead to excessive pressure and to quick destruction and osteoarthritis.

This osteoarthritis is often insensitive or painless due to the lack of innervation of transplanted tissue.

It is however not as a joint tabetic since on the contrary in lesions of tertiary syphilis, only the bones are not innervated. Adjacent tissue, capsule, ligaments, muscles, tendons, subcutaneous tissue and skin have their normal innervation and allow the patient to "feel" their articulation.

In cases of massive joint destruction, a prosthesis is often necessary in the lower limbs (78%). At the elbow there is often (92%) joint dislocation which is sometimes well tolerated and does not justify complementary therapeutic methods.

All total joint transplants, using the ligament allograft, were disrupted and had to be replaced more or less in the short term, with total joint replacements.

However partial grafts which were reattached with ligaments of the recipient were, in order, well integrated and are currently still quite functional.

Infectious Pathology: when one has to deal with an infectious disease, we must first conduct a complete removal of all infected or necrotic tissue and any metal equipment.

This removal is generally very demanding and requires active patient cooperation as they will often remain several months in traction.

The establishment of a cement spacer containing antibiotic is not indicated because only superficial antibiotics are salted and there is more bacteriolytic activity so that the spacer becomes a foreign body that could sustain the infection.

Once the infection is under control we can consider replacing a bulky equipment as shown by a massive prosthesis sleeved by an equally massive bone graft.

Moreover, when reconstruction material is difficult to maintain due to the retraction of musculo-fascial masses, an inflatable balloon, placed in situ will keep stability instead of the future implant.

If one is not patient enough to replace an implant when the VS is lower than 20 and it is the first time PCR and less than 5; we generally obtained an excellent result which is maintained over time.

Indications: when there is a significant loss of substance, we have several opportunities to rebuild the skeleton, either after completing the removal of a bone tumor, in order to rebuild a loss of traumatic or post-operative substance:

A Papineau (technical or induced membrane) that associates after the establishment of an intramedullary nail or more usually an external fixator. *Autologous transplantation of allogeneic grafts* (not more than 50%) if the amount of autologous graft is insufficient. These techniques used a few years ago are long and require great patience on the part of the patient and also the surgeon!

This technique avoided a number of amputations at a price of functional sequelae sometimes incompatible with walking.

A vascularized autograft (vascularized fibula or iliac wing with its pedicle) may, especially in children, allow the reconstruction of a loss of some important bone in excellent conditions. These vascularized bone fragments often integrate well and gradually grow with the growth of the bone. However fractures are sometimes feared, if too early resumption of weight bearing goes unprotected.

A massive allograft may be indicated when the defect is important for an adult in cases of traumatic injury. It will first cover the skin defect with a vascularized myocutaneous flap and connected end-to-side on a artery proximity control after the member of vascularization occurs through several venous and arterial pedicles of sufficient size. Secondarily, when the flap has been well taken (three months later) they consider the takeoff and introduce into the bone bed a massive allograft that has to be fixed with an intramedullary nail and more than one or two plates that promote less revascularization of the graft.

When bone reconstruction follows a tumor resection [1, 5–11] or during multiple operations, you must first perform an accurate adaptation of the graft (or porous titanium prosthesis) and secure it so that the patient can quickly walk around in full support.

Discussion

When addressing massive allografts, with stakeholders often using techniques very different from each other, we notice that we are not necessarily talking about the same tissue

The grafts in place are indeed not the same if they were lyophilized, irradiated, heated or frozen.

They are not even the same if they were frozen at room temperature without cryoprotectant, without a gradual drop in temperature, without protection from antibiotics, and thawed without precautions.

They can not be compared if the establishment of techniques has been approximate and insufficient. If contact with the host bone is not perfect, consolidation will not happen and non-union appears often, causing secondary rupture mounting hardware.

And again we can not blame a graft festering if it was not taken with sterile precautions.

These therapies are an important contribution for gross pathology. There is currently no other sustainable option for replacing lost very important substance; these are not the substitutes of massive bone metal prostheses which will be able to replace a massive graft.

These anatomic allografts make possible a perfect reconstruction of the skeleton and achieve a quick resumption of walking which is often of excellent quality.

Moreover these processes that are heavy to put in place and are expensive, become profitable in the establishment of a transplant that costs about ten times less than custom-made metal prostheses.

It is necessary to keep in mind that although functionally joint upper limb grafts are considered by some patients as satisfactory, due to the absence of sufficient biomechanical stresses on the upper limb, there are often complications from the second to third years.

Methods for the conservation and freezing of grafts has allowed us to return to these techniques in the modern era.

When we speak of allo-transplants and their future, we should always have in mind the circumstances in which they were used and their results should be compared to the techniques that would be proposed to treat this patient.

In the lower limb, the grafts fit well and allow to obtain a satisfactory function very often.

With complete joint transplants, because of poor integration and insufficient mechanical strength of ligaments and capsule, joint stability can decline, which is a leading source of instability or long term destruction of joint cartilage, but then we can only use a small prosthetic resurfacing.

Regarding meniscal allografts and nerve allografts, we have not yet sufficient experience to express our opinion.

The Porous Titanium Implants

Bone grafts, however, are sometimes very difficult to obtain and it is certainly the most powerful obstacle to the development of techniques using allografts.

That is why we planned to complete our range of equipment for reconstruction of a series of metal prostheses.

Porous titanium perfectly reproduces the anatomy of the subject and the porosity is anatomically reconstructed.

Basin prostheses, acetabulum, femur, knee or simple diaphyses were conducted by companies like Adler Lima (Fig. 39.3).

The pore size is reproduced according to the desires of the surgeon and the local anatomy (scanner of the contralateral bone).

The aim is to be placed in the same conditions as when using a massive allograft (especially for rebuilding a hemi pelvis or acetabulum) that is to say, to have the opportunity to perform the bone cuts directly in the operating room to perfectly fit the graft or prosthesis which has the defect that needs to be replaced (Fig. 39.4).

The porous titanium is very easily cut with a diamond circular saw speed steel and its porosity allows the fixing of the prosthesis to the bone recipient by means of screws or plates fixed in the receiving bone.

The titanium pores are filled with autologous bone taken by RIA in the femur or tibia ipsilateral. This tissue comprises bone-forming mesenchymal stem cells which reconstruct the bone quickly within the titanium architecture (Fig. 39.5).

The strength of these prostheses is comparable, due to their conformation, to that of cortical bone, which was confirmed by biomechanical studies; which allows a restoration of early patient load (three to five post-operative days).

Of the 20 completed clinical cases (especially in the pelvis) with a decline which reached six years now we have had a mechanical complication associated with poor design of the femoral prosthetic tail; all other cases were perfectly well integrated.

We choose this as an indication of expensive equipment primarily for oncological surgery for which we do not expect the integration of the graft or reattachment of the muscles on the prosthesis.

Conclusions

These building techniques of massive bone allografts or prosthetic substances by porous titanium, shaped on-site in the operating room, allow us to obtain customized prostheses, which are massive but fit perfectly well to the anatomy

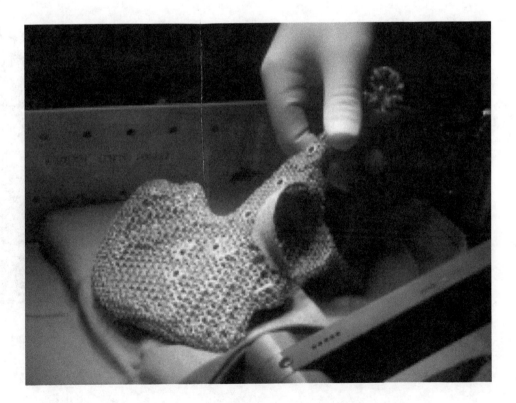

Fig. 39.3 Hemipelvis in porous titanium

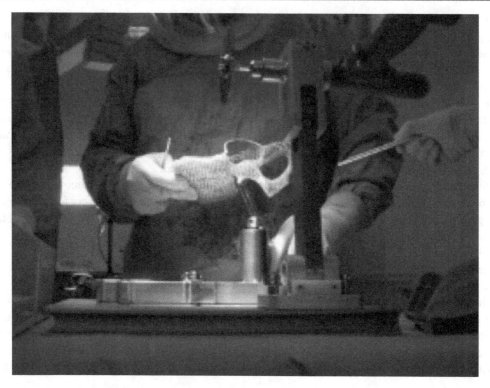

Fig. 39.4 Intraoperative preparation of the porous titanium prosthesis

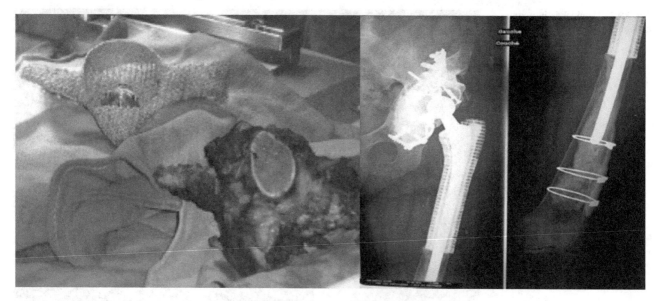

Fig. 39.5 Left porus titanium prosthesis, acetabular and proximal femur with cemented hipprosthesis

of the patients and allow them to regain a satisfactory function in a very short time.

References

1. Jeys LM, Kulkarni A, Grimer RJ, Carter SR, Tillman RM, Abudu A. Endoprosthetic reconstruction for the treatment of musculoskeletal tumors of the appendicular skeleton and pelvis. J Bone Joint Surg Am. 2008;90(6):1265–71.
2. Simon MA, Springfield D, Conrad EU, et al. Surgery for bone and soft-tissue tumors. Philadelphia, PA: Lippincott-Raven; 1998.
3. Avedian RS, Haydon RC, Peabody TD. Multiplanar osteotomy with limited wide margins: a tissue preserving surgical technique for high-grade bone sarcomas. Clin Orthop Relat Res. 2010;468 (10):2754–64.
4. Enneking WF, Dunham WK. Resection and reconstruction for primary neoplasms involving the innominate bone. J Bone Joint Surg Am. 1978;60(6):731–46.
5. Donati D, Di Bella C, Frisoni T, Cevolani L, DeGroot H. Alloprosthetic composite is a suitable reconstruction after periacetabular tumor resection. Clin Orthop Relat Res. 2011;469 (5):1450–8.
6. Ueda T, Kakunaga S, Takenaka S, Araki N, Yoshikawa H. Constrained total hip megaprosthesis for primary periacetabular tumors. Clin Orthop Relat Res. 2013;471(3):741–9.
7. Bell RS, Davis AM, Wunder JS, Buconjic T, McGoveran B, Gross AE. Allograft reconstruction of the acetabulum after resection of stage-IIB sarcoma: Intermediate-term results. J Bone Joint Surg Am. 1997; 79(11):1663–1674.
8. Aponte-Tinao L, Farfalli GL, Ritacco LE, Ayerza MA, Muscolo DL. Intercalary femur allografts are an acceptable alternative after tumor resection. Clin Orthop Relat Res. 2012;470(3):728–34.
9. Raskin KA, Hornicek F. Allograft reconstruction in malignant bone tumors: indications and limits. Recent Results Cancer Res. 2009;179:51–8.
10. Jamshidi K, Mazhar FN, Masdari Z. Reconstruction of distal fibula with osteoarticular allograft after tumor resection. Foot Ankle Surg. 2013;19(1):31–5.
11. Langlais F(1991). In: Limb salvage: major reconstructions in oncologic and nontumoral conditions 5th international symposium, St. Malo ISOLS-GETO. Berlin: Springer-Verlag; 1991.
12. Poitout D. Biomechanics and biomaterials in orthopedics. London: Springer-Verlag; 2016.

Sacral Surgery

40

Peter Rose

Abstract

Sacrectomy is presented to cure sacral malignancies. Indications and contraindications are evaluated. Pre-operative and surgical planning with detailed steps of the anterior and posterior approach is described. Spinopelvis reconstruction with the preferred method of the author, the cathedral technique, is detailed. Finally, post-operative care and analysis of results are presented.

Keywords

Sacral tumors · Sacrectomy · Cathedral technique

Oncologic sacrectomy is a necessary treatment for cure in many primary sacral malignancies. Surgery in these areas is very difficult as a wide oncologic margin can be challenging to achieve because of the direct proximity of neurologic, vascular, and visceral structures (particularly the rectum). As well, high sacrectomy disrupts spinopelvic continuity and may require a significant skeletal reconstruction.

This chapter will address techniques of en bloc sacral resection. The techniques described may be adapted for less aggressive/intralesional techniques for treatment of benign conditions which arise in the sacrum.

Indications

Sacrectomy is indicated in the treatment of primary sacral malignancies with no evidence of distant metastases in which the surgery is anticipated to be curative. Rarely, sacrectomy may be indicated in patients with refractory, aggressive benign tumors (e.g., recurrent giant cell tumor of the sacrum) or if the sacrum is involved by direct extension of pelvic visceral tumors without evidence of metastatic

spread. The most common indication in this category is primary or recurrent colorectal carcinoma with sacral involvement by direct extension with no nodal or distant metastases.

Contraindications

The inability to obtain a wide oncologic margin is a contraindication to sacrectomy. The tumors which are treated in this technique generally require wide resection for cure; if a wide resection cannot be done, it is difficult to justify the morbidity of such a large procedure with an unclear oncologic benefit. That said, compound resections with associated en bloc removal of the rectum, bony pelvis, urogenital, and vascular structures may be pursued to obtain an en bloc tumor resection.

Similarly, in the presence of metastatic disease is a strong relative contraindication for sacrectomy. Barring rare circumstances, these patients are unlikely to achieve cure, and palliative therapy is generally recommended in their care.

Lack of patient acceptance of the procedure is a frequent contraindication to sacrectomy. Depending upon the level of neurologic resection, sacrectomy may require loss of bowel, bladder, sexual, and potentially ambulatory function in patients. Many patients hesitate to proceed with such aggressive surgery given the significant impact on their quality of life.

Finally, medical fitness for surgery is an important consideration in planning oncologic sacral surgery. The nutritional status of the patients is often compromised by the presence of their malignancy as well as disfunction of their lower gastrointestinal tract from the effects of their tumor. Neutropenia is commonly seen in patients who are on chemotherapy and must be reversed prior to surgery. Finally, the stress of the surgery is so great that cardiovascular fitness is a major concern in the pre-operative evaluation of patients. At our institution, a dobutamine stress echocardiogram or

P. Rose (✉)
Mayo Clinic, Rochester, MN 55905, USA
e-mail: Rose.Peter@mayo.edu

© Springer-Verlag London Ltd., part of Springer Nature 2021
J. Paulos and D. G. Poitout (eds.), *Bone Tumors*,
https://doi.org/10.1007/978-1-4471-7501-8_40

equivalent is performed on any patient undergoing consideration for high or total sacrectomy who has preexisting cardiovascular disease or in men over the age of 40 and women over the age of 50.

Pre-operative Evaluation

Pre-operative evaluation begins with proper staging of patients to identify the systemic extent of their disease. Staging for sacral malignancies includes a CT scan of the chest, abdomen, and pelvis, an MR scan of the tumor itself, and a technetium bone scan of the entire skeleton.

There is increasing enthusiasm for positron emission tomography (PET) in the staging of patients with malignancies. We do not routinely employ it at our institution as many patients requiring sacrectomy will have chordoma or chondrosarcoma, and the use of a PET scan is not currently validated in the evaluation of these disease processes.

If staging confirms disease which is isolated to the sacrum, a biopsy is then performed. Biopsy is best performed using CT guidance with a large bore needle inserted directly into the tumor mass in a mid-line or near mid-line approach. It is important that the biopsy be directed by the surgeon who will be taking care of the ultimate malignancy as poor biopsy can easily compromise patient function and oncologic outcome. The biopsy should be planned to appropriately sample the tumor but also minimize contamination of associated soft tissues and the epidural compartment to decrease the risk that a biopsy will spread the tumor.

Once the histology is confirmed, adjuvant treatment is initiated as appropriate.The most common tumors subject to sacrectomy include chordoma, chondrosarcoma, and osteosarcoma. There is currently not an established role for chemotherapy in the treatment of chordoma and chondrosarcoma; the role of conventional radiation therapy is similarly not well defined in the treatment of these tumors [1]. There may be a role for proton beam therapy in the management of sacral malignancies; however, this role is currently in evolution and varies between different institutions.

Local tumor imaging is accomplished with the use of contrast-enhanced MR sequences. Imaging is obtained in three planes (axial, sagittal, and coronal oblique images). The coronal oblique images, which provide coronal images in the plane of the sacrum, are very useful in detecting subtle foraminal extension of tumor. CT angiography is used to assess vascular involvement (Fig. 40.1).

As described above, patients undergo extensive medical testing to determine their fitness for surgery. All patients complete a bowel preparation pre-operatively to minimize rectal contents and the extent of contamination which will occur if the rectum is inadvertently entered at the time of surgery.

Surgical Planning

Oncologic sacrectomy is planned with a goal of a minimum 1-centimeter free bony margin at the site of osteotomy as well as fascial margins containing the tumor in all other planes. The biopsy tract is excised en bloc with the tumor, highlighting the need for careful placement and execution of the biopsy.

Provided there is no rectal involvement, tumors which extend up to the S2-3 vestigial disk (implying an osteotomy through the level of the S2 neuroforamen) are resected from a posterior approach provided that the gluteal vessels are free on pre-operative imaging. Resections at this level do not require bony reconstruction; however, soft tissue flaps are used to help with closure and reconstruction of the posterior pelvic wall. Lesions approach purely posterior utilize bilateral gluteal V-Y advancement flaps.

Resections higher than the level of the S2 neuroforamen or in cases where a compound resection of the pelvic viscera will take place are approached through staged anterior and posterior approaches. In these cases, an anterior approach is used for visceral mobilization, ligation of the hypogastric vessels, anterior pelvic osteotomies, and harvest of a pedicled vertical rectus abdominous flap.

A colostomy is usually formed in the anterior procedure as resections of this nature predictably erase bowel continence.

Approximately 48 h later, posterior tumor resection is performed with associated spinopelvic reconstruction as indicated. The soft tissue defect is closed using a vertical rectus abdominous flap which is pulled through from its position following anterior harvest [4].

Unless the rectum is completely devascularized, the anterior and posterior stages of resection are separated by 48 h. When a spinopelvic reconstruction is necessary (described below), allograft fibula struts are used in the majority of patients. If the patient has had pre-operative radiotherapy, consideration is given to the use of vascularized fibula autografts. This significantly increases the complexity of the surgical procedure however.

In patients undergoing an anterior approach, bilateral external ureteral stents are placed to minimize the risk of ureteral injury around the time of surgery. An inferior vena cava filter is considered pre-operatively in patients undergoing posterior only resection and placed between the anterior and posterior stages of patients undergoing combined resections. This filter device is removed approximately four to six months following surgery when patients are predictably mobilizing well.

All patients are sent to the intensive care unit following their procedures. Most patients will extubate following an anterior procedure but many will require intubation

> > >

ЇЇЇЇ ЇЇЇЇЇЇ ЇЇ ЇЇ

following a prolonged prone procedure because of the magnitude of the surgery and airway edema which comes from the prone position. We do not routinely embolize tumors but rather will formally explore and ligate the vascular structures feeding them in preparation for en bloc resection.

Surgical Technique: Anterior Approach

Robust vascular access is obtained prior to the initiation of the procedure. Patients undergoing anterior approaches have bilateral external ureteral stents placed in position. Positioning is supine upon a regular operating table with the ability to obtain lateral fluoroscopic images if necessary.

A mid-line laparotomy is made and proceeds through a transperitoneal approach. The visceral structures are mobilized, and in the case of colostomy, the colon transected at a safe level with maturation of the colostomy at the conclusion of the procedure. The vascular structures are then explored with ligation of the middle sacral vessels and internal iliac vessels. Careful examination is made of the veins for the presence of tumor thrombus within the vein. If this is suspected, a venotomy is performed and the thrombus sent for histologic analysis. If bland, surgery proceeds. If tumor thrombus is detected, surgery is aborted as the presence of frank tumor thrombus in the hypogastric veins has been seen to herald uniform, rapid development of metastatic disease in patients in our experience.

Once the vascular and visceral structures have been appropriately mobilized, anterior sacral and pelvic osteotomies are performed. Localization is made using the sacral promontory and the sacroiliac joint/sciatic notches which can generally be palpated directly through this approach.

Lateral fluoroscopy may be used to confirm localization if any ambiguity is encountered.

At the appropriate sites, osteotomies are made. Osteotomies through the posterior ilium are generally completed from the anterior approach; osteotomies through the sacrum are unicortical from an anterior approach to minimize the risk of injury to the dural sac from an anterior approach which would be very difficult to control. We prefer the use of a diamond high-speed burr in making osteotomies as it has a low tendency to injury soft tissues and a cauterizing effect upon the bone as it is cut.

We have found it helpful to mark the site of the osteotomy with a small fragment screw placed unicortically. This is helpful because at the time of posterior resection, the screw may be viewed upon a lateral fluoroscopic image to guide the posterior osteotomy into the plane of the anterior osteotomy (Fig. 40.1).

A silastic sheet is placed between the sacrum/tumor mass and the mobilized vascular and visceral structures to mark the plane of the anterior dissection and protect these during the posterior approach. A pedicled vertical rectus abdominous flap is then harvested and tucked into the abdomen just ventral to the silastic sheet. Following tumor resection, the silastic sheet is removed and the vertical rectus flap is then present to assist with wound closure. In rare cases, a transverse rectus abdominous flap may be used if a very large soft tissue defect is anticipated as the transverse flap has slightly greater tissue bulk.

If necessary, colostomy is then developed and the laparotomy is closed in the standard fashion.

Usually on the day following the anterior approach a removable IVC filter is placed as described above. The posterior surgical resection generally takes place 48 h after the anterior approach to allow patient recovery between stages.

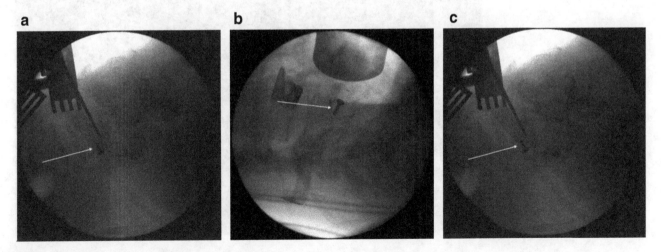

Fig. 40.1 **a** Anterior osteotomy; **b** anterior marker screw; **c** marker screw

Surgical Technique: Posterior Approach

Patients are positioned prone on a radiolucent Jackson table with a Wilson frame to bring the sacrum into the operative field with the hips flexed. Gardner-Wells tongs are placed into the skull and the head is suspended using 15 lb of spinal traction. The anus is sewn shut. Surgical preparation and draping is wide to allow access for gluteal advancement flaps and fibula or sural nerve harvest as indicated. During the procedure, the patient is positioned in maximum reverse Trendelenburg position to minimize intraocular pressure (Fig. 40.2).

A mid-line incision is made excising the biopsy tract. Alternative incisions include a triradiate ("Mercedes") incision or a transverse incision. These alternative incisions have the benefit of avoiding a wound which is directly next to the anus; however, the triradiate incision may make excision of a biopsy tract difficult and at its apex is subject to frequent wound breakdown. The transverse incision similarly may make excision of the biopsy tract difficult and is not extensile along the spinal column in cases where spinopelvic reconstruction is necessary.

Dissection is taken down being sure to avoid any fascial extension of the tumor. Localization proceeds based on a combination of anatomic landmarks and lateral fluoroscopy from cranial to caudal. It is as important to start localization proximally to avoid inadvertent entry into a tumor mass present caudally. If an anterior approach has taken place with placement of a marker screw, this is readily visualized upon lateral fluoroscopy. One useful anatomic landmark in localizing posterior sacrectomy procedures is that the level

Fig. 40.2 Prone positioning

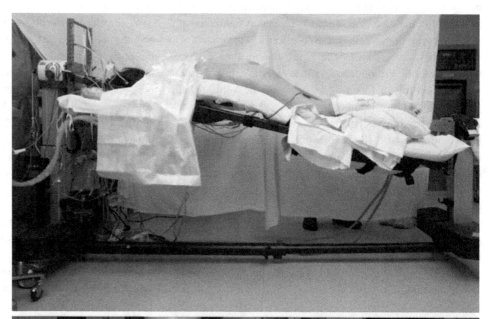

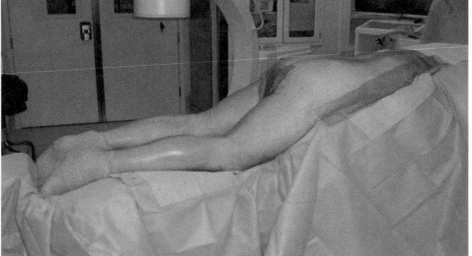

of the caudal sacroiliac joint most commonly falls between the S2 and S3 neuroforamina.

Once the lowest level of the sacrum or spinal column to be saved is identified, lateral dissection takes place. Great care is taken to preserve the gluteal vessels if at all possible as the primary perfusing structures for the gluteal flaps. Dissection comes through the piriformis and coccygeus muscles as well as sectioning of the sacrospinous and sacrotuberous ligaments. If any of the S2, 3, or 4 nerve roots are to be preserved, effort is made to preserve the pudendal nerves to maximize the possibility of bowel, bladder, and sexual function post-operatively in the patients.

As a clear fascial boundary is not always present in the lateral extent of tumors, we seek a minimum 2 cm free soft tissue margin in this extent.

Once the lateral dissection has taken place, laminectomy is performed in the spine or sacrum at a safe level. Nerve roots which will be saved are protected while others are transected. If transsection occurs at the level of the dural sac, it is doubly ligated with a heavy silk suture.

The proximal sacral osteotomy is then performed. Localization of this is critical to avoid inadvertent entry of any tumor mass. Localization occurs through a combination of anatomic landmarks and lateral fluoroscopy.

We prefer to perform this osteotomy using a diamond burr and Kerrison rongeurs to allow delicate extension through the area. Once the osteotomy is complete, care is taken to protect the remaining nerve roots as the tumor is delivered from proximal to distal. The rectum is freed or excised depending upon the extent of the tumor. Final delivery involves sectioning of the ano-coccygeal ligaments for tumors in which the rectum and anus remain in the patient or excision of the anus with the rectum and tumor en bloc for tumors in which this structure is sacrificed (Fig. 40.3).

Pathologic analysis and specimen radiographs are used to ensure that the planned resection has been executed and that margins are free. Once this is done, the posterior abdominal wall is reconstructed either through the use of the vertical rectus abdominous flap pulled through from the previous anterior exposure or with the use of an AlloDerm or similar mesh and bilateral gluteal advancement flaps.

The wound is closed over drains with monofilament and suture. An incisional wound vacuum device is placed sterilely over the closed skin to minimize tension and any post-operative contamination.

Spinopelvic Reconstruction Technique

Biomechanical studies and clinical experience have demonstrated that patients undergoing resections at the level of the S1 neuroforamen or higher will benefit from spino-pelvic reconstruction. In patients undergoing total sacrectomy or greater procedures, the connection between the spine and pelvis is flail; in those undergoing resections which preserve only a small amount of the S1 vertebral body, the remaining structure is insufficient to withstand clinical loads and susceptible to insufficiency fracture.

Our preferred method of reconstruction is the "cathedral technique" [2]. This involves the use of bilateral fibula auto- or allografts spanning between the lowest aspect of the preserved spinal column and the supra-acetabular ilium (Fig. 40.4).

In preparation for spinopelvic reconstruction, the Wilson frame on the operating table is flattened to restore the appropriate lumbar lordosis. Pedicle screw instrumentation is placed in at least the lowest three levels of the spine. We are aggressive in putting large and long screws in and at times even placing these pedicle screws bicortically. Because of the exposure after the sacrum is removed, the surgeon can often place his hand anterior to the spine to be certain that the bicortical screws are going in safely.

Screws are then placed on both sides of the ilium. Ideally, two screws are placed upon each pelvic wing. The docking site for the fibula is made in the dense supra acetabular bone. In cases of very extensive pelvic resection as well, the ischium may be used as an alternative to the supra-acetabular region. This is relatively posterior and a greater distance, so it is not our preferred docking site if the acetabular region is available.

Once this is done, fibular struts are fashioned to span the gap between the pelvis and the spine. These are placed and the pelvis and spine are compressed together over the fibula grafts. Four rods are placed (two upon each side) to minimize the risk that rod breakage will lead to catastrophic failure of the construct.

In the manipulations necessary to place this instrumentation and compress across it, it is very easy for the lowest remaining nerve roots to suffer avulsion injuries. A generous amount of allograft bone is also placed spanning the gap between the spine and the pelvis. It has not been our practice to use bone morphogenetic protein in the setting of oncologic resections.

Post-operative Care

Patients are transferred to the intensive care unit on a specialty air suspension type mattress. The head of the bed is raised as high as practical to minimize the risk of aspiration and to facilitate extubation.

Once patients are extubated, mobilization begins as they tolerate. A ROHO cushion is used to distribute pressure over the sacral wound. Initially patients sit for only 20 to 30 min at a time three to four times per day and gradually advance their sitting as their physiologic state and wound appearance tolerates.

Fig. 40.3 Posterior surgical
approach: **a** tumor dissection:
b sacral osteotomy, nerve roots
are saved and protected

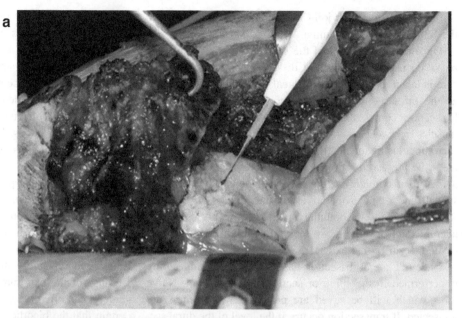

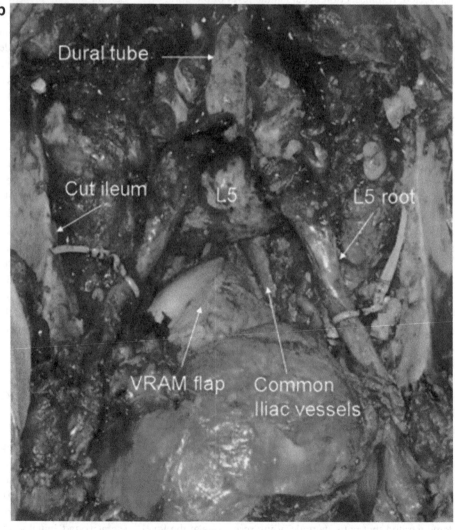

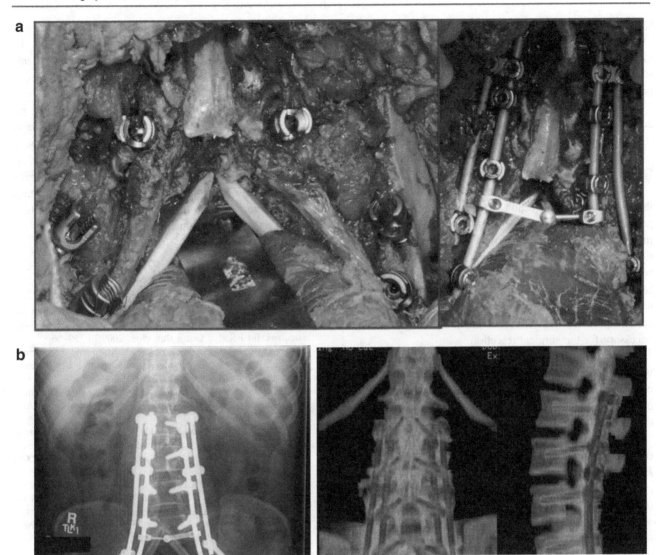

Fig. 40.4 Lumbopelvic fixation after sacrectomy: **a** intraoperative images; and **b** post-operatives images

An incisional wound vacuum is maintained in place to minimize risk of contamination around the incision. This is changed every four to five days for a period of approximately two weeks. Ureteral stents are removed as soon as the anticipated risk of reoperation is low. DVT prophylaxis is provided with unfractionated subcutaneous heparin as soon as the risk of post-operative bleeding has been seen to diminish. The removable inferior cava filter is retrieved approximately four to six months post-operatively.

Antibiotics are maintained for 24 h around the time of surgery. A first-generation cephalosporin is the antibiotic of choice. If the thecal sac is entered at the time of surgery, a single perioperative dose of ceftriaxone is administered as this antibiotic has better CSF penetration. If drains are placed, they are removed by 72 to 96 h. If drains are not adjacent to any instrumentation and have a very high output, they may remain in place for a longer period of time.

In patients undergoing resection at the L3 level or higher, there is a risk of development of chylous ascites post-operatively. Patients judged to be at risk for this are treated with parenteral nutrition until they are tolerating oral intake. At that time, a low fat diet (thoracic duct leak diet) is used and continued for six weeks perioperatively to minimize the risk of complications developing.

Results

Results of oncologic sacrectomy are difficult to establish from the literature as they will vary by histology. Specifically, the outcome becomes dominated by the characteristic of the tumor which is under treatment.

Good information can be gleaned on studies of specific techniques or which group histologies independently.

Oncologic results are most favorable when complete en bloc excision of the tumor is successful. This is best illustrated by the report of Fuchs et al. on the operative management of sacral chordoma from the Mayo Clinic. In this series, patients in whom a wide oncologic margin was achieved had uniform survival; those in which a lessor margin was achieved had a higher risk of succumbing to disease [3].

Neurologic function following transection of nerve roots of the cauda equina has been extensively evaluated by Dr. Gunterberg and by other investigators as well [5–7, 11].

Clinical experience suggests that preservation of either the entire unilateral cauda equina (S1 through S4) or preservation of bilateral S2 and unilateral S3 nerve roots are minimum requirements to have a high likelihood of functional bowel and bladder capacity. Notably, even in patients with preservation of ample nerves to provide for bowel and bladder function, return of this capability often requires four to six months following the procedure as the nerves of the cauda equina are often heavily stunned by the manipulation necessary for the surgical resection.

We favor an instrumented spinopelvic reconstruction when surgery creates a spinopelvic discontinuity [9]. In cases of high subtotal sacrectomy, biomechanical data and clinical experience favor reconstruction when resection is at the level of the S1 disk or higher [7, 8].

Recent reports have highlighted the complications and outcomes in patients undergoing oncologic sacrectomy [12]. Perioperative complications from positioning are seen in patients with morbid obesity or in procedures lasting longere than ten hours [10].

In a large series of patients undergoing a spinopelvic resection (importantly distinguished from lessor resections which do not violate spinopelvic continuity), Rose et al. reported a wound complication rate of approximately 50 percent and a deep infection rate of 35 percent. Approximately 15 percent of patients required revision of spinopelvic instrumentation for pseudoarthrosis and implant failure. Importantly, the majority of surviving patients were independent in the activities of daily living with appropriate assistive devices [9].

Conclusions

Oncologic sacrectomy is a necessary treatment option for many patients with primary sacral malignancies in hopes of achieving a cure. Resections are resource intensive and have significant morbidity associated. Resections up to the level of the S2 neuroforamen may be approached from posterior alone; those which require resection of adjacent pelvic vis-

ceral structures or higher levels of resection most commonly benefit from a staged anterior and posterior approach. In patients requiring resection of the majority of S1 or frank disruption of spinopelvic continuity, an instrumented spinopelvic reconstruction is indicated.

Soft tissue reconstruction following sacrectomy may be performed by bilateral posterior gluteal advancement flaps (in the case of posterior resections) or with a pedicled vertical rectus abdominous flap in the case of an anterior/posterior resection. The magnitude and complexity of these procedures highlights the importance of a team approach in the care of these patients to maximize their functional and oncologic outcomes.

References

1. Delaney TF, Liebsch NJ, Pedlow FX, et al. Phase II study of high-dose photon/proton radiotherapy in the management of spine sarcomas. Int J Radiat Oncol Biol Phys. 2009;73:259–66.
2. Dickey I, Hugate R, Fuchs B, Yaszemski M, Sim F. Reconstruction after total sacrectomy: early experience with a new surgical technique. Clin Ortho Rel Res. 2005;439:42–50.
3. Fuchs B, Dickey I, Yaszemski M, Inwards C, Sim F. Operative management of sacral chordoma. J Bone Joint Surg Am. 2005;87:2211–6.
4. Glatt BS, Disa JJ, Mehrara BJ et al. Reconstruction of extensive partial or total sacrectomy defects with a transabdominal vertical rectus abdominus myocutaneous flap. Ann Plast Surg. 2006; 56:526–530.
5. Gunterberg B, Kewenter J, Petersen I, Stener B. Anorectal function after major resections of the sacrum with bilateral or unilateral sacrifice of sacral nerves. Br J Surg. 1976;63:546–54.
6. Gunterberg B, Norlen L, Stener B, Sundin T. Neurologic evaluation after resection of the sacrum. Invest Urol. 1975;13:183–8.
7. Gunterberg B. Effects of major resection of the sacrum: clinical studies on urogenital and anorectal function and a biomechanical study on pelvic strength. Acta Orthop Scand. 1976;162:1–38.
8. Hugate R, Dickey I, Phimolsarnti R, Yaszemski M, Sim F. Mechanical effects of partial sacrectomy: when is reconstruction necessary. Clin Ortho Rel Res. 2006;450:82–9.
9. Rose P, Yaszemski M, Dekutoski M, Shives T, Sim F. Classification of spinopelvic resections: oncologic and reconstruction implications. In: International Society of Limb Salvage Meeting. Boston, MA; 2009.
10. Sherman C, Rose P, Pierce L, et al. Prospective assessment of patient morbidity from prone sacrectomy positioning. In: American Academy of Orthopedic Surgeons Meeting. New Orleans, LA; 2010.
11. Todd L, Yaszemski M, Currier B, Fuchs B, Kim C, Sim F. Bowel and bladder function after major sacral resection. Clin Orthop Rel Res. 2002;397:36–9.
12. Zileli M, Hoscuskun C, Brastianos P, Sabah D. Surgical treatment of primary sacral tumors: complications associated with sacrectomy. Neurosurg Focus. 2003;15:1–8.

Index

A

Adamantinoma, 135, 137, 189, 190
Adjuvant therapy, 61, 89, 100, 215
Aggressive osteoblastoma, 31, 32
Aneurysmal bone cyst, 12, 27, 29, 31, 67, 143–155, 157, 179, 184, 215

B

Benign bone lesion, 157
Benign bone tumor-like lesions, 4, 215
Benign bone tumors, 4, 5, 8, 21, 27, 47, 57, 67, 87, 115, 125, 129
Benign cartilaginous neoplasm, 57
Benign lesion, 52, 58, 139, 143, 152, 154, 155, 185, 216
Bone bank, 83, 215, 217–219, 222
Bone cyst, 6, 8, 12, 143, 149–151, 157–159, 162, 215, 220
Bone graft, 41, 60, 61, 63, 89, 91, 105, 130, 135, 158, 215–217, 221, 223, 224
Bone hydatidosis, 169
Bone metastasis, 8, 199–201, 209–212
Bone neoplasms, 209
Bone pain, 177, 179
Bone sarcoma, 11, 35, 39
Bone substitute, 215
Bone tumors, 3–6, 8, 9, 13, 19, 21, 27, 35, 47, 57, 67, 73, 87, 88, 97, 105, 117, 121, 127, 131, 143, 171, 179, 183, 184, 189, 193, 199, 210, 211, 224
Brodie's abscess, 171
Brown tumor, 87, 143, 179

C

Campanacci staging, 87, 88, 215
Cancer treatment, 163, 166
Cartilage, 4, 23, 31, 47–49, 51, 52, 57, 58, 67, 73, 76–78, 102, 103, 135, 144, 185, 217–224
Cathedral technique, 229, 233
Chemotherapy, 3, 35, 40–43, 79, 97, 100, 101, 103, 104, 107, 108, 117, 121, 128, 131, 183, 187–189, 193, 194, 201, 209, 222, 229, 230
Chondroblastoma, 11, 27, 29, 57, 63, 67–72, 87, 215
Chondroblasts, 67
Chondroma, 19, 52, 57, 61, 73, 76, 77
Chondromyxoid fibroma, 4, 11, 31, 57, 63, 64, 143, 150, 157, 159
Chondrosarcoma, 4, 5, 7, 9, 11, 29, 35, 49, 51, 52, 54, 57, 58, 73–79, 84, 143, 184, 185, 215, 221, 230

C (continued)

Chordoma, 11, 183–188, 230, 236
Cranial bone tumor, 115
Curetage, 215
Cytogenetic, 48, 97–99, 107

D

Denosumab, 90
Desmoplastic fibroma, 125, 126, 128

E

Enchondroma, 5, 31, 53, 57–61, 63
Equinococosis infection, 169
Ewing's sarcoma, 3, 6, 8, 36, 97–100, 106, 107, 127, 165, 171
Exostoses, 53

F

Fibroblasts, 21, 127, 135, 137, 150
Fibrosarcoma, 8, 35, 102, 125–128, 193, 194
Fibrous bone lesions, 134
Fibrous dysplasia, 29, 31, 125, 128, 133, 135, 137, 143, 149, 150, 157
Fingertip tumor, 195

G

Giant cell tumor of bone, 27, 29, 31, 67, 89, 157
Glomus tumor, 195, 196

H

High degree sarcoma, 193
Hypercalcemia, 179, 200, 209
Hyperparathyroidism, 4, 87, 88, 143, 179

L

Langerhans cell, 163–166
Lipoma, 11, 129, 131
Liposarcoma, 131, 193

© Springer-Verlag London Ltd., part of Springer Nature 2021
J. Paulos and D. G. Poitout (eds.), *Bone Tumors*,
https://doi.org/10.1007/978-1-4471-7501-8

M
Malignant bone tumor, 4, 5, 8, 13, 35, 97, 183, 189
Malign bone tumours, 97
Malign bone sarcoma, 97
Massive endoprostheses, 79, 202, 217
McCune–Albright syndrome, 133
Metaphyseal fibrous defect, 4, 139
Myeloid neoplasm, 163, 165, 166
Myeloma, 4–6, 8, 11, 179, 184, 194, 200, 201, 210

N
Neoplasm recurrence, 32, 47, 48
Nidus, 21–24, 31
Non ossifying fibroma, 139, 143, 150

O
Orthopedic surgery, 106
Osteitis deformans, 177
Osteoarthritis TBC, 173
Osteoblastoma, 9, 27–32, 35, 143
Osteochondroma, 4, 5, 11, 19, 47–54, 57, 73
Osteofibrous lesions, 133, 135, 137
Osteogenic sarcoma, 4, 35, 36
Osteolysis, 29, 31, 39, 98, 167
Osteoma, 4, 9, 19, 20, 36
Osteoma osteoide, 9, 21–24, 27–29, 31
Osteomyelitis, 4, 98, 99, 165, 171
Osteopathia codensans, 175
Osteopoikilosis, 175
Osteosarcoma, 4–6, 8–11, 14, 27, 29, 31, 32, 35, 37–39, 42, 51, 53, 77, 78, 98, 125–128, 143, 145, 150, 152, 155, 171, 177, 193, 194, 230
Osteosynthesis, 24, 57, 60, 158, 162, 221, 222

P
Paget's disease, 4, 5, 177
Pathological fracture, 8, 57, 63, 65, 87, 98, 115, 127, 133, 139, 143, 147, 153, 157, 177, 189, 199, 200, 210–213
Pleomorphic sarcoma, 131, 185, 193, 194
Porous titanium, 217, 224–226
Porous titanium implants, 224
Pseudotumor, 143

R
Radical surgery, 35, 38, 41
Radiofrequency, 21, 24, 187
Radiotherapy, 3, 79, 90, 97, 100, 101, 121, 128, 136, 143, 152, 153, 155, 183, 187, 188, 194, 201, 210, 211, 213–216, 230
Reconstructive surgery, 42, 79, 199, 202

S
Sacral tumors, 101
Sacrectomy, 229, 230, 232, 233, 235, 236
Spine tumor, 29, 32

T
Tumor-like bone lesions, 4, 215
Tumor-like lesions, 4, 215

U
Undifferentiated sarcoma, 194

V
Vascular bone tumors, 4
Vascular tumor, 11